You'll Wish You Were an Elephant
(Killing Cancer Kindly)
By
Dr Mohammad Muneeb Khan

The team at Killing Cancer Kindly is committed to reviewing, revising, and updating our information database in light of new evidence and findings. Your suggestions and opinions in this regard are welcome.

Visit www.killingcancerkindly.com

DEDICATION

THIS BOOK

IS

DEDICATED

TO

<u>YOU</u>

CONTENTS

AUTHOR'S FOREWORD

This is a book to lift your spirits, fill you with hope, and inspire you.

Scientific facts are presented in an entertaining and simple way. You will find dozens of new ideas and theories from 'canproms' and a Pandora gene of cancer to 'cancer motherships' and a new theory of human evolution, which will pave the way for preventing, treating, and curing cancer.

Our aim is to replace information with knowledge so you can understand and be empowered to make free decisions and choices about your life and health. By doing so, we can reduce the risk of cancer from 50% to less than 5%.

I invite you to join us in this global mission to kill cancer kindly (without making mankind suffer) so we can all live in a better, safer, cancer-free world.

You are already contributing to this effort by buying this book, as part of the proceeds will go to our charity, Killing Cancer Kindly with Dr Khan.

This book was inspired by patients and their families, and is an acknowledgment of the amazing courage and dignity that humans can have in the face of adversity.

Dr Mohammad Muneeb Khan

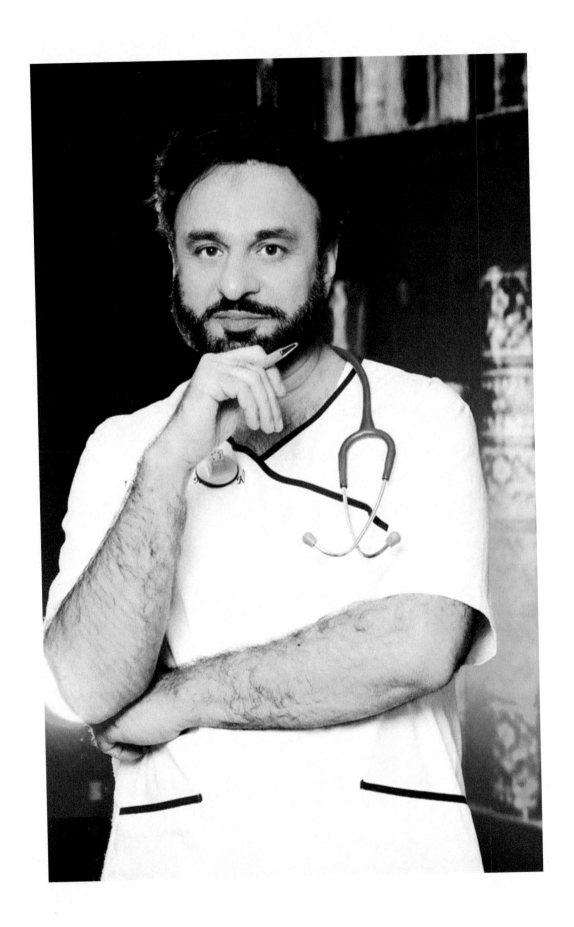

PREFACE

Why Write This Book?

Sir Edmund Hillary was once asked why he climbed Mount Everest and he famously answered, "Because it was there". It's a reply many of us are familiar with. Back in 1953, he and Tenzing Norgay took on that immense climb and triumphed, reaching the peak. Yet, since then, many hundreds have donned their boots and followed in their footsteps. Nowadays, reaching base camp can even be booked as an activity holiday. So, while the climb is still as challenging, it perhaps no longer has that aura of a near-impossible feat. Everest had been conquered and new challenges beckoned. Just 16 years after Sir Edmund looked down from on high, Neil Armstrong set foot on the Moon and looked down upon Earth! A very different perspective indeed, and one made possible by an equal determination to rise to a new, greater challenge.

For many of us, cancer is the Mount Everest of human health. It's there, standing tall above all other illnesses, seemingly insurmountable, challenging, and scary. It's the dreaded 'C' word, the 'He-Who-Must-Not-Be-Named'. We try to ignore it like the metaphorical elephant in the room. And yet, this understandable reluctance to look the beast in the eye is to our detriment because, equipped with a touch of understanding, there is much we can do to avoid or conquer it.

I was 15, already committed to the medical profession, when I had my first encounter with 'C'.

A dear family friend had been diagnosed with it in her mid-thirties and, despite her being one of my favourite aunts, I was not allowed to visit her. The experience intrigued me enough to develop a keen interest in understanding what had happened to her. I went through my teenage years and then medical school in pursuit of getting to grips with the science and art of oncology. From the first days of my job as a junior doctor to working as a specialist in this field, I've witnessed the rapid rise in cancer cases, and the complexity of the disease and its treatment. But most of all, I've been touched by the courage, resilience, and dignity of those who face it; a truly humbling experience.

At the time of writing, I'm working at one of the best cancer centres in the UK. Yet, such is the negative connotation about 'C 'that my hospital baulked at the idea of calling it a 'cancer' centre, so my patients have to look for the Oncology and Haematology Centre when arriving for their appointments.

The 'C' word haunts patients and doctors alike. I want to set about changing this negative mindset.

Without doubt, cancer is a life-changing (if not life-wrecking) experience. But it is made more challenging by the uncertainties and misinformation surrounding it.

We live in the *Information Age* where vast amounts of information, true or fake, lie just a click or two away; zillions of bland facts, overwhelming and overloading our minds. Frequently, our lack of understanding or context causes anguish and agony, especially in relation to medical matters.

Often, it feels to me as if wisdom – that combination of experience, knowledge, and good judgement – is rapidly becoming extinct, or is being swallowed up by an ocean of 'stuff' and deafening 'white noise'. We need to make sense of things, and to do this we need to answer the 'whys', 'hows', 'what-ifs' and 'buts'. These are questions I grapple with every day as a doctor.

Unsurprisingly, then, the motivation and driving force for this book has been my patients and their families, who have guided me all the way. The goal is to create a better understanding of cancer and how to prevent it at different levels, not only before the onset of disease but also after it has occurred.

So, what sort of book is this? The approach I have taken may surprise you. If you're expecting page after page of relentless 'bad news 'or a textbook-like A–Z of depressing symptoms, diagnoses, and frequent summoning of the Grim Reaper, you'll be disappointed.

Likewise, if you're expecting to squirm in your seat, or suddenly worry that the slight-but-perceptible ache in your stomach is something really, *really* serious, you're out of luck.

If you want to be scared witless, I suggest buying a Stephen King novel – he does *scary* so much better than me.

What I do want to do is lift your spirits, fill you with hope, and inspire you.

I want to share with you my never-ending wonder at the miracle that our bodies are, and some of the incredible things that are going on day and night inside us, and which we are oblivious to.

I want to share stories with you. Some are just myths, parables, or legends; others are of great scientific discoveries and mankind's endeavour to understand life itself. There is a good deal we know about what causes cancer, or affects our risk of suffering from it.

These don't just involve the well-known culprits, but also aspects of our diet, behaviour, and the environment. And there is some good news emerging, too. Some things many of us enjoy are actually good for us. Hopefully, along the way you'll be entertained, as well as gaining an insight into a remarkable truth.

Your body – yes, *your* body – is fighting to prevent cancer even as you read this! The thing is, for it to have the best chance of keeping you well, it needs you to do your bit. Hopefully, I can equip you with enough knowledge and wisdom to enable you to do this.

My personal dream is to establish *Preventive Oncology* as a new and separate entity among the medical sciences. This book is a small step in my long journey to conquer this particular mountain.

INTRODUCTION

INTRODUCTION

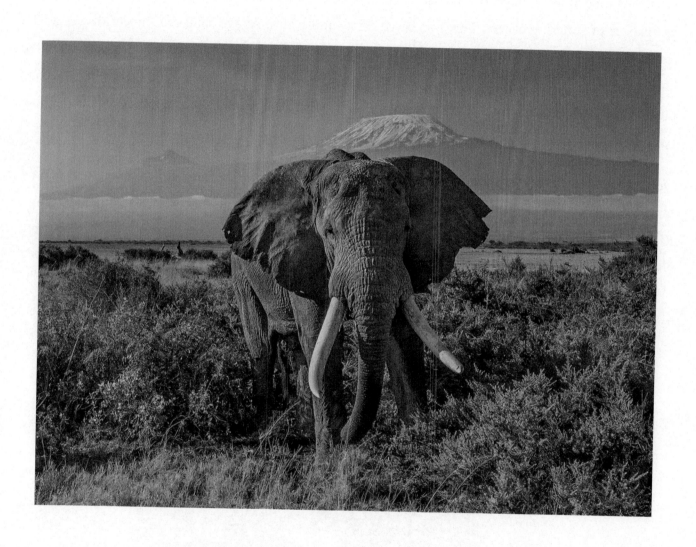

INTRODUCTION

It might come as a surprise to learn that elephants are pretty resistant to cancer. What's more, we have a good idea why this is the case, but we'll come back to that later on in this book.

So, it's good news … for elephants.

For a long time, it was thought that the larger the species of animal and the longer it lived, the greater were its chances of suffering cancer. This was based on a simple idea. As we shall see, cancer occurs as the result of damage to our body's cells, in particular their DNA. Understandably, then, we supposed that the bigger the animal, the more cells it would have (generally true), so the greater the possibility that one might get damaged (also true). And the longer it lives, surely the greater the chances of this happening (yes, quite likely).

On this basis, as the world's largest land animal, living for up to 50–70 years and weighing in at several tonnes, elephants would be expected to have the highest incidence of cancer of all. But they don't. Elephants bust this idea, even when the rates are adjusted for other risk factors such as alcohol consumption[1], smoking[2], and a vegetarian diet.

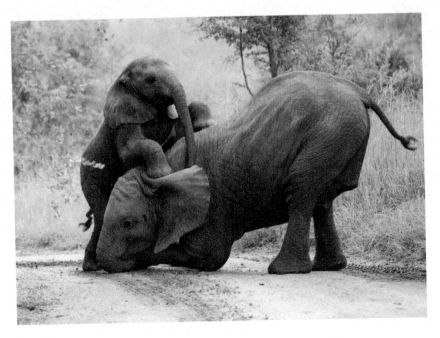

[1]Mind you, not all elephants are teetotal. Domesticated elephants easily pick up the habit of drinking alcohol and seem to enjoy it too. And in case you are wondering if they ever get drunk, the answer is yes, but you need between 10 and 27 litres of 7% alcohol to get a 3,000 kg elephant tipsy. Anything less and it's safe to drive your elephant home.
[2]Again, elephants can be exposed to smoke and there are reports of wild Asian elephants from Nagarahole National Park in South India ingesting wood ash and blowing smoke.

Interestingly, it's true for whales, too. Speaking of diet, even committed non-vegetarians like lions and African wild dogs have a very low rate of cancer compared to humans.

So, are these just exceptions to the rule? The answer is no, they're not.

In Oxford, England, in the 1970s, the eminent epidemiologist Sir Richard Peto formulated what is known as 'Peto's paradox' – basically, saying that at the species level (across different species) the incidence of cancer doesn't appear to be related to the number of cells in an organism (size).

Various studies have lent support to this. For example, using data from San Diego Zoo, California, a survey of 36 mammalian species ranging from the mighty elephant to the koala, llama, lion, and jackal, and down to the tiny striped grass mouse weighing in at an average of a mere 51 grams, no relationship between size and cancer incidence was observed. That's across six orders of magnitude in terms of size or, put another way, the elephant (largest) is about 100,000 times bigger than the striped grass mouse.

And yet, that's only half the story. *Within* a species, including humans, this idea of size and lifespan does have a bearing.

You may have overheard someone say, "If anyone lives long enough, they will eventually get cancer". It's a real conversation killer at dinner parties, and not recommended as a chat-up line for anyone desperately seeking that first date, but there does appear to be some truth to it.

In relation to size, in some studies[3], it has been observed that taller people had a higher incidence of cancer, even after adjustment for other risk factors. Similarly, in relation to bodyweight, being overweight or obese is frequently associated with higher risk.

Are these observations unique to humans? Again, the answer is no. For example, in North America, when the causes of death in over 74,000 pet dogs were investigated, it was found that the lowest incidences of cancer occurred in the smaller breeds. So, in some respects, size does appear to matter.

Although cancer is responsible for between 11 and 25% of human deaths, I think of it as often being a *potentially* fatal disease. Fortunately, not everyone diagnosed with cancer dies of it. Some are cured and, importantly, many have the disease controlled for a long time; sometimes for many years, occasionally for decades.

---

[3] More on this and other risk factors later in the book.

We often speak of 'seeking a cure for cancer'. But, as we'll learn, cancer isn't a *single* entity. Finding a cure-all is therefore improbable. Medicine has made great strides forward in detecting, diagnosing, and treating many cancers. Hopefully, there will continue to be breakthroughs, leading to individual cancer types becoming either curable or controllable, and therefore offering sufferers prolonged survival with a decent quality of life.

But pinning our hopes on breakthrough treatments is, in some ways, missing a trick. We're ignoring something that, when we stop and think about it, is really quite astonishing. You might even call it one of the greatest ever breakthroughs that we've ignored. Time to take a deep breath. Cue the drum roll.

OK, here it is:

We can already prevent almost half [4] of cancers occurring in the first place. And this is a conservative estimate. We might be able to prevent many, many more than this.

Imagine a world where cancer is a relatively uncommon disease. This could actually become a reality. What's more, we have the knowledge to make it so; today, here and now.

There's even better news, too. Our bodies (yours and mine) have inbuilt mechanisms to prevent, stop, and even kill cancer. And it happens every day throughout our lives.

In fact, the body's anti-cancer systems are so effective that most of the cancers are nipped in the bud. Which brings us to the obvious question, 'Why on earth is cancer becoming so common?'

The answer is that, like everything in life, our body's defence system against cancer has some limitations. Ironically, we (unconsciously) keep testing and challenging those limits with our unconventional lifestyle and exposure to environmental risk factors.

Despite all the additional challenges that we have introduced to our life, our amazing body continues to fight vigorously against cancer and in most cases succeeds in avoiding it, at best, or delaying its onset, at worst.

If only we would be a little more kind to our body and reduce the stress on our anti-cancer system, many of us could live a cancer-free life. And there are ways to boost our body's ability to fight cancer, too. Not only by enhancing our inbuilt capability but also by using the world around us to help make it strong.

---

[4] According to the World Health Organisation (WHO), between 30 and 50% of all cancer cases are preventable.

And that is where this book comes in. Its aim is to help you understand how amazing our body is at preventing and fighting cancer, how we can reduce the stress and make it work in our favour, how to boost its cancer-fighting capabilities by making small-but-significant positive and easy-to-achieve changes in our diet and environment.

To achieve this, we don't even have to adopt the lifestyle of elephants – although we can use them for inspiration and a model for a cancer-free life.

Because those big, burly mammals have been doing it for millions of years.

PART I

WHAT ACTUALLY IS CANCER?

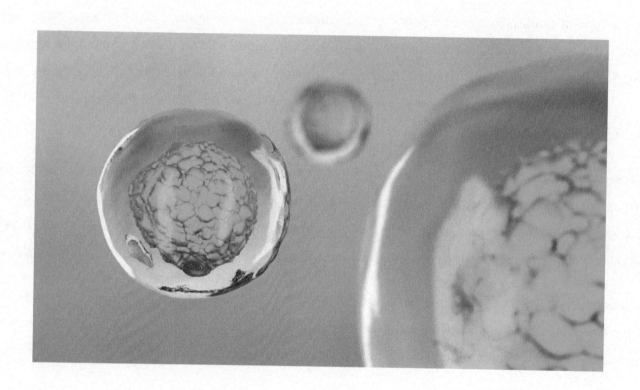

PART 1: WHAT ACTUALLY IS CANCER?

1   Cancer, a Creature in Many Guises

American writer Gertrude Stein[5] once famously said, "Rose is a rose is a rose is a rose is a rose".

Over the years, this sentence has been parodied by many writers and lyricists. Most famously so by a Nobel laureate, Ernest Hemingway[6], who, while describing man's canine best friend, borrowed the phrase from Gertrude, apparently without her knowledge or consent, as they were not on talking terms at the time, and said, "A bitch is a bitch is a bitch …".

People fond of floral language or repetition might find a certain logic in these descriptions. Some might think of them as a kind of 'law of identity', labels given to things, allowing us to group them together. And, yes, that's helpful. Up to a point. The danger is that we come to think of them all as being the same thing. You may be thinking, *"Cancer is a cancer is a cancer…isn't it?"* I have a problem with that. It's too big a generalisation.

A rose is not just a rose but a group of many different plants and hybrids whose flowers vary in colour, shape, size, and other characteristics, depending on the part of the world they come from. There are over 30,000 varieties, wild species having been cultivated and hybridized over thousands of years. If you purchase a dwarf variety or patio rose, don't expect it to grow up the wall of a house like a climbing rose.

And dogs, like roses, come in a multitude of colours, shapes, and sizes. If you want to race your dog and win prizes, buy a greyhound or whippet. A St. Bernard might not make the winner's podium on too many occasions, although I know which I'd rely on if I were stuck on top of a mountain.

When it comes to explaining cancer, the general approach tends to be similar to Gertrude's and Ernest's description of roses and canines. This is because we generalise cancer based on its outcomes: a disease causing suffering and death. However, cancer is not just a disease but a group of diseases varying in their shape, size, form, and characteristics, depending on the part of body they originate from and the kind of environment they grow in. For example, a blood cancer exists in a liquid environment while a breast cancer occurs as a solid lump.

---

[5] Don't worry if you have not heard of this famous writer before. Now, we both have.
[6] I would be slightly concerned if you never heard of him before. Having said that, there's always a first time for everything.

Interestingly, just as dogs have transformed over centuries from being a wolf to a domesticated animal, cancer is the result of a transformation over a period of time. It's a change of a normal functioning body cell to an abnormal, non-functioning, wild and ferociously diseased cell; the transformation from a best friend to a worst enemy.

A good way to think of it is like Robert Louis Stevenson's Dr Jekyll turning into the monster that is Mr Hyde, but with the transformation never wearing off. Mr Hyde stays as Mr Hyde. The monster persists, and has to be confronted, contained or, preferably, destroyed.

Being given the news that you or someone close has the big 'C' is crushing enough, but to be informed that it has 'spread 'often feels akin to being told the Grim Reaper is just finding somewhere to park up outside your front door and will be with you shortly, sharpened scythe in hand. If you stop and think about this, it suggests that having 'C' might not be so terrible, provided it hasn't spread. And this is indeed sometimes the case.

A classic example is the type of skin cancer called *basal cell carcinoma (BCC)*, which grows very slowly, doesn't spread (only invades locally), and is very responsive to treatment, with cure rates approaching 100%. If you're going to get cancer this is the one you want! Really, it is.

Another type of skin cancer, malignant melanoma (MM), however, is not as well-behaved. It doesn't like to stay in the same place like a BCC and tends to go wherever its fancy takes it to. If one has the choice between skin cancers, this is one you really don't want. This idea of spreading, or *metastasizing*, to other sites in the body is often important in terms of treating and curing cancer. Why should this be the case?

The best way to understand this is by drawing on a parable. It's based on one of my favourite childhood stories my grandma used to tell, a tale passed down the generations and found across different cultures in many versions. I will share with you the somewhat-modified version I tell my children. Really, I do, and they enjoy hearing it. Probably because it has the word 'mutants 'in the title.

The March of the Mutants (Grandma's Version)

"Once upon a time, long, long, ago," said grandma, "the human race started from two individuals, a man and a woman." (We will call them 'Adam and Eve'[7] or 'a Man and Woman', depending on one's religious inclination, or lack of it).

---

[7]Genetic analyses have suggested that all humans – the black, the brown, the white, and yellow nations and groups –might be traced back to a common human ancestor.

"They had many children. Over the generations they evolved into a multitude of races[8]. Whether hunter-gatherers or farmers, they lived sustainably and in harmony with nature and with one another ... well, most of the time, with a few exceptions, like the occasional bloody war.

"But over time, among the children of Adam (Man) and Eve (Woman) an unusual change (mutation) occurred, and it gave rise to a race of humans who did what no other humans had done before. They consumed resources without replenishing them and in doing so destroyed the environment around them leaving nothing, absolutely nothing, in their wake. Wherever they spread, they left death and destruction behind, leaving no food, no water, and no resources for any other living creature. This evil race of humans was best at surviving, but at the cost of all other living creatures."

(Grandma had a different name for them but I call them the 'GM[9] mutants'.)

"Their abode was a valley surrounded by unsurpassable peaks and a narrow passage through which they emerged regularly to devour everything around them, much to the annoyance of all other races spread across the hills and plains. Fortunately, there was a kindly king of a nearby land who had an excellent idea for solving the problem. Although his people were all for wiping out the GM mutants with axes, spears, and bows and arrows, he proclaimed there was actually no need to kill their enemies. Instead, he ordered that they be contained within their valley. He reasoned that if the narrow passage could be blocked, the GMs would be isolated from the outside world and no longer pose a threat. Being known as a wise king, his people offered a polite round of applause, each looking at the other and wondering why on earth they hadn't thought of it before.

"It was an ambitious and colossal project. Finally, after a phenomenal effort under the watchful eye of the kind and wise king, his people filled the gap between the mountains with a wall of iron. Job done. They could relax. Or could they?

"The mutant race was confined but not killed. Understandably disgruntled, they nevertheless lived on, moaning and cursing, reproducing within their valley using the available but ever-dwindling resources. And within them grew a burning desire to break out from their valley and wreak revenge. They figured that if they could strike down the iron wall, they'd emerge, wave after wave of them, invading, consuming, gorging themselves, destroying everything in their path, once and for all. Legend has it that these mutants

---

[8] Every generation of humans is slightly different from their parents in shape, size, looks, health, and disease. This variation is due to a slight variation in their DNA and, over long periods of time, this results in a different race or ethnic group.

[9] Gog and Magog according to the Bible, and Yajooj and Majooj according to the Quran, but you can also call them 'GM' for genetically modified mutants (at the risk of being superfluous as mutants *are* genetically modified). But then again, it's a done thing in the English language, like a 'free gift', 'added bonus 'or 'mutual cooperation.'

are still alive in the sealed-off valley, slowly but steadily chipping off at the iron wall, and one day they will manage to break through it, and this event will mark the end of days, the beginning of the final chapter in human history."

All very interesting but what's the story got to do with cancer, I hear you cry? The answer is that the story of cancer is very similar. Every human starts from two cells, a male (sperm) and female (egg or ovum). Over time, these cells multiply into billions and make a body, comprising tissues and organs. During the ongoing process of growth and division over an individual's lifetime, some cells mutate and become abnormal. Most of these abnormal cells cannot survive and die. But, just like the GM mutants in the story, every now and again some mutant cells develop an ability to bypass the body's processes for killing damaged cells, and survive. Over time, they also acquire further mutations giving them additional powers, such as …

1. An ability to grow and reproduce at a faster rate than normal body cells.

2. Gaining the power to damage any bodily barriers in their path.

3. The capability to break off from their body organ and move to other parts of the body to overtake its normal cells and grow a mutant colony.

4. Consuming all food and water available in the body and starving off the normal cells.

5. Damaging the body parts they invade and grow, eventually causing destruction.

These mutant cells are called a *cancer*.

Just like the GM mutant race of humans, every cancer is confined in its place of origin by a physical barrier[10], initially stopping it from spreading. Over time, some cancer cells develop the ability to break free of this barrier and spread far and wide in the body. In doing so, they consume all of its resources, leaving behind a trail of death and destruction, just like the mutant human race.

1.1   Bamboozling the Patient with Clever Words

Before we go any further, I have to apologise. I'm doing so on my knees, and on behalf of the entire medical profession, and I hope you can find it within yourselves to forgive us.

---

[10] For most cancers, it is a barrier known as the *basement membrane*. We will talk about it in more detail in the next sections.

As the great Bard of Avon, Shakespeare, once asked, "What's in a name?"

Apparently, a lot of confusion when it comes to cancer. In my view, the name itself needs re-thinking. What do we call it? Cancer? Tumour? Neoplasia? Malignancy?

All of them are right, but *not always*. 'Cancer' and 'malignancy' refer to the nasty disease we are talking about. Here's what I mean, and why it can befuddle many a patient (and medical student).

A *neoplasia* is a new growth of cells, but so is a *tumour*, and yet neoplasias can be benign, which means they're a lump of cells that grow and divide, but go nowhere. Benign growths are naughty but not nasty fellas. However, when cells become nasty, they divide and grow to invade and spread, and yet they are still referred to as a 'neoplasia'.

Why on earth we have to make it so confusing is beyond me. Apparently, it's done for 'historical reasons', relics of a past when a lump, any lump, was called a *tumour* in Latin, and *neoplasia* in Greek (from the words *neo*, 'new' and *plasma*, 'formation or creation or plastic', meaning 'formed or moulded'). Ironically, the Greeks and Romans did not use these terms for cancer. Greeks called it *karkinos*, meaning 'crab', because that's what it looked like – a mass of tissue spreading out to other structures. The Romans agreed, translating it to *cancer* in Latin.

English speakers decided to use the term 'cancer', but also 'tumour' and 'neoplasia' to sound clever and confuse the public. And I am not kidding you. The main aim for naming diseases and treatments in Latin and Greek, sometimes using terms that even the Latin or Greek speakers did not use, was to keep the common man (and woman) in the dark. By doing so, physicians and the educated elite, who spoke and understood classical languages, could stay aloof[11] and use such knowledge as an extra means of power over the public. So, while the populace worried about lumps and bumps, the higher echelons of society were smug in their knowledge of *neoplasias, karkinos, oncos* (Greek for 'swelling' – that's where the terms 'oncology' and 'oncologist' come from), tumours and cancers, until they ended getting them all mixed up, and couldn't tell one from another.

---

[11] Reminds me of the time when one of my senior doctors left a lot of juniors in confusion by stating, with an emphatic sigh, "Ars longa, vita brevis" and not bothering to explain it. With the use of the first word 'ars', those of us who were only familiar with the classic English language thought he had an anatomical deformity (arse/backside) that might shorten his life, till much later, when we realised it was Latin for 'Art (is) long, life is short'. Thankfully there was nothing wrong with his rear.

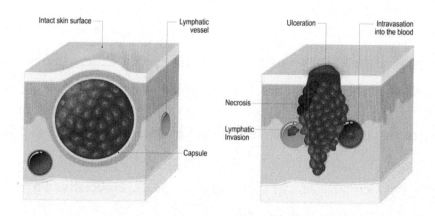

Benign tumour (left) and cancerous tumour (right).

The first thing that a cancer patient, their family members, and even medical students have to confront is the confusion caused by these terms. But if you think this is bad, wait till I tell you the skewed system for naming benign and malignant tumours.

Cancer or malignant tumours are often called *carcinomas*, especially when they arise from skin or cells lining the organs; like squamous cell carcinoma of the skin and renal cell carcinoma of the kidney.

Benign lumps also have names ending in an 'oma' but without the 'carci' bit. Examples of this include a *lipoma*, an innocuous lump of fatty tissue, and a *papilloma*, a harmless growth of skin cells known to you and me as a 'skin tag'. But for some bizarre reason, the nastiest of skin cancers is known as a *melanoma*, as if it was a lump of innocuous pigment-producing skin cells.

Instead of rectifying the mistake, experts have tried to hide their embarrassment by adding the word 'malignant' to it, making it a *malignant melanoma*, as if there was a benign melanoma somewhere, too. There isn't. So, what do we call a bunch of benign melanin-producing skin cells that are not cancerous? The answer is not a 'benign melanoma' but a *mole* (if you are a commoner or feudal peasant) or a *naevus* (if you have a medical degree).

Similarly, 'mesothelioma' should be the name of a benign tumour of the membrane around the lung. It's not. It's a nasty malignant growth of this membrane, the benign form being known as a *pleural plaque*. I know, it sounds like something you might hang on your wall, as if you'd been awarded a prize!

Hepat*oma* is not a liver lump but actually a liver cancer; sarc*oma* is a soft tissue cancer; lymph*oma* a blood cancer ….

I could go on for pages, but you get the idea; the naming system for benign and malignant cell growths is totally 'fudged up'.

It's a mess that needs to be sorted. Only then can we improve public understanding and awareness of this disease. And this has to be done if we, the medical profession, want to gain their confidence.

It's not just the nomenclature (system of naming things) for cancer that is confusing. The anti-cancer drug names are even worse. Firstly, most make no sense. There is a term in the English language for it[12]; 'neolalia', defined by the Merriam-Webster Dictionary as "speech, especially of a psychotic that includes words that are new and meaningless to the hearer".

Need I say more?

So, given that the terminology serves to make understanding cancer difficult, I suggest we look at it from a different perspective.

I have made a conscious effort to keep the language simple and uncomplicated because instead of using technical, foreign terms, what's far more important is having a grasp of what is actually happening when cancers form, develop, and spread.

Which brings us back to a focal point. When talking about cancer, I've mentioned our body's cells on several occasions. This is where cancer begins … and ends. So, time to investigate this further.

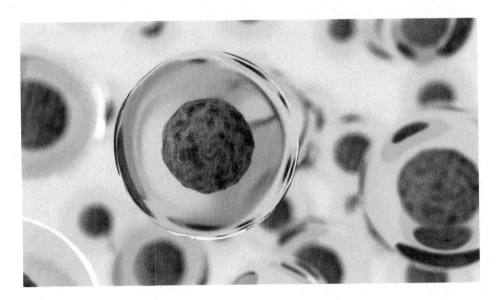

---

[12] Unsurprisingly, the term is a combination of two Greek words, *neos* ('new') and *lalia* ('talk'), chosen specifically for the reason that it could only be understood by the elite and highly educated.

1.2   Building Blocks: The Cell

These little grey cells. It is 'up to them'.

Hercule Poirot, Agatha Christie's famous detective, in her novel, *The Mysterious Affair at Styles* (1920)

The human body, just like all other life forms, is made of basic units, or building blocks, known as *cells*. And there are a lot of these cells in your body. A quite jaw-dropping number, in fact. About ten thousand trillion, according to some experts. Expressed another way, that's 10,000,000,000,000,000 cells in every single one of us. Some are really tiny, others larger. Some live less than a day, while others will live as long as you. Many are highly specialised, forming organs and tissues, and performing incredible feats to keep us alive and kicking.

Given all this, it's hard to imagine that before 1665 nobody had any idea that cells even existed.

In that year, an Englishman, Robert Hooke, discovered small "chambers" in plants while studying them under a magnifying lens. They reminded him of the cells that monks lived in, and hence the name we use today. Hooke was an interesting fellow. Born in 1635 of a humble background, he made a big name and fortune for himself as a scientist and architect. His big break came in 1666 with the Great Fire of London, after which he was given the task of surveying more than half of the razed city.

He was a contemporary of many great scientists of the age, such as Robert Boyle and Isaac Newton. He frequently squabbled with Newton over the credit for many discoveries, including gravity. It's not known whether an apple fell on his head too! Newton had his revenge when he became the president of the Royal Society after Hooke's death, getting rid of Hooke's scientific papers and the only known portrait hanging in the Royal Society in London. Fortunately, Hooke's most famous work, a book called *Micrographia*[13], published in 1665, remained out of Newton's reach.

Although Robert Hooke is credited with discovering the cell, most of the initial progress in the science of microscopy of the cellular world was made by a different "Mr Hook", the uneducated Dutch linen draper, Antonie van Leeuwenhoek. This seemingly improbable contribution came about because Leeuwenhoek was a genius with lenses, and a budding naturalist too.

---

[13] Full name, *Micrographia: or Some Physiological Descriptions of Minute Bodies Made by Magnifying Glasses*. The name says it all.

His initial interest in lenses was simply because he wanted to see the quality of the linen thread close up by magnifying it. But soon he was studying and reporting all sorts of discoveries from the world invisible to the naked eye, including, in 1676, the first observation of a single cell organism. Called 'protozoa', he saw millions of them in a single drop of water. He named them 'animalcules', or 'little animals' at the time.

Remarkably, by the time he died in 1723, he'd notched up quite a number of 'firsts', being the first to observe bacteria and yeast, and accurately describing red blood cells, capillaries (tiny blood vessels), spermatozoa, striated muscle fibres, and the crystalline lens of the eye[14]. His microscopes were small, using just a single lens held close to the eye, with the specimens mounted on a needle in front of it, and which could be adjusted back and forth.

Leeuwenhoek kept his method for making his lenses a closely guarded secret. It wasn't until the 1950s that someone was able to recreate the exact type he was working with.

Progress was slow for the next 150 years. Then, in 1831, Robert Brown, a Scottish scientist, discovered the nucleus in a cell. More on this later, as the nucleus contains something rather important to this book and cancer.

Even then, people did not know the importance and diversity of cells until 1839, when a German, Theodor Schwann, published his book, in which he told the world that all living creatures are made of cells. His 'cell theory' was presented along with other deductions, including that an egg (ovum) begins life as a single cell[15].

Although cells come in a vast range of shapes and sizes – each specialised or *differentiated* to form part of a specific organ or tissue – they all share certain features or structures.

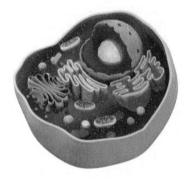

---

[14] He is also thought by some to have been the first to have stained samples to see them better under his lens, doing so using saffron.

[15] He is also credited with coining the term *metabolism* (the chemical processes that occur in a living organism to keep it alive) and also discovered a type of cell that forms the sheath of nerve fibres, and which was named after him (*Schwann cells*).

1.3   Exploring the Cell

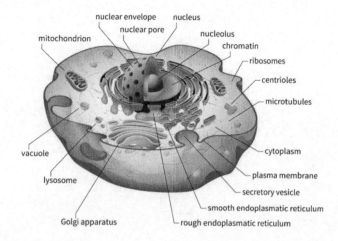

To explore the cell properly, we're going on an expedition. Things could get a little messy, so it's time to put on those swamp boots and helmet, or mask, snorkel, and flippers if you prefer. We're going to shrink ourselves down to something really small – way smaller than a cell, say the size of a virus – and embark on our journey by entering the body's circulation (blood vessels).

Entering a major blood vessel, we hurtle along at speed, a bit like being on a motorway, a network connecting all our body's organs. Eventually, we take a turning onto a more minor road, or smaller blood vessel, and repeat this onto ever narrower roads and lanes until we reach small channels called *capillaries*. Here, finally, we can escape the road, exiting through an open gate (the walls of capillaries are leaky, allowing things to pass back and forth).

Leaving the capillary, we enter the space between cells, aptly called the *intercellular space*. It can be quite wet here and is often flooded with fluid leaking from nearby cells. Bet you're glad of those boots now! Our bodies have pretty good flood defences, however, and excess fluid is carried away by drainage channels known as *lymphatics*[16].

Having splashed about a bit, waded, or swam, we reach the nearest cell. The first thing you see is the cell's outer boundary wall, known as the *cell membrane.* If you expected to be stood before something really solid and impressively protective, like a castle's ramparts, you'll be surprised. The cell membrane is a viscous, double-layered, oily bubble made of proteins and a fatty lipid material containing a lot of cholesterol. This cholesterol wall is studded with receptors that have attachment sites for different chemicals. In addition, there are channels, pores, passages, and pumps, allowing movement of stuff in and out of the cell. And there's much going on. It's a hive of activity.

---

[16] More on them later as these drainage channels play an important role in the escape and spread of cancer cells.

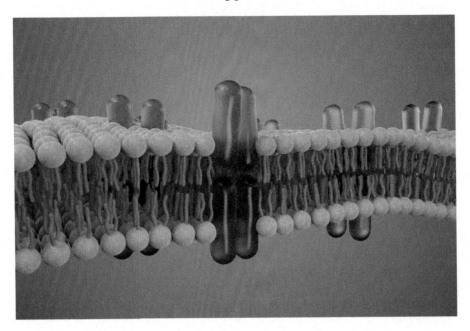

Structure of cell membrane, showing a double layer of fat molecules with transport channels to move chemicals in and out of the cell.

In some tissues, like the outer layers of skin and the gut, called *epithelia*, the cell membrane also keeps cells anchored to a structure known as the *basement membrane*, a delicate layer formed out of protein fibres and polymers of sugars known as *mucopolysaccharides*. If you recall our story earlier about the mutant tribe, and this idea of 'breaking out', the basement membrane is one of those barriers that cancer cells might need to overcome if they are to spread to other parts of the body. Even cancer cells that do not originate from areas with a basement membrane have to face it eventually, because it is found in the walls of the blood vessels, hence making it an important geographical barrier.

Time to go inside. I see you peering around for the equivalent of a front door, as the leaky pores are too small for us to squeeze through. In fact, to enter the cell we need to hitch a ride on a glucose molecule and so, on my instructions, you each grab hold of one. Being your trusted guide, I point to an insulin molecule attaching to its receptor on the cell membrane[17], and you gasp as a channel into the cell suddenly opens. We all groan as some wise guy at the back of our tour party shouts, *"Open sesame!"* (there is always one, isn't there!). But there's no time to waste, and I usher you all inside while the channel remains open.

Stepping into the cell, I spot many puzzled faces among our group. A hand is raised. Ah, you imagined the cell would be full of transparent jelly, did you? I explain that a cell's *cytoplasm* isn't like that at all.

---

[17] Insulin is a chemical made in the body (hormone) which helps get glucose into cells. Glucose and insulin play a vital role in the nutrition and growth of normal and cancer cells.

In fact, we've just entered an incredible maze. It is called the *endoplasmic reticulum*[18] (often affectionately abbreviated to simply the *ER*; 'endoplasmic' refers to its location inside the cytoplasm and 'reticulum' means a network).

The walls of this maze are made of the same double-layered cholesterol-containing lipid found in the outer cell membrane. Just like the internal walls of a house, the ER comes in two sorts: those that are smooth (called *smooth ER*) and those which have appliances attached to them (called *rough ER*).

The rough parts of the ER resemble a gigantic factory complex. Here proteins are made. The appliances attached to the wall are known as *ribosomes*. We huddle round to take a closer look.

Human cells love making proteins. So far, more than 200,000 different proteins have been identified in them. And those are just the ones we've discovered. Perhaps unsurprisingly, we don't know the function of most of them. Those that we do know about are used as structural materials, catalysts for chemical reactions (known as *enzymes*), messengers, receptors, hormones and so on. Among them are proteins that act to stimulate or stop cell growth.

Handing out some magnifying glasses, our expedition party takes it in turns to inspect what's going on in these *ribosomes*. And each sees a production line operating at full tilt. Messengers arrive with templates for protein synthesis, and machinery lines up these templates with the building blocks of proteins, called *amino acids*. The amino acids get joined together in the right order, and finished proteins leave the factory, neatly folded. The sheer variety of proteins emerging from all the ribosomes causes gasps of amazement and favourable comparisons with Willy Wonka's chocolate factory in Roald Dahl's famous children's book. Like Charlie, the main character in the story, we all feel like we've found a Golden Ticket.

The smooth ER has a role, too. It is an expert in making fats known as *lipids*, such as the notorious and ubiquitous cholesterol. As an aside here, given that we so often hear about lowering our cholesterol to help prevent problems like heart disease, you might be quite surprised to think of so much of it being present in our cells. In fact, while excess cholesterol in certain forms is indeed undesirable, the simple fact is that cells need cholesterol in order to exist and function properly. You'd not survive (or even exist) without it.

Time to move on. Gazing about, we can all see many weird and wonderful structures in the cytoplasm which carry out various cellular functions. I point to endosomes, lysosomes, peroxisomes, Golgi bodies, and your mind is spinning. We could spend a lifetime exploring them but, as time is limited, I draw your

---

[18] This is a general rule, and as is the case with all rules, there are some exceptions. In this case, red blood cells and sperm, which do not have the endoplasmic reticulum maze.

attention to some unique and bizarre occupants of the cell, known as the *mitochondria*. There are hundreds of them.

MITOCHONDRIA

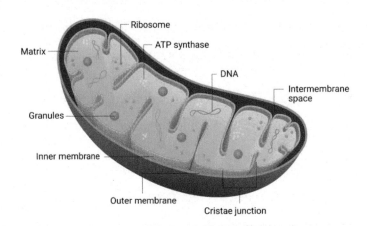

Weirdly, they look like bacteria. And such a comparison might be close to the truth. It is possible that that long, long ago, they may indeed have been free-living bacteria which invaded other cells and decided to stay. Legend[19] has it that when the mitochondria arrived at their new home, they liked the cosy environment as it provided them with protection and food, and the host cell also found them to be very useful. This is because mitochondria are experts in generating efficient packs of energy (known as *ATP*[20]). ATPs are like rechargeable batteries[21]. Mitochondria are the cell's power plants, manufacturing, charging, and recharging the ATP batteries that we run on.

In a typical cell, mitochondria make *one billion* ATP molecules every two minutes. Sounds impressive, but the greedy cell consumes this energy within two minutes too. Yet, mitochondria never complain and have been dutifully doing their job for billions of years. And all that energy has allowed life to evolve beyond a single-cell existence. If it was not for this co-existence of cell and mitochondria, we would not have multicellular life forms on the planet!

Despite co-existing for billions of years, the mitochondria have integrated but not actually assimilated into their new homeland. They retain their own outer and internal membranes and ribosomes, which are as foreign to the cell as any bacteria would be. They also have their own genetic material, comprised of DNA (see below). They remain so similar to bacteria that antibiotics which work by selectively attacking and

---

[19] I say 'legend' but the technical term is 'hypothesis'. The scientific community is divided in their opinion on this matter. One half believes it to be true and the other half doesn't.

[20] ATP stands for *adenosine triphosphate*. Note 'tri' ('three'); hence it has three phosphate molecules attached to it.

[21] Whenever the body needs energy, the phosphates are chopped off, releasing energy and heat. The stripped-down molecule is recycled back to ATP by the addition of phosphates by the mitochondria, and so the cycle continues.

destroying bacterial ribosomes often destroy human mitochondria too, despite sparing the human cell's own ribosomes.

You can also think about mitochondria like a lodger renting your spare room. Apart from providing energy to a cell (akin to weekly rent), they have an independent existence within the cell. They divide and multiply at will, deciding on their own, without consulting the cell (their landlord). But they do it judicially and only increase in number when the cell's energy requirement is high (the thoughtful, helpful sort of lodger – the kind you want).

Continuing through the maze of the endoplasmic reticulum, it leads us all the way to the centre of the cell and our last port of call, its nucleus. The first thing we notice is that the nucleus has its own membrane (*nuclear membrane*) and that it is a continuation of the ER.

The nucleus is the command centre of the cell. The information needed to create and control cell function is located here. One heck of a lot of information needs to be stored, and it comes as no surprise to see it all tightly packed in such a small space. The information is contained within material you've undoubtedly heard of, namely our DNA.

We're going to stick around and examine this DNA closely because it is damage to this stuff that leads to cancer.

The nucleus is full of DNA. And I mean *really* stuffed full with it. It's wound-around proteins called *histones*. When not actively dividing, we call this material *chromatin*. During cell division, however, we see the DNA as aggregated structures called *chromosomes*. If we were to stretch our DNA out, each tiny, microscopic cell nucleus would yield an incredible two metres of this thread. You'd think it would burst the nucleus or break out, but it doesn't. It stays put, preferring to issue orders from its confines, a bit like a general from the safety of headquarters during battle. And these orders are in the form of molecules closely related to DNA, called *RNA* or more specifically *messenger RNA*. We'll examine DNA and RNA a little later.

From our brief expedition into the cell, hopefully you've gained a sense of a scene of organised activity, like a well-oiled industrial city of thriving factories. But this was a healthy cell. Before we step back into the circulation and head home, let's briefly take a peek at what a tumour cell looks like. Anyone fond of chaos and post-apocalyptic worlds should feel right at home.

The first thing you will notice on our approach is that the blood vessels leading to the tumour seem different. They're changing from the smoothly bored pipelines we expected to see to increasingly leaky tubes. The closer we get to the tumour, the more new vessels we spot branching off in all directions too. It's like an untidy mass of tangled wiring in places.

The tumour itself looks like a slum, not a well-ordered industrial town.

Unlike normal cells that stand side by side, attached to each other and their foundation (the basement membrane), here cancer cells are strewn all over the place. Many seem pressed together, overcrowded in the space available. Others have broken off contact from the others. Elsewhere, the basement membrane is being torn to tatters by cells busily making holes in it in order to escape. These tumour cells are intent on seeking their fortune elsewhere.

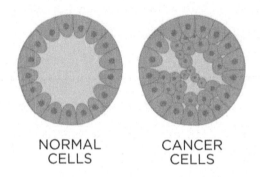

NORMAL
CELLS

CANCER
CELLS

Comparison of normal and cancerous milk ducts in ductal carcinoma of the breast.

Cautiously, I wave you forward for a closer look. The cancer cells are bloated and misshapen with bizarre-looking, massive nuclei[22] occupying most of the internal space. The outer cell membrane is choked full of receptors. We pause to watch what binds to these receptors, and we see different hormones and other growth-promoting chemicals.

Pores, channels, passages, and pumps for exchange of food, water, and other materials are also more numerous compared to a normal cell. As cancer cells love glucose, there are extra receptors for insulin and its partner in crime, a chemical known as *insulin-like growth factor 1* (IGF-1)*,* which open new channels for glucose to enter. This cell is voracious. It wants food and more food. It wants to keep growing, and to do so faster[23.]

One of you asks me, "What did this cell used to do?"

I peer long and hard and find the best reply I can: "Hard to tell. It's barely recognisable."

---

[22] Pleural of *nucleus*.

[23] The role of glucose, insulin and IGF-1 are pretty important, not only in growth of cancers but also in preventing and treating them. We have a whole section dedicated to it later in the book.

41

Someone else asks, "Are they all like this?"

I realise it's time to explain what sets cancer cells apart. We call them the 'hallmarks of cancer', those tell-tale signs. There are 10 of these currently considered the most important. Let's briefly look at each in turn.

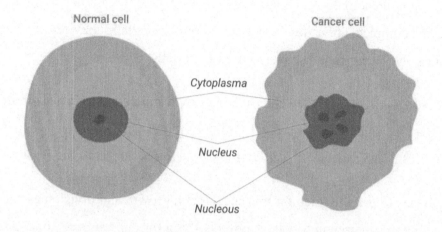

Comparison of a normal cell (left) and cancer cell (right).

1.4   The Hallmarks of Cancer[24]

No. 1   *Unlimited Growth (Self-Sufficiency in Growth Signals)*

NORMAL CELL DEVELOPMENT

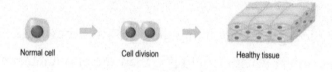

ABNORMAL CELL GROWTH

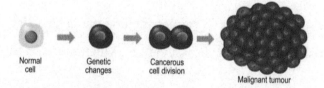

Normal cells follow the body's rules and regulations to grow and multiply only when needed and told to do so. They await signals, in the form of hormones or growth-promoting chemicals.

---

[24] In January 2000, two brilliant scientists, Douglas Hanahan and Robert Weinberg, came up with six characteristics of a cancer cell which makes it stand out among the normal cells. In 2011, the list was updated to 10 hallmarks of cancer. I have taken the liberty of adding three more which, in my opinion, are vital and distinguishing characteristics of cancer cells, and which can play an important role in detecting and treating cancer.

Cancer cells are rebels. They grow and divide at will. In fact, they can motivate themselves by secreting their own growth signals and hormones[25].

Normal cell growth and division is controlled by our genes[26]. Here is something that might potentially confuse you, so take a moment to think about it. One group of genes are known as *tumour promoter genes*. This seems wrong; the complete opposite of what they should be called. They're called 'tumour promoter ' genes simply because they were first discovered in tumour cells.

In fact, when they function normally, they control cell growth and division. However, in cancer cells these same genes are overactive and are out of control. Think of it like a car's accelerator (gas) pedal. You need it for normal driving. But in a cancer cell it is as if it's stuck, pressed flat to the floor.

The rest of the body has to pay the price for this accelerated growth and division as cancer cells consume food and water, including essential nutrients, leaving nothing for the rest of the body. This can starve and lead to the death of normal cells. In a cancer patient this is evident by weight loss and progressive loss of energy and normal body functions.

No. 2   *Not Knowing when to Stop (Insensitivity to Anti-Growth Signals)*

Not only do cancer cells grow at their whim, the rotters also ignore any warnings or instructions from the body to stop growing or dividing.

Every human cell has dedicated genes, controlling their growth. Above, we heard about the somewhat incorrectly named tumour promoter genes. Thankfully, there are also tumour suppressor genes which do exactly what their name suggests. There are three types of tumour suppressor genes:

Caretaker Genes

These take care of any damaged cell DNA. Examples include the genes BRCA1 and BRCA2[27] which, if damaged, can increase the risk of developing breast cancer. Much more on this later.

Gatekeeper Genes

These tumour suppressor genes prevent excessive and uncontrolled growth of cells.

---

[25] A phenomenon known as *autocrine signalling*.

[26] Genes are portions of chromosomal DNA conducting a particular function such as growth or cell division, or making a particular component or chemical for the human body.

[27] BRCA stands for *BReast CAncer gene*. BRCA1 is found on chromosome 17 whereas BRCA2 is found on chromosome 13.

Landscape Genes

Landscape tumour suppressor genes control the environment around the cell. When these genes are damaged, the environment becomes more conducive to unregulated cell growth and multiplication.

Unfortunately, in cancer cells these genes are damaged (mutated) or suppressed and cannot function normally. If we think of them as a car's brakes, then it's easy to imagine the consequences of our brakes failing.

Interestingly, another mechanism of controlling cell growth is 'contact inhibition'. When normal cells divide, they fill up the space available. When they start to push against each other, this gives them a signal to stop multiplying any further. However, cancer cells do not have contact inhibition and continue to grow, regardless of the overcrowding.

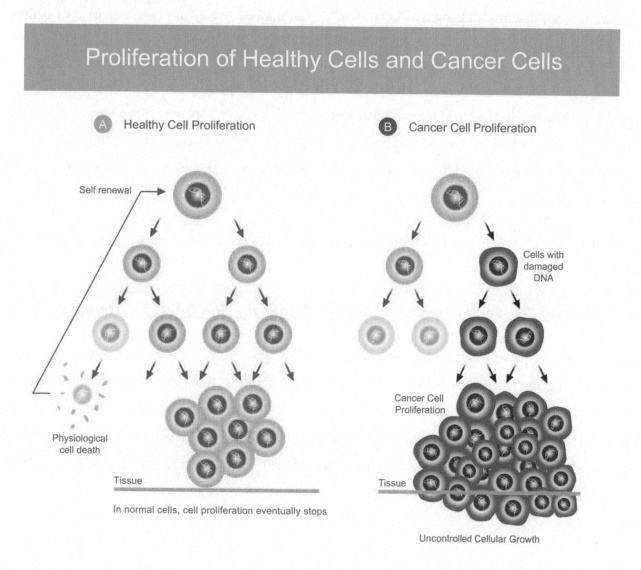

No. 3   Cheating Death (Avoiding Programmed Cell Death)

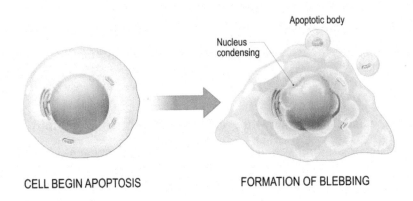

APOPTOSIS
(programmed cell death)

Apoptotic body

Nucleus
condensing

CELL BEGIN APOPTOSIS   FORMATION OF BLEBBING

Programmed cell death, also known as *apoptosis*[28], is an important way our bodies get rid of damaged cells.

It's a cell's self-destruct system for when it develops irreparable damage, especially DNA damage causing hazardous mutations, leading to abnormal functions. Apoptosis is therefore normally a very important way in which we are kept healthy. Our body is able to rid itself of these diseased cells using a highly controlled process. Remember those friendly lodgers in the cell, mitochondria? They play an important role in this process.

Cancer cells often lose this essential protective mechanism, and so damaged cells survive and may go on to form tumours.

No. 4   Living Forever (Limitless Replicative Potential – The Quest for Eternal Life)

Healthy body cells have a normal life cycle; they are born, grow, live, get old and then die. The process of biological ageing is called *senescence*. This might seem obvious. What may surprise you, however, is that mammalian cells have an internal limit, restricting their multiplication to about 60 to 70 doublings. After this they reach a stage of senescence. It is called the 'Hayflick limit', named after Leonard Hayflick whose work, in the 1960s, refuted the idea that a healthy cell, under the right conditions, could continue dividing forever (i.e., was immortal). *It isn't.*

---

[28] From the Greek word *apoptosis* meaning 'falling off'. E.g., like dead leaves falling off a tree.

Senescence is controlled by DNA segments found at the end of our chromosomes (like the plastic tips at the end of shoelaces). These segments are known as *telomeres*[29]. With every cell division cycle, these 'chromosome tips' get shortened. And when they reach a certain limit, the cell gets the signal not to divide any more.

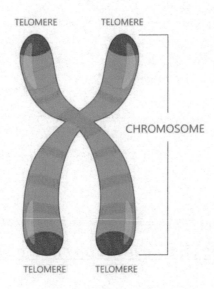

Cancer cells overcome this, producing an enzyme[30] known as *telomerase*, which keeps adding more *telomeres* to the chromosome tips, allowing them, in theory, to divide forever. Some of you might be thinking this is the way to immortality, possibly even to capturing eternal youth. If you're a cancer, maybe it is, but it's not an approach I'd recommend trying!

No. 5   Growing New Blood Vessels (Sustained Development of New Blood Vessels, Angiogenesis)

Normal blood tissue and cells have a limited supply of blood vessels, delivering oxygen and nutrition to them.

As we saw during our expedition, cancer cells are greedy and needy (due to their rapid growth), and this increased demand leads to growth of new blood vessels. Usually, this capability of making new vessels is only active in the body during embryonic development and wound repair.

New vessels increase the flow of blood to the tumour by diverting it from the rest of the body's organs, so not only does it feed the tumour's needs, but comes at a cost elsewhere.

---

[29] From the Greek words *telos* ('end') and *meros* (part).

[30] An enzyme is a protein that helps carry out chemical reactions in the body.

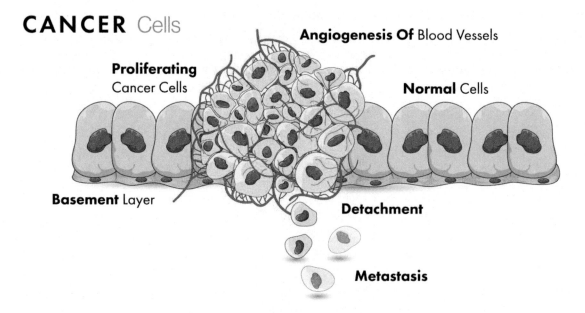

CANCER Cells

Proliferating Cancer Cells

Angiogenesis Of Blood Vessels

Normal Cells

Basement Layer

Detachment

Metastasis

Cancer cells growing a new blood supply (please note how they break out of the basement membrane barrier).

No. 6   Invading and Colonising (Tissue Invasion and Metastases)

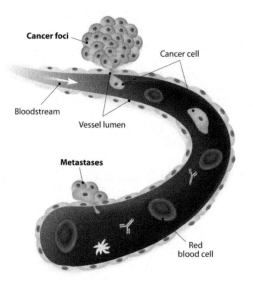

Cancer foci

Cancer cell

Bloodstream

Vessel lumen

Metastases

Red blood cell

The ability of cancer cells to spread to distant parts of the body is a hallmark of advanced disease. We considered this earlier in our story about the mutant GM tribe and their desire to break out of their valley. Escaping involves many processes like breaking off, being able to enter blood vessels, and successfully invading new organs and tissues, so often cancer cells have to accumulate many changes (mutations) before they can spread. Once they reach a new site, they set up a colony and expand, starving and killing off the native cells in the process.

No. 7   Unconventional Eating Habits (Deregulated Metabolism)

Warburg effect

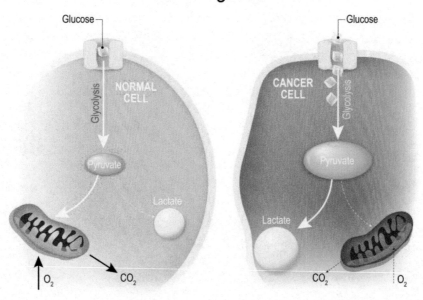

During our expedition into a normal cell, we came across those remarkable interlopers called *mitochondria*, the power plants of our cells, which create those power packs (ATPs) from glucose. We also learnt that usually they replicate themselves in response to the cell's needs for energy. In a bizarre twist, in cancer cells the mitochondria do not participate in providing energy to the cell. It's as if they are refusing to cooperate in the cancer cell's nefarious activities. The exact reason for this is not yet known but might hold an important clue to treating and curing cancer.

Cancer cells sideline the mitochondria and find an alternative way of generating energy from glucose. They instead convert it to a substance called *pyruvate*, which provides energy but is pretty inefficient. This switch is known as the 'Warburg effect', named after the German chemist who observed that in all types of solid tumours he studied, they secreted an unusual amount of a particular type of acid known as *lactic acid*.

Sidelining mitochondria also has an additional benefit for the cancer cells. As mentioned above, mitochondria play an important role in apoptosis, the programmed cell death of damaged cells. They do this by releasing special proteins that initiate this process. Switching metabolism to a process of fermentation causes a shutdown of the mitochondria and the safety system that kills off abnormal cells, like cancer cells.

No. 8   Fooling the Security Forces (Evading the Immune System)

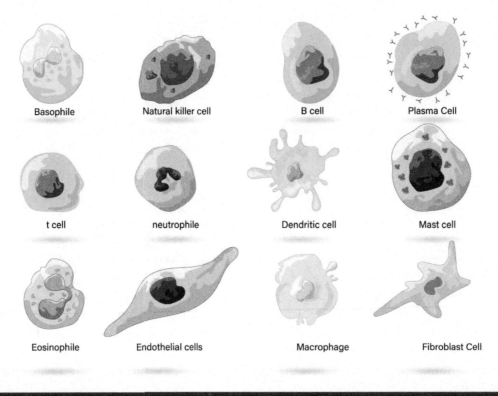

Immune Cells Collection

Our immune system has the capability of identifying and getting rid of abnormal cells. Cancer cells are abnormal but often manage to evade the body's immune surveillance. They do this in many ways, one of which is by continually changing their outer shape and form by shedding cell membrane markers, which the immune system uses as clues to identify them[31].

Sometimes, they hide behind normal cells, using them as a body shield to avoid detection by immune cells. One such hostage is a tiny blood cell known as a *platelet*. While travelling in the blood stream, cancer cells are an open target to the body's security system known as the *white blood cells*. To avoid them, they attract and stick platelets all around themselves, masquerading as a group of platelets travelling normally in the blood stream.

Stimulating and supporting the immune system in fighting cancer is the new frontier and we will discuss it in more detail later in this book.

---

[31] The technical term for such markers is an *antigen*.

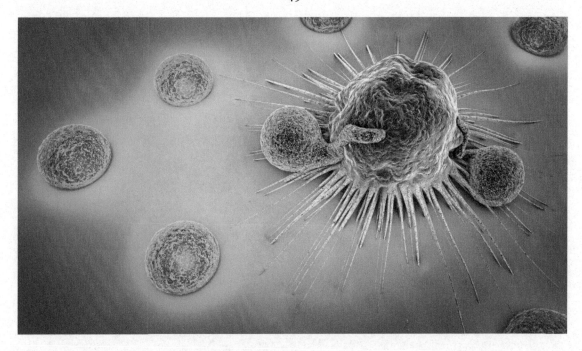

Immune cells attacking a cancer cell.

No. 9   The Born Mutant (Genome Instability)

Cancer cells generally have severe chromosomal abnormalities, worsening the disease as it progresses. These abnormalities are also a source of multiple mutations in the DNA which promote cell growth and invasion.

No. 10   Hot and Sore (Inflammation)

Cancer cells have a highly inflammatory environment around them, encouraging the growth of new blood vessels and helping to spread the disease both locally and far and wide.

* * *

These are the 10 well-recognised and classic characteristics of a cancer.

However, more recently news has started to filter through about some other unique features of cancer which has not only increased our understanding of the disease but given hope that they can be used in detecting and treating cancers early.

I have chosen three of them and added to the classical list of 10. So here they are, Khan's Triad of Additional Cancer Characteristics.

No. 11 Increased Acid Production

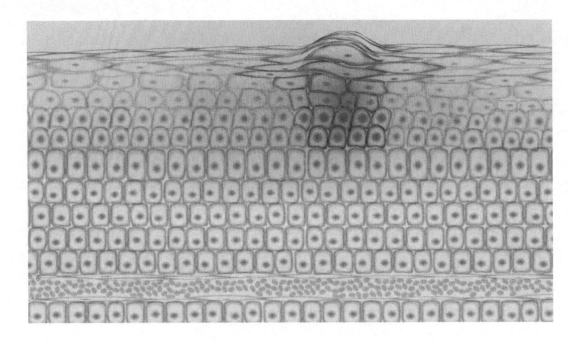

Skin cancer (melanoma) cells growing among normal skin cells.

Cancers love to live in an acidic environment. To do so they produce a lot of acid.

Acidity is measured in terms of pH. A pH of 7 is neutral, like water. Below 7 is acidic and above is base or alkaline. The normal human body maintains a pH between 7.35 to 7.45. Cancer cells create a microenvironment around them with a pH between 6.5 to 6.9. This raises two important questions. Why do they do it and how do they do it?

A. Why they do it? An acidic environment is toxic to normal body cells but not cancer cells, which are resistant to it. It kills off normal cells and also helps the cancer to damage barriers like the basement membrane which otherwise stop them from spreading.

B. How do they do it? Cancer cells make a lot of acid. Normal cells use mitochondria to get energy. Mitochondria are like kitchens with master chefs, they neatly process glucose to generate 36 packets of energy (ATPs) with very little waste. Cancer cells, on the other hand, brutally chop off glucose to get just two packets of ATP and turn the rest into lactic acid.

This is an important difference between normal and cancer cells, and has potential for devising new detection and treatment strategies (more on it later in this book).

No. 12   A Pursuit of Primitiveness (Devolution)

Cancer is evolution in reverse, a process of devolution if you may. Instead of being part of a well-organised multicellular body, cancer cells are eagerly reverting to a primitive, unicellular life.

The genes activated in the cancer cell are not just random genes but the exact primitive genes which allow a cell to grow, live, and divide like a single cellular organism. These primitive genes are usually kept tucked away to be used only at rare moments in life. For example, when the body needs to make a sperm, or a white blood cell needs to move around. But cancer cells activate all these primitive genetic instincts and use them to implement their selfish agenda of self-survival at the cost of other cells.

These behaviours are eerily similar to single-cell organisms, like bacteria. Living with little or no oxygen, breaking glucose by glycolysis instead of using mitochondria, making and secreting acid to 'kill thy neighbour', and destroying the body's infrastructure to expand your territory are typical primitive behaviours.

It's no surprise that when the human genome was studied, it was found that cancer cells showed activation of primitive genes which are found in unicellular organisms, and which in normal cells are kept inactively tucked away in normal human DNA.

No. 13   The Mothership Phenomena

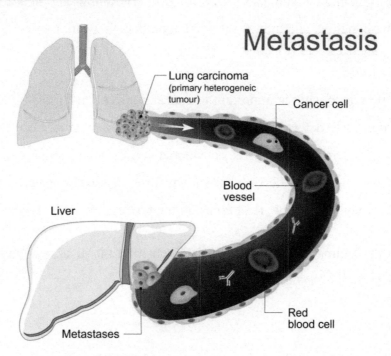

It has been known for a long time that cancer starts in one part of the body and then spreads far and wide. Traditionally, we thought that when a tumour becomes overpopulated with cells competing for food and resources, some of them would break off and travel in search of greener pastures, establishing new colonies at distant shores and live happily ever after.

We were wrong.

Increasingly, the evidence is painting a very different picture.

Cancer cells start breaking off the mother tumour at a much earlier stage, before the main camp becomes overcrowded. They are not desperate but adventurous. These cells enter the bloodstream and circulate around the body and, hence, are known as *circulating tumour cells* or *CTCs* for short. The body in general, and the bloodstream in particular, is quite hostile to them. They get tossed and turned, knocked and hit, bruised and ripped in this process. Special immune cells with a license to kill, known as *natural killer cells* (NK cells[32]) hunt them down. Most if not all CTCs are killed (told you the human body is amazing at killing cancer). However, some might survive and eventually make their way back to the main tumour site. But these survivors are not the naive CTCs that left the tumour earlier. Now they are battle-hardened veterans who have fought the odds and lived to tell the tale. In the safety of their mothership tumour, they grow and divide and venture out again, with more experience and in greater numbers than before. The process is repeated over and over again, sometimes over years until a tough cadre of colonisers is developed that can fight or deceive the body's anti-cancer system.

Cancer cells returning to the mothership also reseed the primary tumour and hence the main colony also becomes repopulated with tougher and more aggressive members that can, more effectively, ward off any attacks from the immune system.

This mothership-satellite relationship is important to cancer survival and spread. I believe it has a major role in cancer prevention, early detection, and treatment. As a general rule, once the cancer has spread, removing the primary (mothership) tumour is considered futile, but in some cancers (such as kidney cancer) removing or damaging the mothership has shown shrinkage of the satellite tumours. We will talk about it in detail at a later point. For now, let's focus on the process of cancer formation.

We have talked about the hallmarks of cancer. What lies behind the disease is damage to our DNA, so let's take a closer look at it.

---

[32] Their official designation is *CD56 lymphocytes*.

1.5   DNA Unravelled

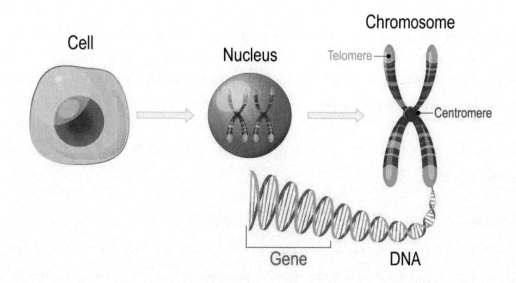

Despite being discovered more than 150 years ago, in 1869, by Swiss scientist Johannes Friedrich Miescher, at the time experts weren't sure what DNA did, or if it did anything useful at all. There was time when it was even referred to as a "stupid molecule". Hard to imagine, now we know so much more.

To his credit, Johannes not only discovered this enigmatic molecule but also suggested that it could be involved in the transmission of hereditary information. He went as far as suggesting that DNA might have something akin to an alphabet to write information. Johannes was way ahead of his time. It was not until 1953 that these facts were accepted.

Despite Johannes' intelligent observations, the experts of his day did not give any importance to DNA. Instead, they fixated on the tiny amount of protein found in the nucleus and considered this to be where genetic information was stored. They thought that DNA was no more than 'packaging material'. Why the cell bothered to create such abundant amounts of this 'filler 'never seemed to have occurred to them. DNA was considered boring. After all, as far as they could tell, it stayed in the nucleus, did not react with any other chemical, and was made up of too few basic components to be meaningful. Proteins, on the other hand, well these were more familiar and exciting. They were found everywhere, moved in and out of cells, and came in an incredible range of structures, sizes, and shapes.

Call it human nature if you like, but so often what we can't understand or associate with is labelled as useless and unimportant. DNA continued to suffer from this ignorance for many decades afterwards.

And, yet, DNA kept stubbornly turning up in every experiment involving a quest for genetic and hereditary information. Be it the discovery of chromosomes in 1888, or the pioneering work of Thomas Morgan

Hunt, who deliberately mutated flies with X-ray radiation like in a sci-fi horror movie. DNA, it seemed, refused to be ignored.

Finally, it caught the attention of a clever Canadian chap, Oswald Avery.

Oswald Theodore Avery Jr was born in 1877 in Halifax, Nova Scotia, but spent most of his career working at the Rockefeller Hospital in the Big Apple, New York City, USA.

He started by studying music but later switched to medicine at college, and in 1912 was awarded a scholarship to work in the USA.

His field of interest was flu and pneumonia. While studying these diseases, he grew fascinated with a type of pneumonia-causing bacteria known as *pneumococci* (*pneumo*, referring to lungs and lung infection; *coccus*, plural *cocci*, meaning 'round-shaped'). The *pneumococci* came in two varieties: rough and smooth. They were designated as 'R' and 'S' strains accordingly. The rough R type was harmless to humans but the smooth S variety, which had a capsule around it, caused fatal infections.

He noted that when grown in culture media, S bacteria produced more smooth bacteria and the R type produced more rough bacteria, suggesting this difference between R and S strains was hereditary, and therefore predictable.

Avery decided to perform an unusual experiment. Having selectively killed the smooth, deadly strain, he mixed the dead bacteria with some living R type. To his surprise, the rough R bacteria transformed into the smooth type. It was as if they had picked up the hereditary information on how to make a smooth coat from their dead friends. Baffling! How could this possibly be?

Next, he designed a clever experiment. He used protein-breaking enzymes called *proteases* to digest all the proteins from the dead S bacteria, and again mixed it with the living R variety. According to the predominant theory of his time, because proteins were believed to be the source of genetic and hereditary information, he expected that the information would be lost, and so there'd be no effect on adding it to living R-type bacteria. To his utter surprise, the R bacteria promptly transformed into the smooth variety, just as before.

Avery rightly concluded that proteins could not be the source of the genetic information. The only remaining candidate was the hitherto much ignored DNA.

But Avery was not in a hurry to shout his discovery from the rooftops. First, he wanted to prove this fact beyond any doubt. To do this, he set about destroying the DNA in the dead S-type bacteria before again mixing them with living R bacteria.

If he was right, with the DNA destroyed, nothing should happen. And guess what? This time, nothing happened. Hurrah! It was the last nail in the coffin of the longstanding 'protein theory of hereditary' and indisputable proof of DNA's role. Time to tell the world.

However, what happened next was something Avery could not have predicted.

Instead of being hailed and lauded, there was a storm of criticism against him, led by eminent scientists who had a blind faith in the protein theory of inheritance.

After publishing his ground-breaking findings in 1944, Avery was nominated for the Nobel Prize many times throughout the 1940s and 1950s, but the protein enthusiasts lobbied hard to make sure that he never got one (feel free to boo and hiss at the injustice of it all). But many had been persuaded. Oswald Theodore Avery Jr passed away on 20th February, 1955, and was eventually declared "the most deserving scientist not to receive the Nobel Prize for his work".

So, finally, and belatedly, there was a growing consensus among the scientific community regarding his extraordinary contributions to modern science.

With this shift in thinking, between 1944 and 1953 there was a frenzy of scientific activity to determine the structure and function of DNA. The race was on and in the lead were three distinguished figures of the scientific world. Linus Pauling of the Caltech Institute, USA, already had two Nobel Prizes and was a pioneer and expert in the field of X-ray crystallography, which he was using to determine the shape of DNA. He was after his hat-trick for the mantelpiece.

Meanwhile, in England, the New Zealand-born Maurice Wilkins and Rosalind Franklin, daughter of a London banker, both experts in the fields of chemistry and X-rays, were the closest contenders to Pauling for the win.

The puzzle they faced was really tricky. On the one hand, chemistry told them what DNA contained, and the proportions of each constituent. On the other hand, 'photographs 'resulting from bombarding DNA with X-rays, showed a distinctive 'pattern'. Different crystal structures were known to give rise to different patterns. So, how could the constituents be arranged in three dimensions to create the same pattern when blasted with X-rays? Quite a mind-boggling problem, and to solve it would require much trial and error, and clever thinking.

So, imagine the shock and surprise when, on 25th February, 1953, the eminent scientific journal *Nature* published a 900-word article titled 'Structure for Deoxyribose Nucleic Acid' which correctly described the double helical structure of DNA, written by two previously unknown chaps: James Watson and Francis Crick.

Both Watson, a young American in his twenties, and Crick, an Englishman in his thirties, were never part of the formal race for discovering the structure of DNA, and neither had specialist training in chemistry or X-ray crystallography, either. But to their advantage, they had direct access to both Wilkins and Franklin, and hence their work, and indirect news of Pauling's progress in USA through his son, who worked in the UK.

They further took advantage of the fact that Franklin and Wilkins, who worked in the same department, "did not get along", which could be an understatement of the century. Actually, they were bitter enemies and often not on talking terms. Watson and Crick played this to their advantage. Through Pauling's son they found out that his father was obsessively fixated on the idea that DNA was a triple helix (it isn't; it's a double helix, but gosh he nearly cracked it) and was stubbornly and frustratingly trying to fit all available information into his preferred model.

On the other hand, Wilkins and Franklin were on the right track but jealously guarded their secrets from one another, so neither saw the whole picture. Franklin, on one occasion, even announced the "death of the double helical structure theory", despite having evidence to the contrary, just to mislead Wilkins.

Wilkins was a more willing partner for Watson and Crick than Franklin, sharing both his, and at one crucial point, Franklin's, X-ray crystallography findings with them. Inadvertently, he'd passed on crucial information to these two young men whom he found quite non-threatening in the competitive world of scientific discovery.

By early 1953, Watson and Crick had completed their model using bolted metal plates, which accurately showed a double helical, spiral structure of the DNA molecule. In 1962, Watson and Crick were awarded the Nobel Prize for their work. A third person shared the prize. Maurice Wilkins was rewarded too.

An interesting fact about us is that if we compare human DNA from different races, it would be very difficult to tell us apart. Incredibly, we all share 99.9 percent of our DNA. This means that an Australian Aboriginal's DNA is 99.9% identical to the DNA of a Northern European, a Canadian Inuit or an African from the Congo. Despite all of our apparent differences, deep down we are all very similar, almost identical.

Yet, despite scientific progress, 97% of our DNA is still an enigma. Some scientists think that it has no function and call it 'junk DNA'.

Is this likely? Remember, before Oswald Avery's findings, DNA was considered to be 'packaging material for proteins' in the nucleus because scientists could not make sense of what it did. The same ignorance seems to still prevail among some.

I personally can't believe that the human cell goes to all this effort, making up to two metres of DNA, for no good reason. It's a ludicrous idea. It's simply our current ignorance about what most of it does.

Being the essence of life, and of inheritance, we might have guessed that nature would come up with a truly elegant, beautiful, and remarkable solution. And, for our purposes, we need to look at DNA a little more closely, as this will enable us to see how damage to it can lead to many diseases, especially the one we are talking about: cancer.

1.6   Our Amazing DNA

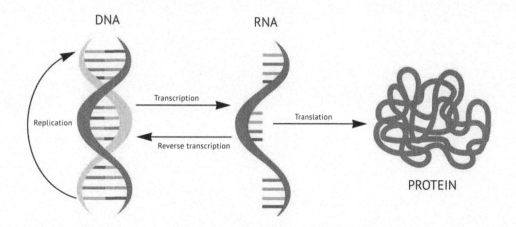

DNA and RNA making proteins.

Not only is DNA an elegant solution, it is also a surprisingly simple one. So, how does it actually work?

DNA sits in the centre of the cell (nucleus) like an army general and sends its orders as coded messages via a messenger rightly known as a messenger RNA (mRNA[33]) to the cell.

The mRNA takes the orders to protein-making factories known as ribosomes.

Human cells make hundreds of thousands of proteins[34], each capable of carrying out a different type of function ordained by the DNA.

The whole process is not only amazing but also surprisingly accurate.

You might be wondering why we've taken such a detour into the basic processes in our cells. This book is about cancer, isn't it? Yes, exactly. If you think about the process outlined above, it is quite easy to imagine that if our DNA was damaged in some way then problems might arise. Suppose, for example, something caused a DNA strand to break. Or something led to the deletion of a section of DNA. The genetic code[35] would be changed too, and it might give a wrong message to the mRNA. This could lead to errors in protein synthesis, and the resulting protein wouldn't function properly. What if the error occurred in a protein that controlled cell division, maybe resulting in the cell thinking it needs to continually replicate? And what do cancer cells do? They replicate, forming colonies of defective cells … see what I mean?

Later, we'll have a closer look at some of these errors or *mutations* in relation to cancer.

---

[33] RNA stands for *ribonucleic acid*; mRNA is a single-stranded mirror version of one of the DNA strands which can easily slip out of the nucleus.

[34] Proteins are made of subunits known as *amino acids*.

[35] The part of DNA that carries the code to insert a particular amino acid in a protein chain is known as a *codon*.

1.7   Damaging Our DNA

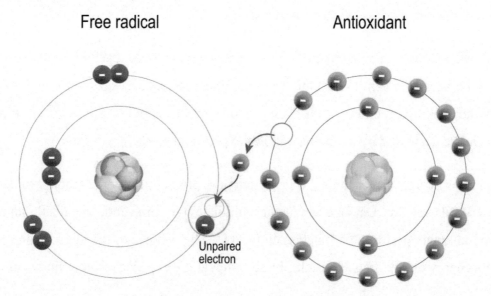

Free radical   Antioxidant

Unpaired
electron

Antioxidant (anti-cancer chemical) detoxing a free radical (cancer-causing chemical).

Any change[36] in our DNA (known as a *mutation*) can affect its function. For example, making the cell grow out of control or divide continuously, or lead to defective protein synthesis etc.

You might think that instances of damage are thankfully rare but, in fact, they are common. A bit too common if you ask me. Here's an incredible fact. Each strand of DNA can be damaged up to 10,000 times a day! This damage can be due to toxic products made in the body or found in the environment. For example, chemicals known as *superoxide radicals*, which have very toxic, negatively charged oxygen atoms, react with normal cell structures, including DNA. Luckily, nature also has some very helpful chemicals known as *antioxidants* such as vitamin C and vitamin E, which neutralise them. We will talk about these later in the book.

But chemicals are not the only things to damage cells and their DNA. Radiation, X-rays, and ultraviolet light can also cause this damage.

DNA can have damage to just one strand or both strands. As might be expected, single-strand damage is easier to repair than double-strand damage.

Errors and damage can also occur when cells divide (duplicate), with faults arising during the copying of the chromosomes.

---

[36] A change in DNA (mutation) can occur due to many reasons. The most common are physical damage or errors during cell division, when DNA is doubled in size and then split between the two cells. Sometimes, parts of DNA get dislocated and reattached to a different segment, which results in malfunction.

As we saw above, DNA is a twisted, double strand. In cell division, it first needs to be untwisted into a straight ladder and then the two strands are unzipped.

Once unzipped, each strand is copied and this process is prone to error, causing mutations. Fortunately, our cells have a robust mechanism to heal this damage. There are special enzymes which check the DNA for any errors and make corrections, both during and after the copying process[37]. If that fails, often defective cells can be destroyed by the body, helping to prevent disease.

However, sometimes the repair mechanism is defective or overwhelmed by the amount of damage and the resulting mutated cells survive. Damage can also accumulate over time and, as a result, an abnormal cell emerges. It may no longer perform the functions it used to. The damage to its internal controls might lead it to focusing its energy on dividing and multiplying, often at the expense of other body cells.

Such mutants or *transformed cells* are called *cancer cells*.

When you consider the complexity of DNA and the sheer opportunity and frequency of damage, it's not a surprise that cancer occurs. In fact, the real surprise is how often it does not happen. Every day *each* strand of our DNA suffers more than a thousand[38] cuts which can potentially cause a cancer (and that's just one type of damage). Credit has to go to the excellent repair mechanism our cells have.

---

[37] The copying process is known as *DNA replication*. There are many enzymes involved in DNA repair such as DNA polymerase, exonuclease, endonuclease, and DNA ligase.
[38] Up to ten thousand cuts depending on the number of damaging factors we are exposed to.

1.8   How Cancer Spreads (Metastasis)

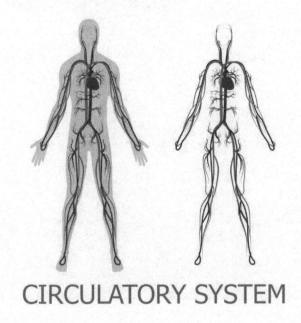

CIRCULATORY SYSTEM

Human circulatory system showing arteries and veins.

Imagine a modern city. Its basic units are houses where people live. The houses are connected to each other by streets. Streets are connected by small roads within neighbourhoods. Larger roads and motorways connect cities throughout the country.

Within the cities there is another network of underground connections linked to every house, draining away water and sewage, the sewerage system being connected to filtration plants in every town.

The human body is very similar in layout to a modern city.

Its cells live in clusters called *tissues*, within different organs. Cells and tissues are connected to each other by capillaries, like streets. Capillaries join to form larger vessels called *veins* and *arteries*, one-way roads with unidirectional flow of blood. Veins and arteries join from different organs to make larger veins and arteries.

Just like the sewerage system in the cities, the human body also has a drainage system known as the *lymphatics*[39]. This drains excess water and waste from cells into channels connected to filtration plants known as *lymph nodes*. Lymph nodes are located in every region of the body. They filter out any debris and pour the filtered fluid into the main blood circulation.

---

[39] We briefly touched on it earlier and I promised to tell you more, so here it is.

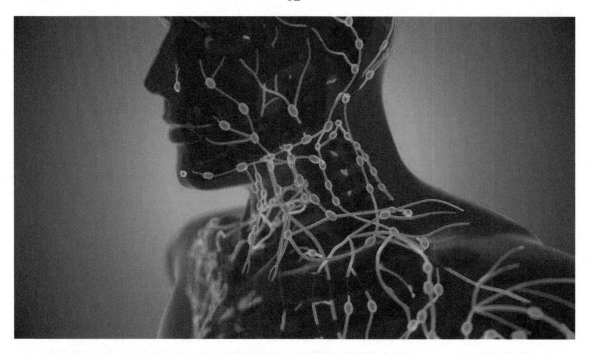

Human lymphatic system with lymph nodes and connecting channels (lymphatics).

When cancer cells start to grow in any part of the body, they soon run out of resources like food and water due to overpopulation. Hence, they need to move out to new areas where there is more space for them to grow.

They do this by using the network of blood vessels. In addition, they also use the lymphatic system to escape. As lymphatics are connected to the lymph nodes for filtration, cancer cells get trapped in the lymph nodes, making them swell and become visible.

Lymph node

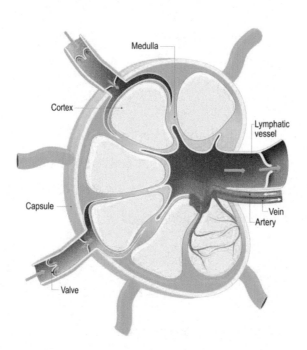

These are often the earliest sign of cancer spread, presenting as palpable lumps. However, the entrapment is temporary, with many cancer cells escaping the lymph nodes to spread, while others stay, turning the lymph nodes into new growth centres.

Once the cancer cells reach a new site, they set up a colony and start to grow at the expense of the native cells. This causes a slow and steady destruction of the normal cells and, eventually, the organ invaded fails to perform its normal function. The choice of organ depends on the cancer type. Curiously, certain cancers have a particular affinity for specific organs.

For example, prostate cancer cells are very fond of growing in the bone. This has given rise to the 'seed and soil' theory of cancer spread, stating that certain cancer cell types are suited to grow in the environment of a particular organ and preferably metastasise (spread) to it even if it is far from their site of origin. So, a prostate cancer cell would often bypass nearby organs such as bowel, bladder, kidney, and spleen, preferring to grow in bone as distant as a rib or the skull.

Evidence is emerging that metastatic cancer cells don't always develop in response to overpopulation at the site of origin. Some cancer cells are 'born adventurous'. They have mutations that give them the ability to break off from the primary tumour and spread to distant sites early in the course of disease. These cancer clones migrate much earlier and start growing as a new colony in far-off parts of the body, sometimes even before the primary tumour becomes visible.

Although the primary site of cancer development acts like a mothership, launching metastatic cancer cells, once the migrant cells have colonised the new site, they start to evolve differently from the parent cells. Over time, new 'clones' are formed that are more suitable to growing in their new environment, and these behave differently from the original tumour [40]. Last but not least, as we discussed earlier the colonisers/settlers keep revisiting the motherland and enriching its genetic pool. This makes treating and curing cancer more challenging.

---

[40] This phenomenon is known as *cancer clone phylogenomics* and has been demonstrated in colon cancer cells by Christina Curtis at the Stanford University School of Medicine in California, USA.

WHAT
MAKES CANCER
SO DIFFICULT
TO TREAT?

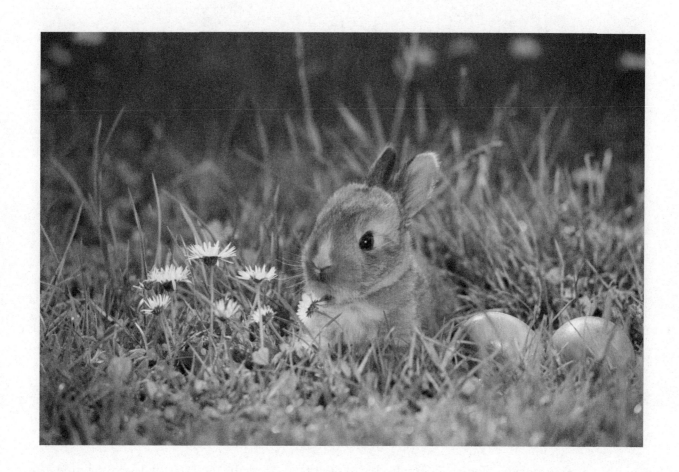

PART 2: WHAT MAKES CANCER SO DIFFICULT TO TREAT?

2   The (Australian) Rabbit Analogy

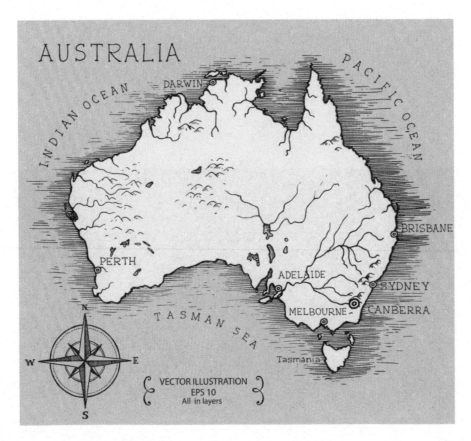

Trying to treat cancer is a bit like killing rabbits in Australia. It sounds simple but is actually one of the biggest challenges ever faced by mankind. To understand it, let's talk about rabbits first.

There was a time, long, long ago when there were no rabbits in Australia and everything, flora and fauna, man and kangaroo, lived (relatively) happily.

Then along came European colonists who introduced rabbits to Australia, and this had a devastating effect on the country.

Initially, it looked like a harmless exercise; rabbits shipped in and bred in captivity, sold for meat and fur. Then, one fateful day in 1859, a gentleman by the name of Thomas Austin (of Barwon Park near Winchelsea, Victoria) made a terrible mistake. He asked his nephew, William Austin, in England, to send him some rabbits. The idea was to let them go wild and breed freely, so they could be hunted for game. His nephew hurriedly collected two dozen rabbits of various breeds and sent them to Australia.

Now everyone knows that rabbits breed like ... well, like rabbits.

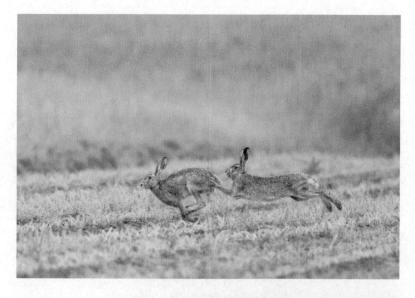

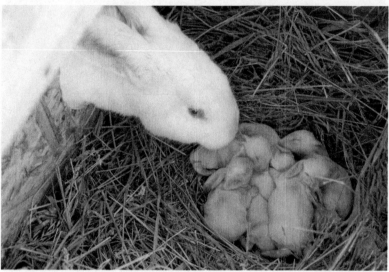

And that is exactly what happened.

These furry little terrors spread like a cancer, invading and destroying the Australian landscape. They consumed everything in their path: trees, herbs and shrubs, let's say any vegetation in sight[41], used holes and tunnels to hide, survive, grow, and breed, expanding their territory to hundreds of square miles. The milder Australian winters encouraged them to breed all year round. By 1869, 10 years after Thomas Austin had released his 24 rabbits, Australians were hunting up to two million rabbits a year and the total population was still expanding[42].

---

[41]The method applied by rabbits in destroying the plants, especially the trees, is called 'ring barking' or 'girdling'. Girdling is the complete removal of a strip of bark from around the entire circumference of a plant and results in death of the area above the girdle. A branch completely girdled will fail and when the main trunk of a tree is girdled, the entire tree will die, especially if it cannot regrow from above to bridge the wound.

[42]It is the fastest spread ever recorded of any mammal in the world.

Things were made worse by a prolonged drought, causing widespread destruction of plants and trees. Soon, the fertile topsoil turned to dust and blew away, never to be replaced, turning vast regions of the country into an expanding desert[43].

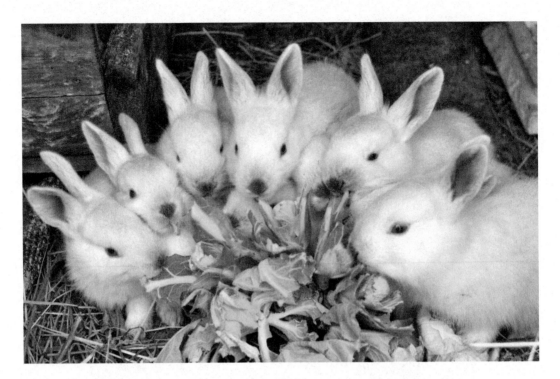

Unlike other continents, Australia had no natural predators to hunt the rabbits and keep their population in check. Some people tried to introduce predators to control their spread, but these new animals found it much easier to catch and kill the local animals rather than the crafty rabbits, which were fast on their paws and good at hiding underground[44].

Others used poisons and toxins, but these again killed more native animals than the pesky pests[45].

What they needed was a bunny-specific treatment that would only kill the rabbits and spare other living creatures.

And finally, the magic cure was found ... or was it?

---

[43] Australia is mostly desert, especially in the centre, but around the rim there are thousands of miles of fertile regions which became the target of the rabbit epidemic.

[44] One way of doing this is hunting using ferrets, where ferrets are deployed to chase the rabbits out to be shot or into nets set over the burrows.

[45] Australians used all kinds of gruesome methods to kill rabbits. Destroying warrens through ripping (a procedure where rabbits are dismembered or buried alive as a bulldozer dragging sharp tines is driven over their warrens/burrows). Other methods included ploughing, blasting, and fumigating.

In the 1950s, a virus known as 'Myxoma virus' was discovered that selectively caused disease (myxomatosis) in rabbits. The disease was very lethal, killing 99% of its victims[46].

It wasn't long before there were millions of dead bunnies all over the landscape where once they had run amok.

It seemed like the curse was over, but it wasn't long before the rabbit population started to recover.

And here's the catch.

In his rush to send rabbits to his uncle, Thomas Austin got hold of a potpourri of different breeds. That meant a lot of genetic variation among the rabbits, and even more in their offspring due to reshuffling of genes (just like when you shuffle a deck of cards, you get dealt a different hand every time). This interbreeding often creates tougher animals, more resistant to the challenges of their environment – especially disease – compared to thoroughbred animals.

The disease killed 99% of the rabbits, which sounds astonishing, but also meant that one out of every hundred survived the plague. Australia had hundreds of millions of rabbits (600 million by one estimate in 1950s) meaning millions survived.

Combine the two factors and you get multi-million disease-resistant bunnies who went back to their business of eating, growing, hiding, mating, and reproducing. Soon the population was replenished, and the destruction of the Australian environment resumed.

To date, the rabbit epidemic in Australia is controlled but not cured.

The story of cancer is very similar.

It starts with a bunch of mutated cells undergoing genetic reshuffling with every generation, multiplying into a large number of cells that invade and consume one organ after another, expanding their territory over time.

---

[46]In 1950, after research was conducted by Frank Fenner, myxoma virus was deliberately released into the rabbit population, causing it to drop from an estimated 600 million to around 100 million. Genetic resistance in the remaining rabbits allowed the population to recover to 200–300 million by 1991.

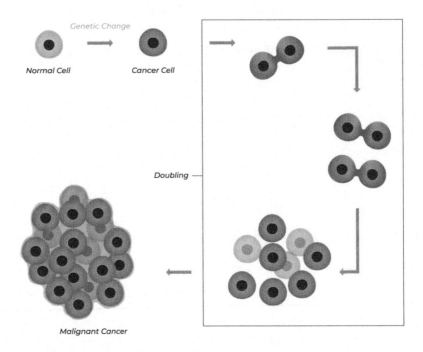

Genetic Change

Normal Cell　　*Cancer Cell*

Doubling

Malignant Cancer

PROCESS OF CANCER CELL DEVELOPMENT

Like the rabbits in Australia, they face few threats from natural predators. The human body's defence system is best designed to kill bugs like viruses, bacteria, parasites, and fungi.

Like rabbits, cancer cells are good at hiding and breeding.

One can use poisons and toxins to kill them (it's called 'chemotherapy') but just like their use in Australia against the rabbits, these chemicals are often more toxic to the normal body cells than the cancer cells. Even when they kill the cancer cells, it comes at a cost of damaging the body and hence very high doses can't be used.

Sometimes, cancer-specific drugs are found which selectively target and kill up to 99% of the cancer cells. But a small pea-sized cancer can comprise hundreds of millions of cells, and so millions survive the treatment. Even a very effective and targeted treatment that could kill 99.99% of cancer cells would leave behind hundreds of thousands of survivors which are resistant to the same treatment and soon start to replace the dead cells and even outgrow their predecessors.

Last, but not the least, the carnage committed by the rabbits in Australia was made worse by natural disasters such as the prolonged drought. Similarly, often the human body is not hit by cancer in isolation. Other health problems such as heart disease, infections, and diabetes reduce the ability of our body to recover from the devastation of cancer and its complications.

So, the best way to deal with cancer is to prevent it, like not letting any bunnies loose in Australia in the first place.

If it does develop, the next best strategy is to detect it and treat it early. That is, kill the bunnies before they start hiding underground and spreading like wildfire. Treating cancer in its early stages is often very effective and sometimes curative (for example, early-stage testicular cancer can be cured 97% of the time if caught early. Compare this to treating other diseases such as a stroke or heart disease, where the *cure* rates are around zero).

Even when not cured, early-stage cancer can usually be controlled effectively for a long period of time.

As we've seen, cancer is a disease of genetic mutations. These mutations accumulate over a period of time, and the more the mutations – in quantity and quality – the more aggressive the disease. What helps in treating cancer is having fewer mutations and less genetic variation among the cancer cells. That sounds difficult but is actually easy to achieve. By avoiding the agents that damage genes and cause cancer (known as 'carcinogens', a combination of two words, *carcinos*, 'cancer' and *gen*, 'genesis/birth'), even if cancer does develop it has less resistance to treatment compared to cancers in a body exposed to a lot of carcinogens. And, importantly, this continues to be the case after a cancer has started.

In other words, someone who smokes fewer cigarettes and drinks less alcohol would have a less nasty and more treatable cancer than a person who smokes and drinks excessively, and who continues to do so after their diagnosis.

More importantly, avoiding carcinogens can delay the onset of cancer, even if one is destined to have it due to a genetic defect by birth.

This is a message I give to all of my patients, especially those who end up with cancer when they have lived a healthy lifestyle, and in some cases have never smoked cigarettes or drank any alcohol. If they did so, they would have had the cancer many years or decades earlier, and it would have been of a nastier kind. Hence, avoiding carcinogens is always beneficial when it comes to cancer and its treatment.

2.1   Can Cancer Be Cured?

Many cancers are curable, but with the current treatment options it is not possible to cure all types. It is sometimes possible to cure cancer even when it is in its advanced stages. The best example is testicular cancer. When in its initial stages, it can be cured 97% of the time, but even when it has spread to other parts of the body the cure rates can be around 40%. For most of the other cancers, it's easier to treat and cure them in an earlier stage.

As a general rule, cancers are classified into four stages:

Stage 1 and Stage 2 are localised to the site of origin.

Stage 3 is locally advanced disease, often involving the regional lymph nodes.

Stage 4 is metastatic disease which has spread to other parts of the body.

Treating cancer is less challenging in the early stages and for many types a cure can be achieved if diagnosed. But the catch is that cancer is quite … *quiet* …in its early stages and only becomes evident when it has started to spread.

The fact that so many cancers currently either cannot be cured, or have very low rates of cure, often gives the impression that medicine has failed here where it has succeeded in other areas of disease. In fact, this isn't true.

Speaking about truth, I'll let you in on a well-kept medical secret … one which doctors won't tell you. It's the metaphorical elephant in the room that all medical professionals avoid.

And, by letting it out, I risk upsetting my community and falling out of favour with them. On second thoughts, I am no blue-eyed boy of the medical fraternity to start with (brown-eyed, I confess) so here goes nothing.

"Modern medicine is great in diagnosing illness but not very good at curing most of them."

There, I said it. That's a load off my chest.

Don't get me wrong, we might not cure many diseases, but we do control them reasonably well.

Our record in curing diseases is … well, how should I put it … not brilliant. For example, high blood pressure (hypertension) can be controlled with medications, but has a *cure* rate of … wait for it … A BIG FAT ZERO. Here are some more examples to illustrate. Starting with heart diseases, like angina, ischaemic heart disease, heart attacks (myocardial infarctions), and cardiac failure, all can be controlled effectively for decades but have a cure rate of ZERO%.

Lung diseases – the likes of emphysema, asthma, pulmonary fibrosis, cystic fibrosis – all can be managed and controlled to a variable extent, but the cure rates are unanimously ZERO%.

For many metabolic disorders, including diabetes, autoimmune diseases (like rheumatoid arthritis), Crohn's disease, ulcerative colitis, and degenerative problems like osteoarthritis, percentage cure rates are ZERO. Inherited diseases, hormonal imbalances, connective tissue disorders, likewise, and the list goes on and on.

However, it's actually easier to point out the few diseases that we *can and do* cure. Ironically, the one category of diseases that do have a reasonable cure rate for, and continue to improve it by having more curative treatments available, is cancer!

With advances in diagnostic and treatment strategies, there is hope that more types of cancer will be curable in the future. Even without a cure, new treatment modalities have made it possible to control cancers for a longer time, like a chronic disease. Targeted treatments are also making it more tolerable to have anti-cancer therapy with fewer or less severe side effects. What's more, it is leading the way for other medical specialties in seeking and developing better management strategies and potential cures for non-cancer disease.

But as long as we are still waiting for effective treatments to come through, prevention remains of paramount importance. Even when we have curative treatments available, it makes sense to prevent cancer from developing in the first place. Ask any young man who has been cured of testicular cancer by use of surgery and chemotherapy. If given the choice, they would have preferred to have avoided it in the first place.

2.2   Cancer Myths and Why They Were Born

Cancer is a weird and wondrous disease. Its behaviour is unpredictable, at best ranging from the mild and mundane to the fast and furiously fatal. Not only does it behave differently from one type to another but also acts differently in every person depending on individual variations and factors. Add to it the fact that it can behave differently from one day to another in the same patient and you get an idea of how unpredictable it can be.

Take, for example, kidney cancer; a well-known aggressive tumour, richly supplied with blood vessels, notorious for growing and spreading; with every indication that it is there to stay. However, in some cases it starts to shrink, on its own, and might even disappear, without any treatment, only to reappear after a long period of absence, sometimes five to 10 years later. The exact cause of this phenomenon is not known but suspected to be immune-mediated. And this is exactly the kind of situation which gives birth to cancer myths.

Anyone whose cancer has behaved favourably, shrunk, or disappeared on its own might attribute the 'miracle' to a coincidental factor: a herbal remedy, a spiritual experience, a new exercise regimen, or food ingredient etc. However, when the same intervention is tried in a different patient and the same benefit is not achieved, it leads to disappointment. The danger of these myths is that people abandon conventional treatments of proven efficacy in pursuit of the mirage created by the myths, and often with disastrous results.

Sometimes, these myths are due to an honest error of judgement. For example, in the 1970s it was noticed that the incidence of stomach cancer was lower in Japanese who watched television, which at the time was a relatively new form of entertainment and had taken the country by storm. This was a bizarre phenomenon which could not be explained rationally.

It took some time for the researchers to realise that those watching TV were prosperous enough to buy televisions and refrigerators. In fact, they bought the refrigerators first, which helped preserve food and reduced the risk of carcinogens in non-refrigerated, traditionally preserved food.

Food contaminated with bacteria or preservatives were a major risk factor for developing stomach cancer, and using a refrigerator reduced the risk.

Speaking of cancer myths, here are some common myths and the misconceptions about cancer.

(i) Cancer Is a Manmade Disease

Fortunately, not. Nature made it without any help from us. It occurs due to mutations that can be caused by anything which causes irreparable damage to the DNA. The confusion arises from the fact that cancer is more common in the developed world compared to societies who are living a natural lifestyle. The fact is, manmade factors do increase the incidences of cancer, but it affects all kinds of animals and has been around for hundreds of millions of years. Almost all multicellular animals have been found to have cancer, from the primitive hydra to the ferocious shark.

(ii) Chemotherapy Kills Patients, Not Cancer

Cancer kills patients. Chemotherapy kills cancer cells.

Some types of cancers can be and have been cured by chemotherapy. Chemotherapy can have serious side effects which can kill a patient but so can drinking water (choking) and driving (road traffic accidents). Overall, chemotherapy kills many more cancer cells and saves many more lives compared to the lives it puts at risk.

For some cancers such as testicular cancer, chemotherapy does an amazing job of melting the tumour and often curing it. For others, it has better control of disease than cure rates. At times it shrinks the cancer, occasionally sending it into remission, but mostly it tends to stop or slow down the cancer growth, hence improving survival and quality of life.

There are many ways we can help the human body get more benefit from chemotherapy and we shall talk about them later in this book. But before we move on to the next section, I would like to share with you some rather great news from the frontline in the war against cancer.

Newer, better targeted, and more effective drugs are being developed for almost all type of cancers. These are different from conventional chemotherapy drugs. Some target the proteins involved in cancer growth and spread (for example, a category of drugs known as 'tyrosine kinase inhibitors' or TKIs for short); others strengthen our immune system to engage and destroy cancer cells. And the good news does not stop here. Research is being carried out to combine these drugs (TKIs with immunotherapy or even traditional chemotherapy) or use them in tandem, and the outcomes have been very positive in most cases, with some of the notoriously hard-to-treat cancers now being controlled for years. For example, in one trial of combination therapies for an aggressive brain tumour known as *glioblastoma multiformae* (GBM), not only did the treatment work well but in two patients the tumour disappeared altogether, something which was unheard of before.

(iii) Cancer Is Caused by Vitamin Deficiency

Vitamins are vital to human health.

The best source of vitamins is nature: fruits, vegetables, meat, eggs, and sunlight to name but a few. Without vitamins, our body systems are unable to function properly, and this includes our in-built anti-cancer mechanisms such as the immune system.

So, it was natural that scientists thought cancer might be occurring due to vitamin deficiency. Over the decades, a lot of effort and money has been poured into research studying effects of vitamins on cancer. What scientists found was astounding. Natural vitamin supplements *did* reduce the risk of cancer (we will talk about them in detail in the coming chapters), but synthetic preparations did the opposite by increasing the risk of cancer growth. With hindsight, this should not come as a surprise. Vitamins are vital to all types of cell growth, including cancer cells. Natural sources also have other beneficial elements along with vitamins, including antioxidants, and provide a slow and steady release of vitamins as per the body's requirement.

Supplementation with synthetic preparations can overwhelm the system and cause more harm than benefit.

But the myth of preventing and curing cancer by vitamins has survived and flourished for one big reason: manufacturing vitamins is a big, multibillion dollar business.

The worst of the 'vitamin deficiency cancer 'myth is the story of cancer being caused by deficiency of a mythical vitamin known as 'vitamin B17'. This is the newest gimmick for selling a product that is alleged to be a magical cure for cancer.

Firstly, there is no such thing as vitamin B17. There is a chemical known as 'amygdalin' (from the Greek word *amygdale* for 'almond') from which a chemical named 'laetrile' has been derived. Laetrile, a synthetic compound, is not a vitamin but has been nicknamed vitamin B17. Amygdalin is actually a toxic chemical (a *cyanogenic glycoside*) found in the seeds of apricots, bitter almonds, apples, peaches, and plums. It releases cyanide, one of the most poisonous substances known to mankind and other animals[47]. Its 'deficiency' is a blessing, not a problem. The human body definitely does not require this poison. In fact, our bodies have developed a system of identifying its bitterness fast so we spit out the nuts or seeds (like bitter almonds) that contain it.

And it has no practical role in killing or controlling cancer, either. Low doses of both amygdalin and laetrile are ineffective against cancer cells, and high doses would kill the patient before they kill any cancer cells.

(iv) Sodium Bicarbonate (Baking Soda) Can Cure Cancer

This myth arises from the fact that cancer cells have an acidic environment around them. But this environment is the result of cancer growth and metabolism rather than a cause of it. It's like looking at pictures of battlefields and bombed cities (e.g., Hiroshima and Nagasaki) and concluding that destruction leads to war. Hence, if we can regularly repair buildings, there would be no war.

The human body has a very effective system[48] of neutralising any acids or alkali bases (like sodium bicarbonate) that we consume. Taking sodium bicarbonate will not have any significant effect on the acid-base balance. The human body will neutralise it immediately. If it wasn't neutralised, it could prove fatal because we can only survive in a strict pH range of 7.35 to 7.45 (which, ironically, is already a non-acidic pH). Any attempt to make the human body pH more alkaline would result in a swift death.

---

[47] For example, a few bitter almonds are enough to kill a horse, but it rarely happens because horses hate the taste and spit it out no matter how hard you try to convince them of its alleged health benefits.

[48] Known as *homeostasis*.

It's extremely unlikely for any alkaline product like sodium bicarbonate to reach the cancer cells and affect their acidity. Think of cancer cells as small, hot water springs (deep-sea vents) in the ocean spewing out acidic material. They are unlikely to raise the temperature of an ocean and adding icebergs into the ocean will not cool down or neutralise the deep-sea vents as the sea water will dilute the effect very quickly (this process is known as 'ocean homeostasis' and is similar to the homeostasis system within the human body, which is essential to keeping all physical systems stable and functioning properly).

(v) Cancer Is Caused by Acidic Food

This myth once again stems from the acidic micro-environment around the cancer cell. Acidic food cannot significantly add to the body's pH. The body's neutralising system (homeostasis) immediately restores the balance. In fact, when it comes to cancer and acidic food, the opposite is true. Contrary to the myth, most acidic foods, like citrus fruit, have antioxidants, including ascorbic acid (vitamin C), which can neutralise cancer-causing chemicals and reduce the risk of cancer.

(vi) Drinking Hot Water Can Cure Cancer

Hot water is a good laxative but has little additional health benefits. If hotter than 65 degrees Celsius it can cause heartburn in the short term and oesophageal cancer in the long run. The temperature required to kill cancer cells is exactly the same as that required to burn the human body to a crisp. It's akin to killing your garden weeds by bombing your house. Not recommended.

(vii) Enemas Cure Cancer

This myth goes back to ancient Greece, before the times of Jesus Christ. The ancient Greeks believed that cancer was caused by an excess of a mysterious dark humour known as 'black bile' and one way of ridding the body of its excess was using laxatives. Over the centuries, patients have been subjected to brutal and often lethal doses of laxatives in an attempt to cure cancer. Needless to say, the technique failed but unfortunately the myth's survived.

(viii) Coffee Enemas Cure Cancer

Drinking coffee is known to reduce the risk of cancer (more on it in a detailed discussion in a dedicated section) but has no curative effects. As for coffee enemas, based on millions of years of mammalian experience, it is clear that all kinds of food and drinks in general, and coffee in particular, are best consumed through the mouth. Absorption through the large bowel is much less than when consumed by mouth.

(ix) Shark Liver Oil Cures Cancer

This myth developed from an earlier myth that sharks don't get cancer. They do, and have done so for millions of years as seen in the fossil record. But we found this out quite late. Unfortunately, by then the myth had been established, and there was nothing sharks could do to save their lives. They were hunted relentlessly for a magic cure rumoured to be made by their liver.

Unsurprisingly, the spectrum of benefits was extended to curing the common cold and swine flu (probably based on the observation that sharks don't have runny noses) and human immunodeficiency virus/HIV (maybe because, despite the fact that sharks never use condoms, not a single shark has been sighted at an STD clinic). And why stop there? So, more recently, the therapeutic spectrum has also included haemorrhoid medications on the basis that … yes, you've guessed it right … no shark has ever gone to a pharmacy asking for haemorrhoid cream.

Needless to say, the use of shark liver oil is only limited by the extent of human imagination and, ironically, so are the supposed beneficial effects. In fact, there is a risk. Some shark liver oils are contaminated by polychlorinated biphenyls (PCBs) and polybrominated biphenyl ethers (PBDEs), cancer-causing, toxic compounds that contaminate sea water.

(x) Charcoal Cures Cancer

This myth is both sad and seriously funny at the same time. It started with the myth of the 'shark oil' cancer cure and spread like a Chinese whisper until the 'shark oil' became mispronounced beyond recognition to 'charc oel' and finally 'charcoal'. Soon, people were sharing the news. This misunderstood message, which was never true to start with, has no substance to it. But people have been consuming charcoal in many forms, pure or supplementary, in the hope to treat cancer.

(xi) Cannabis Is the Cure For Cancer

Cannabis is the commonest weed in the northern regions of Afghanistan, Pakistan, and India. It is well-suited to the mountainous regions of Hindu Kush and the Himalayas. The two common types are *Cannabis indica* and *Cannabis sativa*. For centuries, local physicians have used them as a painkiller, anxiolytic and sedative. There has been a lot of misinformation about cannabis in general, and its role in cancer treatment in particular. So far, there has been no evidence to suggest that it has any benefit in controlling cancers. It does have an important role in cancer symptom control, however. More on this in section 5.6.

(xii) A High-Fibre Diet Prevents or Cures Cancer

Despite sounding good, alas this is another dietary myth.

It is based on two common observations:

A. Cultures with a high-fibre diet have lower incidence of cancer.

B. A high-fibre diet results in regular bowel movements and this has always been associated with health benefits (remember the ancient Greeks getting rid of the mythical black bile by purgation in a hope to cure cancer).

Multiple large trials across the world have been conducted to study the benefits of a high-fibre diet and, although the results confirmed the role of dietary fibre in regularising bowel movements, it did not reduce the risk of any cancer, not even bowel cancer.

It appears that the cultures which have a high-fibre diet also tend to have other important dietary practices such as a diet low in sugar and high in fruits and vegetables, which work together to reduce the risk of cancer. Dietary fibre on its own has no added benefit apart from a regular bowel movement.

(xiii) Cancer Is Caused by a High-Fat Intake

Dietary fat has a bad reputation and gets blamed for almost all ailments known to mankind. This would not have been the case if fat production was an industry with lobbying powers like tobacco and alcohol.

This fact was not lost on the tobacco and alcohol industry who used it as a scapegoat for the rising rates of cancer for many decades.

Despite clear evidence from across the world showing a low incidence of cancer among cultures consuming a largely fat-based diet (Inuit of Greenland and Canada for example, whose main source of nutrition is whale and seal blubber) dietary fat got blamed for heart disease and cancer. However, repeated trials have shown that increased fat in diet does not increase the risk of cancer or heart disease. Being fat does, but eating fat doesn't, and the two are not the same. In fact, the biggest risk factor for obesity is not fat but sugar intake, which can have a detrimental effect on human health.

Obesity and sugar intake do play an important role in the risk of developing cancer, a topic we shall discuss in detail at a later point.

Now it's time to lift the lid on what causes cancer in the first place.

PART 3

LIFTING
THE LID ON
PANDORA'S BOX

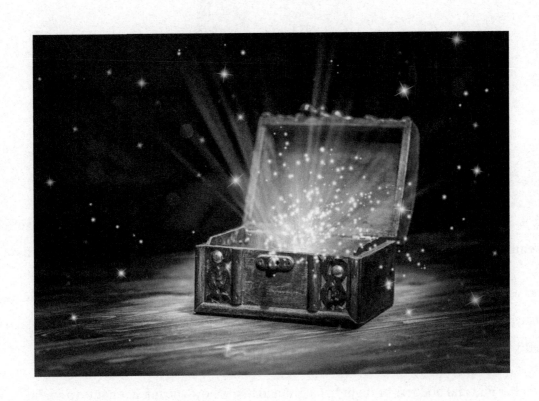

PART 3: LIFTING THE LID ON PANDORA'S BOX

3   Pandora's Box: A Metaphor for What Triggers Cancer

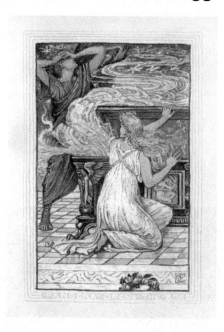

Pandora, says the Greek legend, was the most gifted woman of her time.

Not only that, she was the most beautiful, the most desirable, exquisite, charming and enchanting female on earth. Being the first woman, that's hardly surprising. It helps when you have no competition.

Her creation was a joint venture by the Greek gods Zeus, Athena, and Hephaestus. Zeus gave instructions while Hephaestus handcrafted her, moulding the earth into her body. Athena dressed her in a silvery gown, embroidered veil, garlands, and an ornate crown.

Then every other god and goddess brought her a gift and that's how she got her name (*pan*, 'all' and *doron*, 'gifted' = Pandora).

Before Hermes, the herald of Greek gods, carried her down from Mount Olympus, Zeus gave her a large storage jar (*pithos*[49] in Greek) and entrusted her with it.

Unbeknownst to Pandora, the jar was full of evils: envy, illness, ignorance, poverty, remorse, scorn, worry, hate, and crime. You name it, the jar had it. But among all those evils, Zeus added *elpis* ('hope' in Greek), as a caretaker, to keep them in check and stop them from breaking out of the jar. Pandora was made the

---

[49] The Greek word *pithos* got mistranslated to the Latin *pyxis*, meaning 'a box', by the 16th century Dutch priest, scholar, and philosopher Erasmus (Desiderius Erasmus Roterodamus). Since then, much to the annoyance of the Greeks, the story has been retold as 'Pandora's box' rather than Pandora's jar.

minder, the gatekeeper, and had to make sure the lid remained in place. Zeus also told her not to look inside the jar, *ever*, which if you ask me was a recipe for disaster because, by saying this, he made her curious.

And, curious as a cat, Pandora could not contain her desire to look inside the jar. One day she broke the seal to take a peek.

As soon as the lid was lifted, a swarm of evils flew out of the jar and spread all over the world. Poor Pandora sat in shock, looking at the empty jar but then realised something still fluttered within, trying to escape. It was hope (*elpis*), hopelessly stuck under the lid and unable to fly away.

And since that day, humanity was left with a jar filled with hope to deal with all the unleashed evils. All thanks to the greatly gifted Miss Pandora.

As we saw in the previous section, our cells' DNA is under constant attack, resulting in a wide variety of types of damage. And yet, our remarkable cells set about repairing this damage. Well, most of it. Sometimes the systems are overwhelmed, and as a result damage accumulates. We can think of these as the evils in the jar.

The Greek myth inspired me to look for a 'Pandora of Cancer' – whether there's one culprit that lifts the lid on the DNA mutations causing this disease, releasing them to wreak their havoc.

By analogy, we can think of our cells 'defence mechanisms like Pandora, *elpis* and the jar. They are our tumour suppressor genes. They were mentioned in Part 1 of this book ('Hallmarks of Cancer') and can be grouped as follows:

A. **Caretaker genes are like the *elpis* (hope) in the jar.**

These take care of our DNA by repairing the damage. If more time is needed, they tell the cell to stop growing and attempt repair again. If they fail, they give a signal to the cell to kill itself by apoptosis, instead of allowing it to transform into a cancer.

B. **Gatekeeper genes are like Pandora, the guardian of the jar.**

These genes are the guardians of the DNA, preventing excessive and uncontrolled growth of cells.

C. **Landscape genes are like the jar itself.**

Landscaper genes control the environment around the cell. When these genes are damaged, the environment becomes more conducive to unregulated cell growth and multiplication which helps a cancer to thrive.

Could it be that, among these genes, one or more might actually be responsible for cancer? If, that is, they become damaged and unable to undertake their protective role?

I believe the answer is YES. It is my theory of carcinogenesis. Let's call it the 'MK Theory of Carcinogenesis'. In a nutshell,

The Pandora of cancer is a mutated tumour suppressor gene.

Had this book come with sound effects, I would have accompanied the previous sentence with a fanfare of trumpets, or at least a drum roll followed by a crash of cymbals, and then added a space on the page to allow for a light ripple of applause among readers. If my theory is right then all those other genetic mutations (the evils in the jar), are essentially secondary to the main 'change 'needed to actually transform a cell into a cancerous one.

"Whoa," I hear you cry. *"Hang on a minute. Didn't you tell us earlier that usually cancer occurs as a result of accumulated damage over time?"*

Yes, I did. And it's true. But think about it like a revolver. You can load bullets into the chambers, cock the hammer, and squeeze your finger on the trigger, but the gun won't fire while the safety catch is still on. But should the safety catch be turned off, or fail, then the gun will go off. Just like Pandora and her jar, everything can be safely 'contained 'until one fateful change or error.

There is strong evidence to support my theory, implicating a mutated tumour suppressor gene as the main culprit in causing cancer. The strongest comes from studies done in patients with colon cancer, or more commonly referred to as *cancer of the bowel.*

Scientists have studied the growth and evolution of bowel cancer for decades[50] and have identified the following stepwise process:

1. A normal cell in the lining of the bowel has damage to a gene at chromosome number 5. This is a gene[51] controlling cell growth. Once mutated, the growth control is lost, and the cell starts dividing and growing into a small clump of cells known as an *early adenoma*. But it's not yet a cancer. Far from it. It's just an innocuous (benign) lump, often called a *polyp*.

---

[50] Pioneering work was done in the 1980s by Bert Vogelstein, Clayton Professor of Oncology and Pathology at John Hopkins Medical School in the USA.

[51] Known as the *APC* (adenomatous polyposis coli) gene, which is a fancy way of saying that this gene, when mutated, causes polyps known as *adenomas* in the colon/bowel.

2. As the cells continue to grow and divide over many, many years – decades in fact – they might have additional damage that makes the clump of cells grow into a bigger lump known as an *intermediate adenoma*. This is still not a cancer, though.

3. Two to five years pass, during which the intermediate adenoma acquires more DNA damage, especially to genes at chromosome number 18, and this triggers a growth spurt, making the lump even bigger in size. Now it's called a *late adenoma*. Crucially, however, it's important to note that even this isn't a cancer. Not yet.

4. The defining moment for this big lump of abnormal looking pre-cancerous cells comes in the next 2–5 years when a gatekeeper gene, the Pandora of the genetic cellular world, known as *TP53*, and found on chromosome number 17, gets damaged or mutated. The TP53 stands for 'tumour protein p53', a protein that has been called the *Guardian of the Genome,* and for good reasons.

In its normal form, this protein is integral to repairing damaged DNA strands. Not only is it able to repair damaged DNA, it also has a lot of clout over the command-and-control centre of cell growth. It can tell a cell to stop growing or dividing and then keep the growth button pressed at 'pause' until all the DNA damage is repaired. If the DNA is irreparable, it signals the cell to self-destruct[52]. When the DNA for the TP53 gene is damaged, the cell makes an abnormal protein which cannot perform its functions. The lid is lifted off the jar.

Those pre-cancerous adenoma cells that had been simmering for decades now come to the boil. With the loss of function of TP53, the *Pandora of the Genome*, adenoma cells, quickly accumulate mutations in different genes, encouraging rapid growth – allowing the cells to break the attachments keeping them anchored to the bowel wall, to make enzymes to break barriers, to sprout new blood vessels, to invade blood vessels, and to then travel around the body, invading and colonising new territories. An incompetent Pandora has unleashed a cancer.

Mutations of the gene for tumour protein p53 are known to be involved in more than 50% of human cancers[53]. The rest result from the failure of different tumour suppressor genes, which have similar caretaker or guardian roles as TP53. Growing evidence is indicating that the 50% of the cancers not showing direct damage to TP53 do have some obstructions to the tumour suppressor pathways controlled

---

[52] The cell is induced to release specific enzymes which destroy the cell from within.

[53] I like to think of TP as the 'Tumour Pandora' gene. According to my theory, every cancer has its own Pandora gene that lifts the lid off mutations, setting them free, and the most common culprit in most cancers is a mutated TP53. I also suspect that the other Pandora genes might be regulating the same pathways which TP53 controls. If my hypothesis is proven to be true then we would be able to identify the common genetic stem from which all cancers branch off.

by TP53. In other words, lack of TP53 control is involved in *every* human cancer, making it a true Pandora of cancer. Among the millions (one study found 10 million different mutations in different cancers) of mutations found in cancer cells, the one that stands out is TP53. The elusive needle in the haystack.

We humans have been blessed with two copies of the TP53 guardian genes, one on each of the paired chromosome 17 (you get one copy from your mum and one from your dad, undoubtedly the best inheritance gift a child can have). If one gets damaged, the other steps in to take over, like a tag team. How lucky, I hear you say, feeling blessed. Wait till you hear this.

Elephants, those *oh-so-lucky* pachyderms, have 40 (that's FORTY copies) of TP53 genes. It's like having 40 Pandoras to guard the jar. No wonder their cancer rates are so low, even if they were to drink like a fish and smoke like a chimney. It would take so long to mutate all 40 TP53 genes that one would die of alcoholic liver failure or smoke asphyxiation before a cancer sets in.

And there is evidence to back this up.

Elephants rarely develop cancer despite the fact that they have 100 times as many cells than humans. These animals should be developing and dying from cancer, but they don't.

Dr Schiffman from the University of Utah and colleagues analysed necropsy data from a database of the San Diego Zoo ('necropsy' is another term for autopsy, or post-mortem examination). They also obtained data for cancer rates in elephants from the Elephant Encyclopaedia Database, capturing global elephant deaths and their causes (yes, really, elephants even have their own encyclopaedia!).

Remarkably, despite their size, the cancer rate calculated from 644 elephant deaths was similar, between 3.11% and 4.81% across both sources of information. This is in contrast to humans for whom estimates of cancer mortality are between 11% and 25%.

Next, they compared the response to DNA damage in humans with African elephants. They studied certain human cells (lymphocytes from the blood and fibroblasts from fibrous connective tissue) which undergo P53-dependent apoptosis (cell death) when exposed to DNA-damaging agents such as radiation, and a chemotherapy drug called 'doxorubicin'.

The results provided clear evidence that DNA damage is better managed in elephant cells compared to humans.

For example, the apoptotic (cell death) rate after exposure to radiation was 14.64% in elephants versus 7.17% for healthy human cells. By getting rid of the affected cells, this helps prevent elephants from developing cancer, given that TP53 plays a major role in suppression and response to DNA damage.

Now this raises an interesting question.

If having more TP53 guardian genes against cancer can make a species more resistant to developing cancer, does the number of functional TP53 *within* the same species have an effect on the cancer rate too? For example, if a baby is born with a defective pair of TP53 genes, one functional, the other dysfunctional, would he/she grow up having a higher risk of developing cancer?

In 1969, a Chinese-American physician, Dr Frederick Pei Li, and his colleague, Joseph F. Fraumeni Jr, came across 24 families with a very high risk of cancer over the generations compared to the general public.

Li and Fraumeni were baffled by the variety of cancers among the family members. It was not that they were prone to a particular cancer but seemed to be susceptible to any cancer. There were tumours in their brains and breasts, bones and blood, kidneys and liver, bowel and bladder, prostate and pancreas and so on. Another peculiar feature was that they all occurred at a relatively young age, childhood or young adulthood, compared to the general public, who generally develop the same tumours at a much later age.

Li and Fraumeni called it *Li-Fraumeni syndrome* (not unsurprisingly) and followed the family's medical history for 20 years.

In 1990, the culprit gene for this condition was finally discovered, and it turned out to be none other than the Pandora of the genetic world, the Guardian of the Genome, the tumour suppressor gene, TP53.

Patients with Li- Fraumeni syndrome inherit one defective and one normal gene from their parents. Unlike the general public, who need damage to both genes to lift the lid on cancer mutations, Li-Fraumeni patients only need one hit before cancer is let loose (remember that they already have one defected gene, so a damaging hit to their only other functional TP53 gene unleashes 'the evils in the box'). Depending on which organ gets the DNA damage – e.g., the breast in a female or prostate in a male – a cancer develops.

For example, the risk of developing an invasive cancer by the age of 30 years is only 1% among the general public but about 50% in the families suffering from Li-Fraumeni syndrome.

By the age of 70 years this risk increases to 90% in such families.

The earlier experiment using elephant and human cells has been repeated, replacing the elephant cells with cells from Li-Fraumeni syndrome patients and the results were startling.

When exposed to radiation, damaged normal human cells have an apoptosis rate of 7.17% but Li-Fraumeni cells only have an abysmal 2.71% rate of self-destruction. So, in patients with Li-Fraumeni syndrome, the cells have a reduced ability to protect themselves by removing damaged/mutated cells that may go on to be cancerous.

Once again, this supports my theory of carcinogenesis, that *the Pandora of cancer is a mutated tumour suppressor gene (e.g., TP53)*. It's not until the tumour suppressor gene is damaged that the cancer is born.

As we saw earlier, every strand of DNA can undergo damage tens of thousands of times a day. If you multiply this by the number of cells and days (over decades), you get some idea of the colossal and continuous feat of DNA repair that our guardian genes undertake. And this goes on throughout our body. Incredibly, our in-built anti-cancer system almost always fixes them *all*.

Equally remarkably, if they're unable to fix them, our anti-cancer system kills off the abnormal cells that may lead to a cancer. The amazing truth is that every day our body stops many cancers from happening. And we're completely unaware of this tremendous feat.

And it's not just the tumour suppressor genes[54] like TP53 that make it possible; it's teamwork by all parts of the cell. For example, the mitochondria supply the enzymes needed to kill off any defective cells, and the cell itself triggers the self-destruct sequence of apoptosis, killing itself honourably before it becomes a danger to the body.

So, why and when does this system fail? What makes Pandora lift the lid on cancer?

The risk is present in almost all animals. However, humans stand out as a group. Our cancer rates are exceptionally high. Although genetics plays an important role, because each cancer has a degree of inherited genetic susceptibility, and although there's always an element of chance or bad luck, the human rates are rising due to environmental factors and lifestyle choices.

This is quite a sweeping statement – *environmental and lifestyle choices*. How do we get a handle on it? One way is to think about how the world has changed so rapidly in the past couple of centuries or so. The

---

[54] We are really blessed with an almost perfect system for repairing DNA damage. Apart from TP53, scientists have identified many other gene-based repair systems, and there might be many more that we don't yet know of. Four major and well-known systems are base excision repair, nucleotide excision repair, homologous recombination and non-homologous end joining repair systems.

agricultural (agrarian) revolution was followed by the industrial revolution across much of our world, as man's innovations and discoveries allowed us to create the societies we have today. Prior to this, change came slowly, over thousands of years. So, when thinking about how mankind evolves or adapts (genetically), for most of mankind's history gradual change allowed us to evolve to cope well with our challenges, including cancer. Here's an example.

Migration from Africa to Europe some 50,000 years ago gradually led to those humans evolving depigmented, lighter skin, in contrast to their black ancestors. This adaptation allowed them to secure sufficient vitamin D from the diminished solar ultraviolet B radiation found in cloudy, northern climates. The downside with reduced pigmentation is that the skin is less protected from the risk of the harmful effects of ultraviolet (UV) light, such as skin cancer. But, given the reduced UV light in northern climes, the adaptation achieved its aim with regard to gaining the essential vitamin D. After all, it wasn't as if people spent their days lying in the sun, exposing their fair-skinned, nearly naked bodies, was it?

In fact, prior to Victorian times (1837 to 1901), the notion of a seaside holiday, or lying on a sun-drenched beach under the blazing summer sun, would have led to many a puzzled look. It simply wasn't done; well, not deliberately by most people. In the 1970s, the package holiday was born, and it led to profound changes in how people viewed travelling around the world and using their increasingly available leisure time. It became commonplace for those in northern climes to seek their *fortnight in the sun*. A 'natural 'tan became fashionable – a complete reversal of prior attitudes – and when that wasn't possible, artificial tanning under a 'sun lamp 'became available on many High Streets. That we have ended up with increased risk (and occurrence) of skin cancer is hardly surprising. We simply haven't had the time to genetically adapt to this new way of life. It's all happened too quickly.

You might be surprised to learn that a similar thing is true with breast cancer. Human females are unique among primates in having year-round (non-seasonal) regular menstrual cycles. This increases their chances of pregnancy and helps increase the numbers of humans compared to other species competing with us for food and resources. So, as a species competing with others, it's a favourable adaptation. However, often in today's way of life, pregnancy is not a priority. In the absence of pregnancy, or with delayed pregnancy and breastfeeding (and shorter periods of breastfeeding – it used to be two to five years), there is an increased exposure of the breasts and ovaries to pulses (cycles) of hormones, causing proliferative stress between the ages of 13 and 50. This greatly increases the risk of breast cancer.

In general, our exotic social evolution has not kept pace with biological evolutionary adaptability. The good news is that by understanding this, it also makes most of the cancers preventable.

3.1   Peto's Paradox and Khan's Axiom (Does Size Matter After All?)

Across different species, the incidence of cancer does not appear to correlate with the number of cells in an organism. This, as mentioned earlier, is known as 'Peto's paradox'.

And Peto was right. *At the species level,* this is a fact. Among different species it's not the number of cells and their size but the number of tumour suppressor genes (guardian genes) they have that majorly determines the risk of cancer. The higher the number of genes, the less chance they'll *all* be damaged, and so the lower the risk, and *vice versa.*

However, *within a particular species,* the number of guardian genes is fixed; for example, two TP53 genes in humans, and 40 in elephants. Because the number is fixed, other factors come into play. Here, the risk of cancer *does* depend on the number of cells in an individual. So, size does matter *within the same species.* This is because, the greater the number of cells, and the more they divide, the greater the chances of unrepaired DNA damage and more the risk of developing cancer.

I call it 'Khan's Axiom'.

3.2   Carcinogens

So, based on our current knowledge, we can view cancer as being the result of accumulated damage to our cells' DNA over time, and with, in most cases, a final 'pulling of the trigger' or 'lifting the lid of Pandora's box' to unleash the disease when the guardian genes are damaged.

The next question is, what kinds of things can cause this damage to us and our DNA?

Any substance or factor that can damage cell DNA and start a cancer is known as a 'carcinogen'[55].

From our understanding of cancer, everything in our world can be generally divided into categories.

- *The Good Guys – these stop cancer from developing.*

- *The Bad Guys – these can start a cancer (carcinogens).*

- *Cancer Helpers – bad guys that don't start a cancer but help it grow.*

---

[55] A combination of two words, *carcinos* (meaning 'cancer') and *genesis* (meaning 'to start/generate' or 'begin something', originating from the root word *genno*, which means to give birth').

- *The Indifferent – those which neither start nor stop, or help, a cancer. These are spectators that just watch from the sidelines, and we will talk about them if they are being wrongly accused and implicated.*

- *The Confused – turncoats which switch roles, sometimes stopping, sometimes starting or helping a cancer, and at other times being silent spectators.*

Carcinogens are many and varied, and include environmental, dietary, and behavioural factors (e.g., smoking), as well the consequences of our modern way of life in terms of the things we make and surround ourselves with, and which we use or consume. By examining each of these in turn, it is possible to see where there are significant opportunities for us all to avoid these hazards. And equally importantly, we can identify those things – e.g., certain foods and beverages – which might also protect us. So, it's not all bad news. There are some nice surprises along the way.

Before examining these, though, it is probably best to try and answer another question I'm often asked by patients and their families, and by a good many others. That is, the extent to which our inherited genes protect or predispose us to cancer.

INHERITED
GENES

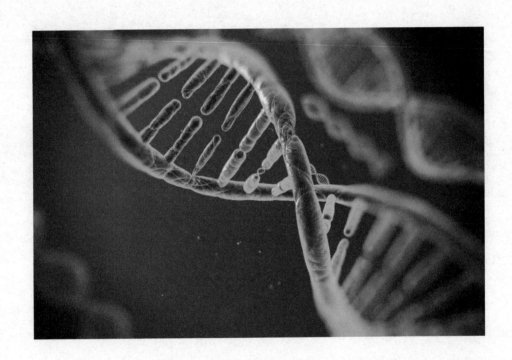

PART 4: INHERITED GENES

4   Inheriting Cancer (Can You Blame Your Parents?)

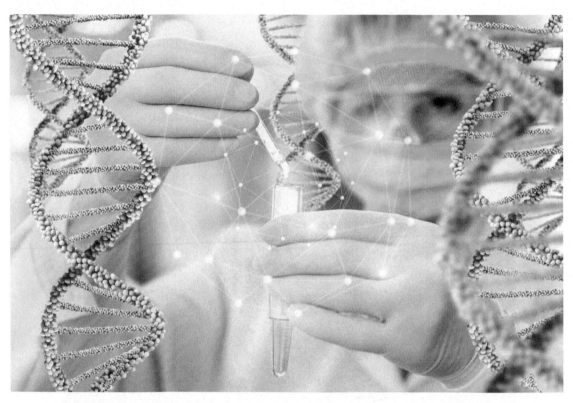

From the day we are born, we are destined to develop a myriad of diseases, one or some of which will eventually spell the end of life.

Everyone has their own Achilles'[56] heel (or heels). For some it will be heart disease, some may succumb to a stroke, and for others it could be cancer. And yes, our genes play a role. But often other factors greatly influence the outcome. So, destiny comes paired with free will and personal choice. In other words, where someone's genetic make-up is known to place them at greater risk of cancer, there are often ways of lessening the likelihood that it will actually occur within their lifetime. But to achieve this may require changes to their behaviour and lifestyle. And this is where, ultimately, it is up to the individual, provided of course that they are equipped with the right knowledge and wisdom to make informed choices (and, hence, I hope this book will help readers to develop a good strategy for life).

---

[56] According to the Greek legend, Achilles (also known as Achilleus), the greatest of all the Greek warriors, had only one vulnerable body part: his heel. His mother had dipped him in the magical river Styx when he was a baby in a bid to make him immortal and invincible. However, his heels, by which his mother held him, remained dry and hence vulnerable throughout life. He was killed in the battle of Troy when, Paris (of Helen, not of Hilton fame) shot him in the heel with an arrow.

Fortunately, the inheritance of cancer-causing, previously damaged genes from our parents is very rare (only 5% of all cancers). Where they occur, they lead to hereditary cancer syndromes passed from one generation to another.

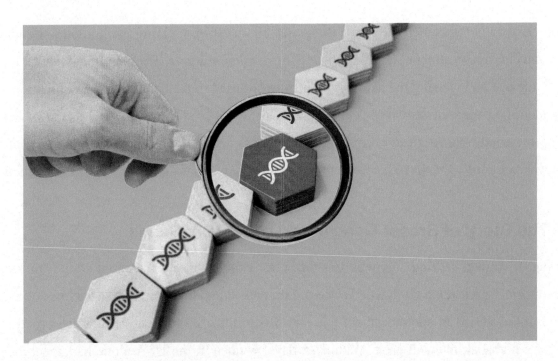

4.1   Heredity and Cancer, a Historical Background

The first ever documented case of an inherited risk of cancer occurred in Brazil in the 19th century. Perhaps surprisingly, it occurred in the field of ophthalmology.

Hilario De Gouvea & His Trusty Ophthalmoscope

Hilario de Gouvea was a brilliant Brazilian ophthalmologist who came from a humble background but had the good fortune of being able to study through a scholarship in Europe. Once back in Brazil, he became a renowned doctor and political figure, participated in the civil war, got imprisoned, escaped through the window of his prison by making a rope out of his bedsheets, disguised himself as a mentally ill homeless person, went into exile in France, and when the French refused to allow him to work as a doctor, he did what no doctor had ever done before – he enrolled in a medical school for several years and got another certification.

In 1872, de Gouvea came across a family with a rare form of eye cancer known as *retinoblastoma*.

De Gouvea had originally removed the eye tumour in the father when the latter was a two-year-old boy by successfully operating on the tumour before it could spread to the brain and cause fatal damage. The boy grew up, married at the age of 21 and went on to have seven children. Many years later, his two daughters presented with the same condition, although their mother had no family history of this disease. One daughter was diagnosed aged two years and the other at five months. Their other (five) siblings were unaffected.

Today, de Gouvea is remembered for two things. In his quest of studying eye tumours, he made early diagnosis and curative treatment possible by using the *ophthalmoscope*. This hand-held device for shining a light into the eye and viewing the inside is an instrument used in all standard eye examinations. And he correctly identified the inheritance of retinoblastomas. To his credit, he was way ahead of his time in identifying the condition, surgically removing the tumours and studying them in detail to confirm their nature. It was not until 1971 that the complete genetic mechanism of this disease was understood.

4.2   The Story of Breast Cancer and the BRCA Genes

The number of women seeking a genetic test for breast cancer sharply increased after 14th May, 2013, when an editorial by a leading Hollywood actress, film maker, and humanitarian, Angelina Jolie, endorsed the testing, followed by an announcement that she was to undergo preventive mastectomy after testing positive for a high-risk mutated gene. Within 15 days, women in the USA alone had spent a collective $13.5 million dollars on the test.

The genes tested for are known as breast cancer or *BRCA* (BReast CAncer) genes.

BRCA genes are tumour suppressor genes (like the TP53 guardian gene mentioned earlier) involved in the repair of damaged DNA. If these genes are damaged, cells are unable to effectively repair genetic damage, leading to the formation of tumours at an earlier age compared to the normal population.

There are two types of these breast cancer genes, known as BRCA1 and BRCA2.

About BRCA 1

The BRCA1 gene is located on chromosome 17. If damaged, this gene can cause increased risk of breast and ovarian cancer. The risk of breast cancer is increased to between 55–70%, and subjects having this defective gene are likely to develop cancer at a very early age compared to the rest of the population. The risk of ovarian cancer is increased to between 40–45%.

The BRCA1 gene makes a protein known as the 'BRCA1 protein'. Whenever a DNA strand is broken, the BRCA1 protein is recruited to the broken edges to repair the gap. In patients with the normal gene, the protein launches a chain reaction, recruiting dozens of proteins to the broken edge, swiftly plugging the breach. In patients with a mutated gene, however, the BRCA protein is not properly recruited, and the breaks remain unrepaired. This permits more mutations, like fire fuelling fire, until the growth and metabolic controls on the cells are snapped, ultimately leading to breast cancer.

But even in BRCA1-mutated patients, cancer requires multiple triggers. The defective BRCA1 gene alone is not sufficient. The environment clearly plays a role, such as radiation, and DNA damaging agents, like carcinogens, which add to the mutation rate. BRCA1 hence predicts a future, but does not determine it.

About BRCA 2

The BRCA2 gene also increases the risk of both breast and ovarian cancer. The risk of breast cancer is increased by 45–70%, once again occurring at a younger age compared to other types of breast cancers. The risk of ovarian cancer is between 15–20%. In addition, if the gene is damaged in a *male*, the risk of breast cancer increases to 7–8% and the lifetime risk of prostate cancer increases to about 33% (a five– to ninefold increase compared to the normal population). In comparison, the BRCA1 gene mutation in males increases the risk of breast cancer by only 1%. In the normal population, who do not have any BRCA mutations, the risk is about 0.1%.

Thankfully, the BRCA gene mutations are comparatively rare. For example, in the USA they are found in about one in 400 people. However, in certain ethnic groups and races the risk is much higher. Among the Ashkenazi Jews, for example, the frequency of BRCA1 or BRCA2 mutations is up to one in 40 people (2.5%). Similarly, in the Icelandic population the BRCA tumour mutation is 0.6%.

4.3   Genetics and Environment: A (True) Story of Destiny and Free Will

It's a cold and wet summer's day (English weather, what can I say?). I am about to meet Mr H.E[57], my first patient of the day. Mr H.E is new to my clinic but has been known to the department for decades. He's a regular customer. Mr H.E is a 72-year-old.

He is seeing me because he was recently diagnosed with an aggressive brain tumour affecting his ability to speak. This was surgically removed but a rim of tumour cells was left behind which could not be removed safely (cutting any further into the brain would have damaged vital centres, putting him in a wheelchair).

---

[57] Not his real name, his real name is … just remembered …I am not supposed to give away his identity due to patient confidentiality, so we will have to settle for his detailed medical history instead.

Looking at his post-operative brain scans, I plan to offer him a combination of chemotherapy and radiation treatment over a period of nine months. Without treatment this type of tumour tends to be fatal in six months.

With treatment, half of the patients (50%) survive beyond 15 months.

At five years this number drops to less than 5% surviving the disease.

Mr H.E knows the treatment is not curative but we both hope that we can control the tumour for as long as possible, and that new treatments might become available in the future which can control it better, and might even cure it.

But Mr H.E is different from the other patients I am meeting that day. Twenty years ago, he first presented with localised bowel cancer which was removed surgically. It didn't come to him as a surprise, as cancer has been in his family for generations. His sister died of breast cancer in her 40s. A younger brother also died of cancer. Another sister had a brain tumour in her 50s. His son died of bowel cancer in his 30s. A niece died of brain tumour in her 20s.

Genetic analysis showed that the family has an inheritable disease known as *Lynch syndrome.*

Lynch syndrome, also known as *hereditary non-polyposis colorectal cancer* (HNPCC for short), is an autosomal dominant genetic[58] condition associated with a high risk of colon cancer, as well as other cancers. The increased risk of these is due to inherited mutations that impair DNA repair[59] (based on the preceding chapters, you've probably guessed this already!).

Mr H.E has had multiple cancers too. Sixteen years after his first cancer, his bowel cancer came back and was once again operated on successfully. One year later he was diagnosed with cancer (transitional cell carcinoma) of his right ureter[60] and this required surgical removal of the ureter and a stent insertion.

The following year the ureteric cancer recurred, this time found growing in the local lymph nodes and the side wall of his pelvis on the right side. Surgery was not possible, so he was given chemotherapy. It worked

[58] We all have a pair of genes, one from each parent. The one which expresses its function while suppressing the other gene is known as a *dominant gene*. An autosomal dominant genetic condition, or disease, is a pattern of inheritance in which the patient has two copies of genes, one abnormal and one normal. The damaged gene is dominant over the normal one and expresses the disease in the body. This is in contrast to autosomal recessive genetic conditions, in which the patient will only express the disease if both parents have passed on defective genes. One gene by itself does not dominate if its second counterpart is normal.
[59] The exact fault is with the DNA mismatch repair system (MMR) which is a system for recognising and repairing erroneous insertions, deletions, and mis-incorporation of bases into the DNA during the process of cell division.
[60] Ureters are the tubes that connect the kidneys to the urinary bladder.

and the cancer shrunk. Ten months later it started to grow again. This time a new treatment, immunotherapy, was tried and the cancer once again shrunk. Midway through this treatment he developed difficulty in finding words when speaking and his brain scan showed the brain tumour we have now met to treat.

I am pleasantly surprised to meet Mr H.E. He is a tall gentleman, very steady on his feet, showing no signs of damage from his brain surgery or tumour except a difficulty in finding words to express himself.

For someone with Lynch syndrome, whose family members have succumbed to cancer at a much younger age, Mr H.E had managed to evade his first cancer until the age of 52, and since then has survived five more cancer incidences.

There must be something, or many things, he is doing right. At 72, he is otherwise fit and well, fully active, has a healthy lifestyle, never smoked with no plans to start now, and has long vowed to drink alcohol only at Christmas, which fortunately happens only once a year.

My first impression is that he will not only tolerate the treatment well but also benefit from it.

But it's a gamble. We are putting the ureteric cancer treatment with immunotherapy on hold while giving him chemotherapy and radiotherapy for the brain tumour. He is willing to take the risk and he proves me right. As of writing, he has successfully completed the treatment, his brain tumour is under control, and the ureteric cancer is also behaving itself despite being off immunotherapy.

Mr H.E is a textbook case of the balance between destiny and free will.

His inherited genes destined him to develop multiple cancers, but his choice of lifestyle reduced the risk of exposure to additional carcinogens, delaying the onset and intensity of his cancers, making them more amenable to treatment.

A large Scandinavian study of twins came to the same conclusion; that despite having similar genes, the incidences of cancers differed among twins. "How much?" I hear you ask. Genetics only accounted for around 27% whereas the environmental factors accounted for a whopping 73%.

It reminds me of a well-known saying by a great scholar[61] from the 7th century who, when asked by his student to explain destiny and free will, told the student to lift one foot off the ground. He duly obliged. "This," said the scholar, "is free will! Now raise the second foot."

---

[61] The famous Imam, Ali, nephew and student of the Prophet of Islam, Mohammad (may peace be upon him).

"I can't," replied the student.

"This, my dear friend, is destiny," explained the teacher.

A Brief Note on Lynch Syndrome

Lynch syndrome is a well-studied genetic cancer risk. It was first described by American boxer and physician Professor Dr Henry Thompson Lynch (also known as Hammerin' Hank[62]), in 1966.

It is estimated that approximately 2% to 7% of all diagnosed cases of colorectal cancer are due to Lynch syndrome (HNPCC).

Most people inherit the condition from a parent. However, not all people with the HNPCC gene mutation have a parent who had cancer. Some people develop HNPCC de novo in a new generation without inheriting the gene (as the old saying goes, "There's always a first time for everything").

Preventing cancer in Lynch syndrome patients depends a lot on screening[63]. Genetic counselling and genetic testing are recommended for families that meet the suspicion criteria known as the 'Amsterdam criteria' (because it was decided at an international meeting held in Amsterdam!). The diagnosis criteria are as follows:

1. Three or more family members with HNPCC-related cancers, one of whom is a first-degree relative of the other two;

2. Two successive affected generations;

3. One or more of the HNPCC-related cancers diagnosed under the age of 50 years; and

4. Excluding familial adenomatous polyposis (FAP), another inherited condition which causes polyps in the bowel and mimics Lynch syndrome.

The exact fault in Lynch syndrome is with the DNA mismatch repair system (MMR). This is a pivotal system for recognising and repairing erroneous insertions, deletions, and mis-incorporation of bases into

---

[62]Before becoming a professor of genetics, Lynch dropped out of high school at 14, joined the US Navy as a gunner at 16 using false identification papers to hide his age, served in the Second World War and, after the end of the war in 1946, became a professional boxer, nicknamed 'Hammerin' Hank'.

[63] Pre-cancerous or early malignant lesions can be detected by colonoscopy and the patient can be offered prophylactic surgery to remove the section of bowel growing the cancer. It prevents the pre-cancerous lesions from becoming cancerous and progressing to an advanced stage or spreading to other organs.

the DNA during the process of cell division. Think of it like spellcheck software that automatically detects and corrects any spelling mistakes in a text.

Without a fully functional DNA spellcheck, the chances of mistakes in the genetic text that codes information increases. With every cell division, these mistakes accumulate. If and when this mistake occurs in a *growth promotor gene*, the message could be misread and the cell go into a vicious cycle of continuous growth, the first step towards becoming a cancer.

Over the years, other errors occur which can trigger the pre-cancer cells to develop into a full-blown cancer.

How often and quickly this happens in a patient will depend on how frequently the DNA is damaged in an individual. Random mistakes, just like random errors in typing a text, happen at a regular rate and usually the body has the capacity to deal with them effectively. Even if one of the repair systems is impaired or totally breaks down, there are alternative systems which can step in. The problem occurs when the frequency and amount of DNA damage spirals out of control due to additional insult by environmental carcinogens, such as those arising from smoking and consuming alcohol. This more readily overwhelms the repair system in patients who have inherited an impaired system to start with.

So, it's not just about the cards that we are dealt with but how we play them that decides the final outcome.

PART 5

SEX
DRUGS &
ROCK & ROLL

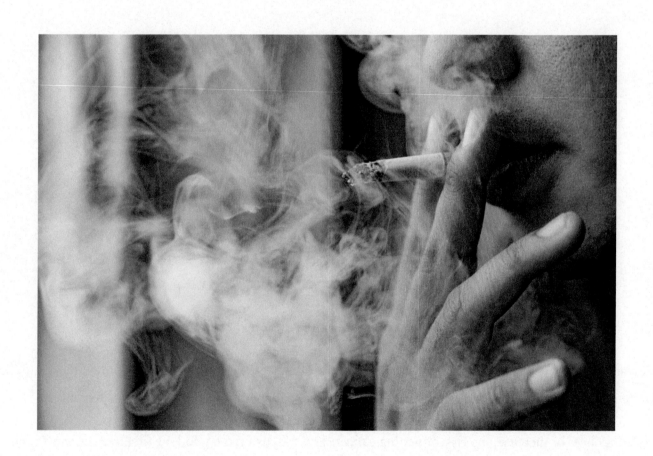

PART 5: SEX, DRUGS, & ROCK 'N' ROLL

5   Sex, Drugs, and Rock 'N' Roll

Good news! As far as we know, rock 'n 'roll is safe when it comes to cancer. So, turn up the volume, sit back and relax. But don't get too comfortable. If romance is on your mind, you might want to make sure precautions are to hand, and if you're a little thirsty then go brew some fresh coffee rather than reaching into the fridge for that bottle of fizz you've got on ice. Call me a party pooper if you like, but I've got your best interests at heart. I want you to have fun. Really, I do! Just … well, read on and make up your own minds.

5.1   Sex

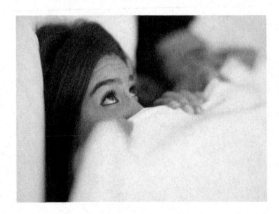

Life, as someone[64] once defined, is a sexually transmitted, terminal condition.

Fortunately, this is not the case for most cancers but in some cases it holds true. Sex (or having sex, to be more precise) is a metaphorical, double-edged sword that cuts both ways when it comes to cancer.

It can reduce, or increase, the risk of getting cancer. Let's focus on the good bit first, reduction of cancer risk with regular sex[65].

The basic principle of 'preventing cancer by promoting sex 'is simple. Having sex burns calories, the longer the better, and burning calories regularly, also known as 'exercise', is proven to reduce the risk of cancer, along with other health benefits.

---

[64] The origin of this phrase is attributed to Ronald David Laing (7th October, 1927 to 23rd August, 1989), usually cited as R. D. Laing (a Scottish psychiatrist who wrote extensively on mental illness, especially psychosis) who said "Life is a sexually transmitted disease". However, I prefer the adulterated version ('terminal condition' instead of 'disease'), which sounds and makes you feel better about life (I prefer not to think of life as a disease').

[65] Kindly note that lighting a cigarette at the end of a session would negate any benefits.

So, how much of a benefit is it, I hear you ask (while no doubt tearing off that sweater and limbering up). Well, it's estimated that while having sex we consume 4.2 calories per minute for a man and 3.1 calories per minute for a woman[66]. I leave you to do the sums for how long a session needs to be to burn enough calories. In addition, it improves your mood (usually), and having sex at least once a week has shown to boost the immune system. A strong immune system is an effective deterrent against cancer.

And then there is a direct benefit in reducing the risk of cancer, too. Men who ejaculate more frequently are at a lower risk of developing prostate cancer compared to those who ejaculate less often.

The biological outcome of sex, *pregnancy*, also protects women against breast and ovarian cancers. We will discuss them in detail later.

Now to the other side of the coin, the darker one.

Sex can increase the risk of developing cancer. It may come as a surprise to many that some cancers are actually *sexually transmitted diseases*. The culprits in most cases are viruses that can cause DNA damage.

The commonest is cervical cancer, which used to be a major cause of death in young women before effective treatment[67] was introduced. It is spread from an infected partner by a virus known as the *human papilloma virus* (HPV for short, and you will hear a lot about it in this section). It's similar to the virus that causes the common skin wart. It usually takes many years for the viral damage to transform, by a stepwise process, into a cancer.

Next is anal cancer. Its most common type, called a *squamous cell carcinoma*, is due to a sexually transmitted virus known as … HPV.

Penile cancer, or cancer of the penis, is also a sexually transmitted disease caused by none other than HPV.

The other genital cancers, vaginal and vulvar, are also caused by a sexually transmitted virus, and yes, you guessed it right this time too, the notorious HPV.

For a long time, it was considered that sexually transmitted cancers are only limited to certain parts of the body, 'where the sun don't shine', but then doctors started to notice a strange pattern of head and neck cancers in the late 1990s, and which may have begun as early as the '70s.

---

[66] Please don't ask me why this difference exists between men and women, but if you find out the reason then feel free to share it.

[67] The treatment is potentially curative even without surgery. Chemotherapy with external beam radiotherapy followed by high-dose internal radiotherapy (brachytherapy) has a good rate of curing this cancer.

Usually, head and neck cancers are associated with people in their 50s who have a long history of smoking, or using other forms of tobacco like chewing tobacco, and increased alcohol consumption. But since the seventies, more and much younger patients, both men and women, between the ages of 30 and 50 started developing cancers of the mouth, especially the tongue, tonsils, and throat. And the numbers continued to rise. Further research showed that these patients had a history of engaging in oral sex. Laboratory tests found evidence for the usual suspect, a virus: HPV.

This was probably the first time in history that a change in human sexual behaviour had led to the development of a new form of human cancer. This doesn't mean that oral sex was invented in the 1970s. It has been around for thousands of years[68], just like French kissing has been in vogue long before the French discovered it. But the sexual revolution of the 1960s and 1970s made it more prevalent.

Although we are, so far, unable to establish the who, how, when, where, and why of oral sex (or French kissing for that matter), we do know that the credit for discovering that the human papilloma virus causes cancer of the cervix in women goes to Herald zur Hausen, a German virologist.

Hausen was a brilliant scientist who gained his degree in medicine in 1960 from the University of Dusseldorf and who then moved to Philadelphia, USA, to do research on viruses. His first discovery was to find the link between a virus (known as the *Epstein-Barr virus*) and a type of cancer known as a *lymphoma*. In 1972, he moved back to Germany and started his work on different types of HPV. He correctly identified HPV in almost 75% of cervical cancers but faced strong criticism from other scientists, who presented their own candidate, the *herpes simplex virus*, for the dubious honour. Finally, Hausen was vindicated and awarded a Nobel Prize in Medicine in 2008, 32 years after he had first reported his findings.

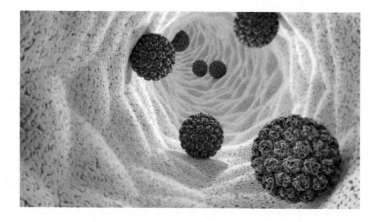

The notorious human papilloma viruses.

---

[68] Some ancient temples in South Asia have erotic sculptures depicting the act of oral sex, and evidence is also seen in ancient Egyptian religious myths of Osiris, erotic frescos in the city of Pompeii, and ceramic pots from ancient American civilisations.

HPV is not the only culprit when it comes to causing cancers. Another sexually transmitted virus (which can also spread by blood, e.g., contaminated needles, or breastfeeding) is HTLV or *h*uman T-*c*ell *l*ymphotropic *v*irus, and this can cause a type of blood cancer (T-cell *l*eukaemia/*l*ymphoma, ATL or ATLL), which is fortunately rare.

For years, researchers tried to find a link between infections of the urogenital tract and prostate cancer. Initial studies did not show any link regarding infections, including those by *N. gonorrhoea*, chlamydia, trachomatis, the syphilis-causing bug (*Treponema pallidum*) and the notorious HPV. However, the final culprit was found to be a sexually transmitted bacterial infection, *Trichomonas vaginalis*. The study, reported in the *Journal of the National Cancer Institute* in 2009, showed increased risk of cancer and its progression to bony metastases. Prostate cancer-specific death also tended to be higher in patients who had trichomonas vaginalis infection (trichomoniasis).

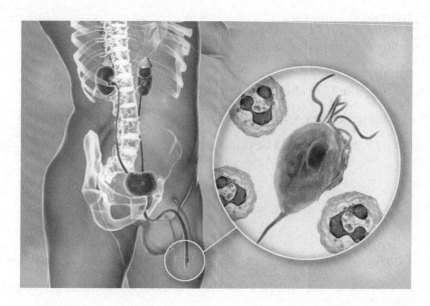

Trichomonas vaginalis bacterium which increases risk of prostate cancer.

Trichomoniasis is believed to affect some 275 million people worldwide and is the most common sexually transmitted bacterial infection. It often presents with itching in the genital area, burning sensation on passing urine, vaginal or penile discharge, and painful intercourse. Women might have a foul-smelling yellow-green vaginal discharge that is often described as having a 'fishy' smell. Infection can be passed from men to women and vice versa. It is suspected that a quarter of men with prostate cancer showed signs of past trichomoniasis, and these men were more likely to have advanced tumours. Research has shown that this sexually transmitted infection can make men more vulnerable to prostate cancer.

The parasite that causes trichomoniasis (trichomonas vaginalis) secretes a protein causing inflammation and increased growth and invasion of benign and cancerous prostate cells. This suggests a possible way in which the parasite trichomonas vaginalis[69] could encourage the prostate cancer cells to grow and develop more quickly.

Fortunately, it is easy to cure with a short course of antibiotics, sometimes a single dose curing 95–97% of the infections.

Other sexually transmitted viral diseases, especially HIV (causing AIDS), also play an important role in increasing the risk of many cancers, if not causing them directly. The virus causing AIDS weakens the immune system, leading to an increased risk of many cancers such as Kaposi's sarcoma, a type of fleshy cancer mostly effecting the skin, non-Hodgkin lymphoma (a blood cancer), lung, bowel, anal and cervical cancer.

More research into the link between cancers and sexually transmitted infections is needed. I suggest using the term *STCs* (sexually transmitted cancers[70]) to create more awareness, and if I had my way, they'd be incorporated into sex education and awareness programmes everywhere.

And this brings us to the important question about sex and cancer. How can we avoid STCs? Do all people exposed to sexually transmitted cancer viruses develop cancer? What can be done to reduce the risk after one has been exposed to it? And what could be done to reduce the damage once a diagnosis of an STC has been made?

So, let's tackle them one by one.

Avoidance through celibacy would seem to be the simplest solution but is not very practical for most people, unless you are committed to spending your life in a monastery, nunnery, or an otherwise deserted island.

For the less religiously committed, being in a monogamous relationship, reducing the number of sex partners and, most importantly, using barrier protection in the form of condoms, will reduce the risk of STCs significantly. Condoms are the key to prevention.

Interestingly, if you are not using a condom, you might be more promiscuous than you think, and I don't mean it in the fun sense. Researchers in the UK surveyed 6,000 sexually active individuals and developed an algorithm to calculate the risk of exposure to sexually transmitted infections. The principle is simple:

---

[69] The infection can be diagnosed very easily by lab tests and treatment with antibiotics has a very high cure rate.
[70] And claim a copyright protection for it.

when you have unprotected sex with another person you are being exposed to infections that person *might* have contracted from all the sex partners they have had until they met you.

Using the six degrees of separation theory (which says that we are all connected to each other through six other people), having unprotected sex with someone is like having unprotected sex with everyone they've slept with, and everyone that those have slept with slept with, and so on.

So how 'promiscuous' is a typical, sexually active individual, if they are engaged in unprotected sex?

According to the online calculator[71] devised by the team, a typical person with an average of nine lifetime sex partners is exposing his/herself to … brace yourself … 3,917,918 (that's three million, nine hundred and seventeen thousand, nine hundred and eighteen) indirect sexual connections.

So, how much indirect sexual exposure does one have in a monogamous relationship? The answer depends on the number of sexual partners and encounters of your partner. For a man having sex with a 20–24-year-old female, the number of indirect sexual partners is estimated as 239,600, and if the partner is aged 25–34 it's 381,586 (based on the observation that with increasing age, the average number of sexual partners and encounters tends to increase). And yet, it's still defined as a "relatively safe, monogamous" relationship.

Taking these numbers into one's stride, the mere thought of potential infections might make a person reach for a box of condoms, or head for the nearest monastery/nunnery.

And it's not just the infections one has to worry about.

Unprotected sex also causes us to pick up many genital floras (bacteria, viruses, and fungi) and pass them on. In one study, women in relationships with promiscuous men were found to have more types of vaginal flora compared to those in relationship with non-promiscuous men, and the types of bacteria changed frequently depending on the men's promiscuity.

Apart from using condoms, another method of reducing risk of sexually transmitted cancers is to have immunisation against the cancer-causing infectious agents. So far, the only successful vaccine available is

---

[71] The aptly name 'Sex Degrees of Separation' Calculator The calculator is meant to give a generalised potential estimate, not an accurate figure.

against the human papilloma virus (HPV), which causes many cancers including cervical cancer. The vaccine is offered to young girls and boys[72] in the hope to develop immunity against the virus.

The vaccine targets up to nine types of HPV viruses, especially type 16 and type 18, which cause the greatest risk of cervical cancer.

The success rate of preventing cancer is high: 70% for cervical cancer, 80% for anal cancer, 60% for vaginal cancer, and 40% for vulvar cancer. There is also evidence that it protects against the mouth and throat cancers caused by HPV, and genital warts (that's a bonus).

Two or three doses, given between the ages of nine and 13, give protection for up to 10 years.

The vaccine is quite safe, and the most common side effect reported was "pain at the injection site", which is less of a side-effect and more stating the obvious, if you ask me.

Last but not least, the age-old tradition of circumcision has also shown to reduce the risk of all sexually transmitted diseases, but this is not as effective as using a condom. Circumcision reduces the risk for HIV by 60%, herpes simplex virus (HSV) by 34%, the notorious cancer-causing HPV by 35%, and trichomoniasis by 48%. Being circumcised and using a condom would definitely confer more protection for both partners.

And this brings us to the next question. Do all people exposed to sexually transmitted cancer viruses develop cancer?

Fortunately, the answer to this question is no.

Not all people end up with a cancer after exposure to a cancer-causing virus. But it's like playing Russian roulette. The risk is there and increases with repeated infections. Also, other carcinogens need to be taken into account. The more the risk factors, the higher the chance of developing a cancer.

Luckily, the process takes many years if not decades, leaving open a window of opportunity for screening to detect and treat the cancer at any early stage, resulting in a high chance of curing it.

So, what can be done to reduce the risk of sexually transmitted cancers after one has been exposed to a sexually transmitted disease?

---

[72] Initially, boys weren't offered the vaccine in the UK because it wasn't deemed 'cost effective' to prevent penile cancer, which is a rare cancer. The fact boys carry the HPV infection to girls, which causes cervical, vaginal, and vulvar cancer, and that vaccinating girls does not develop immunity in all those vaccinated, was totally ignored.

The answer is to reduce further risk. First and foremost, get the infection treated as early as possible. The longer it festers, the greater are the chances of DNA damage that could lead to cancer.

Secondly, avoid getting the same or different infections in future. Preventive measures would reduce the risk of developing the cancer. Multiple exposures and high-risk behaviour would increase the chances.

It's also important not just to focus on the sexually transmitted infections but to avoid other risk factors (like smoking, alcohol, and other carcinogens) that can cause cumulative DNA damage and mutations leading to cancer. And that brings up the last question of our discussion on sex and cancer. What could be done to reduce the damage once a diagnosis of a sexually transmitted cancer has been made?

Believe it or not, preventing the risk factors is still relevant. Continuing the exposure to infections and carcinogens would not make the situation better and most likely would worsen it. Cancer is a mutated cell and adding more mutations to it would only make it more difficult to treat. Fortunately, most sexually transmitted cancers can be detected early through screening programmes.

Effective screening followed by radical treatment often results in a cure. If the disease is advanced, and cannot be cured, there are options for active treatment and controlling the cancer with an aim to improve survival and maintain a good quality of life.

5.2   Oral Contraceptive Pills

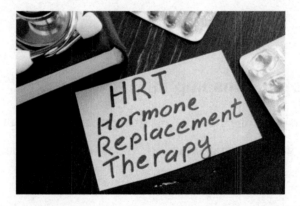

The Swinging Sixties gave us a decade of counterculture, sexual revolution, flower power, The Beatles, John F. Kennedy, Martin Luther King Jr, Che Guevara, Yuri Gagarin (the first man in space), bell-bottom jeans, and a four-letter word, the 'pill'. Of these, only the latter has survived and proliferated since.

And proliferated it has, spreading across the globe, overtaking land and water. Today, one hundred million women worldwide take the oral contraceptive pill voluntarily, and a much larger number of fish and men take it involuntarily.

The synthetic oestrogens are excreted in the urine and faeces of women, ending up in the water system. They pass through water treatment plants unfiltered and end up being consumed by fish and men. Consequently, the number of intersex fish (with both male and female characteristics) has increased with a subsequent decrease in the fish population. Among men, the sperm count has been progressively falling due to contamination of drinking water with female hormones. Whether it has contributed to the rise of the metrosexual male is still a matter of research[73].

Exposure to more oestrogen and progesterone is a risk factor for cancer. Women who take hormone replacement treatment (HRT) for menopause are also at greater risk of developing breast cancer. This is due to the proliferative effects of female hormones on cells, increasing the chances of developing cancer cells. Using birth control pills may also increase a woman's risk of developing cervical cancer.

5.3   Breast Implants

There has been a lot of suspicion about foreign objects that are put into the body, like silicone breast implants or other metals and ceramics. A lot of researchers suspect that these might lead to cancer due to chronic irritation and inflammation. A recent review of documented cases of BIA-ALCL (breast implant-associated anaplastic large cell lymphoma) in the United States between 1996 and 2015 showed that the incidence of BIA-ACAL was two per one million women with use of a textured breast implant, according to the Mayo clinic. So, the risk is present, but the good news is that it is very unlikely to happen.

5.4   Alcohol

5.4.1   History of Alcohol Consumption

We all use alcohol in one form or another, be it as an antiseptic or solvent, not to mention the more familiar form of drink that many if not all are accustomed to. We wouldn't be where we are today, for better or worse, if it wasn't for alcohol and its derivatives.

Allow me to explain.

Humans and alcohol have known each other for thousands of years. There is evidence suggesting that humans started to ferment food as early as 10,000 BC and the knowledge spread fast from one civilisation to another. This is also evident by the fact that races that had moved to farther parts of the globe before

---

[73] Probably because no one else has thought of it and I have been busy writing this book.

this period, such as the Native Americans[74] and Australian Aboriginals, did not have the knowledge to make alcohol and were only introduced to it after European colonisation. Ironically, these races also have a reduced ability to detoxify alcohol and hence suffered from significant problems of alcohol toxicity and addiction once exposed to it.

The first evidence of brewing alcohol comes from around 7,000 BC in northern China. Chemical residues in pots from Jiahu region near the Yellow River show that Chinese were making and using wine on regular basis. There were two important aspects of Chinese alcohol culture.

Firstly, alcohol was simply alcohol to them. They didn't bother differentiating between wine and ale, and called them both *jiu*.

Secondly, they had a complex love-hate relation with alcohol. They loved making the stuff but were scared of its side effects and tried very hard to regularise and sometimes even ban it. They probably made more laws regulating its use than the types of alcohol available.

For example, drinking alcohol was mostly restricted to formal occasions such as religious gatherings, funerals, meetings etc. You just couldn't throw a booze party because it was illegal for more than three people to drink together for 'no reason'. At one point, having more than five drinks was punishable by death. However, drinking at a funeral was acceptable, but complaints have been recorded about people who went from funeral to funeral, mourning and drowning their sorrows in alcohol.

From China, the know-how of making alcohol or *jiu*, was quickly passed on to neighbouring regions. By 6,000 BC, the South Caucasus and Georgian regions were making wine.

From here it went to Mesopotamia, what we now call 'Iraq'.

Around 3,000–4,000 BC, the Mesopotamians discovered the skills of writing and making beer which was known as *kash* in the Sumerian language.

The Sumerians had their own goddess of beer, Ninkasi. Making beer was a female speciality and it was sold at taverns owned and run by women. The goddess of alcohol, Ninkasi, had a close link to the goddess of sex, Inana. The former's commodity was sold inside the tavern and the latter outside, although common sense would dictate it the other way around. The reason for this odd arrangement is that despite the taverns being owned and run by women, no women were allowed inside. Not even the sex workers. If a noble

---

[74] There are a few exceptions, such as the Aztecs of South America who discovered alcohol in the fermented sap of agave plant but most Native Americans remained unaware of alcohol till arrival of the European colonisers.

woman, for example a priestess (known as a "sister of a god" in the Code of Hammurabi) was to be found in a tavern, her punishment was to be burnt alive. So, making and selling alcohol was an exclusively female occupation while drinking it a male one.

Sumerian alcohol also helped the human race to discover an important tool, one that has become an integral part of almost every human household today: the drinking straw. The reason why alcohol was served in jars with a straw is that ancient beer was more like a sludgy porridge and to get to the bottom part, where all the alcohol rich liquid was, a straw was quite handy. It probably also reduced the risk of choking on the sludge when the customer was drunk and trying to gulp down the contents of the jar.

The most important step in refining alcohol production was the process of alcohol distillation, which was started as early as 2,000 BC in the Indus valley civilisation, in present-day Pakistan[75].

Egypt joined the alcohol revolution quite late. But once they did, they made it a central part of their civilisation. Beer was made from barley around 600 BC in Egypt. They also imported wine from other countries. The Egyptian goddess of alcohol, Hathor, actually lived in (present-day) Sudan and was said to have visited Egypt once a year, coinciding with the flooding of the Nile. This occasion was marked by a major festival where Egyptians got drunk and naked to party all night. Unlike the Mesopotamians, Egyptians were more inclusive and allowed both women and men to drink, especially at festivals. For ancient Egyptians, there were two important aspects of drinking alcohol, vomiting and sex, preferably in that order.

Now, all cultures are familiar with the act of vomiting after drinking alcohol but ancient Egyptians took it to another level. For them, it was essential to vomit while drinking and, to make sure of it, they added emetic herbs to their alcohol which made people throw up and then reach out for more beer. This ensured that the stomach was regularly emptied to make room for the next drink. Getting hammered (pun intended) was considered to be a mystical experience that was often followed by the physical act of having sex.

They were also the first to document the effects of alcohol on increasing the chances of having sex on a date. There are ancient Egyptian poems that advise using strong wine and ale to help confuse and seduce the date. A recent American study confirms the Egyptian experience. Chances of an alcohol-free date ending with sex is just 10% compared to 24% with three drinks, 41% with four, and 51% with five drinks. Anything above that follows the laws of diminishing returns as both parties are too drunk to do anything

---

[75] It might come as a surprise that the name 'India' has historically always referred to the region along the Indus River which is in present-day Pakistan. That is the reason why when, in 326 BC, Alexander the Great gained control of the region that is present-day Pakistan, he returned because he had ticked off 'conquer India' in his bucket list. He never bothered venturing any further to present-day India, which was historically referred to as 'Bharat'.

productive (or reproductive). Interestingly, having more than four drinks on a date also lowers the chances of a second date.

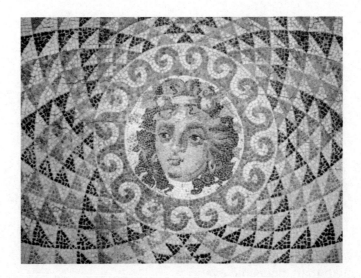

Mosaic depicting Dionysus, an Arab immigrant from Pakistan who became the Greek and Roman god of alcohol.

Back to the ancient world.

The European (Greek & Roman) god of wine/alcohol was an Arab immigrant from Pakistan.

Dionysus was born and raised in Arabia but spent many years wandering along the river Indus in present-day Pakistan, where he learnt the art and science of making wine and also laid the foundation of at least one city.

With his newfound knowledge and friend, Dionysus headed for Europe. He arrived in Greece in a chariot with a large group of exotic immigrants that paraded through the streets singing and dancing. How they made it through Greek border control and immigration is not known.

These included humans and animals, and half-humans and half-animals. Lions and tigers were accompanied by drunk and ecstatic female devotees of Dionysus, a bit like modern-day groupies, known as 'maenads'; centaurs, who were half-man, half-horse; satyrs, who were half-human, half-goat and Dionysus' wise friend and tutor, Silenus, who was mostly drunk and almost human except having a tail and horse's ears. This group of singing and dancing Dionysian devotees was called a *thiasus* by the Greeks.

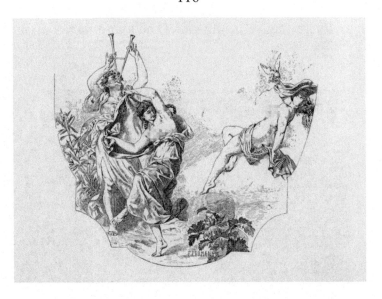

Maenads, the drunk, ecstatic devotees of Dionysus.

But there is more to this myth than meets the eye.

Dionysus' arrival heralded a big change for Europe. Alcohol/wine was newfound pleasure. But there are three important aspects of the Dionysian *thiasus* which have been overlooked by historians:

1. The Centaurs: Half-human, half-horse, centaurs were actually horse-riding humans. The concept of one species taming and riding another is unique to the human race, and it all started with domestication of the horse in Arabia around 9,000 years ago. The chance finding of a statue of a birdied horse in the Al Magar valley, along with petroglyphs (stone carved images) of mounted riders, show that the Arabs had domesticated and ridden horses long before any other nation. This was a revolutionary concept as horses were hunted for food like other game animals, such as deer and antelope. The idea of riding one's food was as unimaginable then as using a banana as a mode of transport today. The early horse riders seemed to have maintained this monopoly for many thousands of years as they hunted, raided, and pillaged neighbouring nations without giving away their secret. The non-riding victims thought these were half-human, half-horse creatures because they appeared at dawn with the sun behind them, shooting arrows and disappearing in a cloud of dust before the victims had a chance to come out of hiding. The Greeks called them *centaurs/ kentauros*, a combination of *ken* ('piercing') and *tauros* ('bull'), as these mounted archers chased and hunted bulls with ease.

The Indians were equally puzzled by their appearance and called them *kinnara*, from the ancient Sanskrit words *ki* (is it?) and *nara* ('human'). The *kinnara* riders established a whole kingdom in the north of India, looting, pillaging, and terrorising the bipedal humans. The Kinnara Kingdom had both male and female accomplished riders, with the females specialising in attacking trade caravans. The psychological aspect of it was so deep that even today the long-haul truck drivers in Pakistan have paintings of half-woman, half-horse *kinnari* females on their vehicles in hope of protection from looters.

So, when Dionysus decided to immigrate with his centaurs, he also brought the art and skill of horse riding to Europe.

2. The Chariot: We all know that the two most important milestones in the history of mankind have been the discovery of fire and the invention of the wheel. But what we almost always overlook is the fact that the wheel was only used in the societies that rode horses. For example, the Native Americans never used the wheel despite having built toys with wheels for kids. This is because they never learned to ride horses which would have led to chariots and carriages.

Ironically, there were horses in North America when humans arrived, crossing the Bering Straits. Known as the Hagerman horse, the Native American horse was similar in size to an Arabian horse. The early humans were delighted to find this handsome animal and hunted it to extinction around 10 thousand years ago. The next time they saw the animals was when the Spanish conquistadors arrived in the new world and were mistaken for – surprise, surprise – half-human, half-horse creatures.

Similarly, the Australian Aboriginals and the Sub-Saharan human tribes never discovered the use of the wheel, either because they never domesticated or rode horses.

Dionysus riding a chariot to Europe heralded not just the introduction of horse riding but also the discovery and use of the wheel, which was to revolutionise the Western world.

3. The Maenads: These were the female worshipers of Dionysus who were very, and I mean *very*, fond of alcohol. They would go into the mountains wearing next to nothing, get drunk and dance and rip animals to pieces. The maenads cult became very popular in ancient Greece and Rome. This was the earliest expression of female empowerment, eventually leading to the concept of feminism in 1837 so women could have the same rights as men, and the RSPCA (Royal Society for the Prevention of Cruelty to Animals) in 1824, so those rights could be exercised without ripping animals limb from limb.

Hence Dionysus' arrival heralded a revolutionary change for Europe, in particular, and the future world in general.

But Dionysus struggled to be accepted by Greek society because he was a foreigner. People often failed to acknowledge that he was a god and he had to convince them by turning them into animals. Whether he used wine in the process is not known.

Dionysus also performed miracles of biblical proportions, literally. He turned water into wine. But the Greeks were not impressed and diluted their wine by a ratio of three parts water to one part wine, which made it no better than beer. Undiluted wine, they said, was a drink of barbarians. This must have upset Dionysus, who was already struggling to be accepted.

The Romans went a step further and diluted their wine by mixing it with hot water. This hideous tradition is almost dead now, except around Christmas time when the wine is heated and mixed with spices like cinnamon, cloves, cardamom, and nutmeg. This is known as 'mulled wine' and is consumed as a reluctant yet religious yearly chore.

Needless to say, alcohol soon became the newfound love from Athens to Amsterdam and beyond. The rich drank wine, the poor ale and beer, but almost everyone drank alcohol in one form or another. All thanks to an Arab immigrant from Pakistan.

So, it's no surprise that the next major innovation in alcohol refinement that was to take Europe by a storm also came from the East and involved an Arab.

The modern form of alcohol distillation was perfected by Muslim chemists during the 8th century. The Arab chemist al-Kindi conducted distillation of wine to create stronger spirits with a higher concentration of alcohol. This opened the gates for more refined forms of alcohol such as brandy, gin, champagne, vermouth, and vodka.

Pure ethanol was discovered by the Persian physician, polymath, philosopher, and probably the first psychologist and psychotherapist, al-Razi (known to Europe as Rhazes, 854–925 AD).

Ironically, for a teetotal religion[76], Muslim scientists were big fans of alcohol; not for drinking it, but for using it in their experiments as a chemical reagent and disinfectant.

So, it is no surprise that the word 'alcohol' actually comes from Arabic language and was initially used for a very refined powder, *al-kuhol*, used as a cosmetic and eyeliner. Later on, this meaning was extended to distilled substances, including different types of alcohol.

---

[76] It's a little-known fact that Prophet Mohammad (may peace be upon him) allowed Muslims to make alcohol so it could be converted to vinegar, which he highly recommended as part of the diet.

Worldwide, on average every human being consumes the equivalent of approximately 6.4 litres of pure alcohol annually, equating to one alcoholic drink per day. However, there is a huge variation in the intake of alcohol, with some not consuming any at all. The top position for alcohol consumption is held by Lithuania with 3.32 drinks per day, closely followed by Belarus (3.00 drinks per day), and in third place, the Republic of Moldova (2.9 drinks per day).

The definition of a standard drink size varies widely within and between countries. For example, in the United States it's about 14 to 15 grams of alcohol. In Great Britain, 8 grams of alcohol is a standard drink (called a 'unit 'in the UK, and defined as the amount of alcohol an average adult's body can process in an hour). In Japan, a whopping 19.75 grams of alcohol represents a standard drink.

The levels of drinking are also defined differently. In the United States, for example, moderate drinking is defined by the CDC (Centers for Disease Control and Prevention) as women having fewer than two drinks per day or men having fewer than three drinks per day. For people aged 65 and above, it is fewer than two drinks per day. Heavy drinking is defined as women having more than seven drinks per week, or three drinks per occasion, and for men more than 14 drinks per week or four drinks per occasion. Binge drinking is defined as women having four or more drinks in one drinking occasion, and men having five or more drinks in one drinking occasion.

Generally, a safe dose of alcohol is considered to be no more than two drinks daily for men and one drink daily for non-pregnant women (see below). The reasons for this gender difference include a lower body size, body water content, and activity of gastric alcohol dehydrogenase enzyme levels which, among women, results in a heavier effective alcohol exposure (alcohol stays in their body in its active form for a longer time compared to men) for a given consumption of alcohol.

Of course, for many, moderate alcohol consumption is an integral part of socialising with friends, whether at dinner parties or just informal get-togethers at home, the pub, or local wine bar. Champagne corks pop on special occasions, and most need little encouragement to raise our glasses for a toast … any excuse will do. Some just like to relax with a glass of their favourite tipple after work, feet up on the sofa, the TV on or a good book in their hands. And our warm, and sometimes fuzzy, relationship with alcohol is served by a huge industry from mega-international companies which have brands of wine, beer, and spirits known the world over, down to small micro-breweries creating niche beers. Then there are the fearless and intrepid who brew their own beer at home, or who create wines from virtually anything growing in their gardens. Who can forget their Aunt Gladys's elderberry wine or Uncle Joe's sloe gin that had quite an unnerving kick to it?

The Munich Oktoberfest is the world's largest folk festival, often attended by more than seven million visitors. With seating for 100,000 and consuming about 15% of Munich's total electricity requirement, this vast annual party gives rise to some pretty impressive figures on alcohol consumption, including approximately seven million litres of beer and 95,000 litres of wine (Cheers! Or *Prost!* as the locals shout).

Those who have ever over-indulged will know all too well the immediate price paid for their excess: the throbbing head, nausea, leathery tongue, and occasionally the desire to stay in bed in the dark until the middle of next week. Often vowing 'never again', curiously never again frequently occurs the following Friday night! And there are the more serious negative social consequences as well, as we're all too familiar with. According to the US National Institute on Alcohol Abuse and Alcoholism, in 2014 there were about 16 million heavy alcohol users and 61 million binge drinkers in the US. Over 10,000 people died in car crashes in which alcohol was involved, alcohol played a role in a third of cases of violent crime, and the total annual cost or burden was estimated at $249 billion.

So, we know drinking too much isn't good for us, and that alcoholics can have a tough time kicking the habit before their liver throws in the towel and gives up. Yet, such is the love of our favourite tipple, we all too readily seize upon any 'good news' of supposed health benefits. And some have indeed made headline news, like, for example, that moderate alcohol consumption may be good for the heart and circulatory system, and might protect against gallstones and type 2 diabetes. Studies do support these claims in relation to moderate alcohol consumption, and scientifically there are suggested mechanisms behind them. For example, the protective effect against cardiovascular disease may be related to an increase in HDL (high-density lipoprotein, often referred to as 'good cholesterol), or increased insulin sensitivity, and possibly the effects alcohol has on the blood's clotting factors (the theory being that it prevents the formation of small clots that can block arteries etc.).

When discussing any potential benefits, it's important to emphasize that they are usually observed in studies of subjects with moderate alcohol intake. Heavy drinking can, for example, increase blood pressure and damage heart muscle, so it not only nullifies any possible benefits but causes harm too.

No discussion would be complete without mentioning the past medicinal uses of alcohol. Pure alcohol (ethanol) has been used as a life-saving drug. It was injected into a patient's vein (bloodstream) as an antidote to treat life-threatening poisoning with methanol (found in disinfectants and windshield-washer fluid) or ethylene glycol (found in antifreeze, often ingested by children because it looks like a 'cool, colourful drink') up until 1997, when fomepizole, a new drug, was approved for this purpose by the US Food and Drug Administration (FDA). Dr Jeffrey Brent, who led a successful ground-breaking trial of the drug, reported that fomepizole did the job as well as ethanol without the risk of getting the patients drunk. Spoilsport!

OK, so what about alcohol and cancer. Well, there's some good(ish) news and some bad news. Let's deal with the bad news first. Recent data indicates that the proportion of cancers attributable to alcohol worldwide has increased. In 2012, alcohol consumption caused 5.5% of all cases of cancer and 5.8% of all cancer deaths. The increase is believed to be attributable primarily to an increase in the prevalence of drinkers and in the amount of alcohol consumed, particularly by women, who are more susceptible to the effects of alcohol, both as occasional or regular drinkers. Binge drinking also tends to have worse outcomes in women than men. The International Agency for Research on Cancer (IARC) considers alcohol as a group 1 carcinogen (meaning there is damn good evidence that it causes cancer). And alcohol consumption is associated with an increased risk of quite a range of cancers, too, including (brace yourself) cancers of the mouth, throat, oesophagus, breast, bowel, stomach, liver, pancreas, lung, and skin.

"Please," I hear you cry, "give us some good news!" Well, I'll do my best. Firstly, there is the possibility that consuming up to two alcoholic drinks per day (up to 30 grams of ethanol but no more) might reduce the risk of kidney cancer. The exact mechanism is not known, but some experts believe it is due to the diuretic[77] effect of alcohol, reducing the transit time of carcinogens through the kidney.

Red wine contains some beneficial ingredients. One of them is known as resveratrol (3, 5, 4-drihydroxystilbene). This is a substance produced by plants in response to stress and is found in grape skin. Resveratrol was found to extend the life of non-mammalian organisms and improve the metabolism and lifespan of mice fed high-fat diets. That all sounds very promising for fat mice but there is a catch. The resveratrol concentration in red wine is about 1.5 to 3 milligrams per litre. An average (70 kg) person would need to consume over 1,000 litres of red wine daily to achieve the resveratrol concentration used in the study on mice. In addition, a clinical trial of resveratrol among 24 patients with multiple myeloma, a kind of cancer of the white blood cells, showed minimal efficacy and an unacceptable safety profile, with five cases of kidney failure. Resveratrol supplements are available, but tablet doses are not standardised and side effects are unknown, and hence their use is not recommended.

I know, good news seems a bit thin on the ground, doesn't it. Having said this, there is something else worth explaining, and which, when you think about it, is actually very good news.

While it is true that alcohol is associated with an increased risk of a range of cancers, in many instances there is a dose relationship – meaning the more you drink, the higher the risk. So, this begs the question

---

[77] Increased urine production

whether there is a 'safe' level. In other words, can you enjoy your favourite tipple while avoiding the risk? It would be easy to simply recommend abstinence, but for many this isn't a lifestyle change they would willingly entertain, and so the question of a 'safe' level takes on a special significance. So, to try and answer this, let's take a look at some numbers.

Based on a combined analysis of over 200 studies assessing the link between alcohol consumption and cancer, here are some headline figures. These are described as 'relative risk' factors (RR) where anything above 1.0 represents an increased risk (e.g., 2 indicates twice the risk, and so on). For each cancer site, the RR is shown for three different levels of daily alcohol consumption (25/50/100g/day, approximating to three, six, and 12 'units' in the UK).

Cancer Site	Pooled RR (relative risk) associated with alcohol intake of:		
	25g/day	50g/day	100g/day
Oral cavity	1.73	2.77	5.72
Oesophagus	1.51	2.21	4.23
Stomach	1.07	1.15	1.32
Colon	1.14	1.21	1.32
Liver	1.2	1.41	1.83
Pancreas	0.98	1.05	1.18
Female breast	1.31	1.67	2.71

Firstly, it is clear that the relative risk increases with the more alcohol consumed, and can lead to almost a sixfold increased risk with cancers of the oral cavity. But examine the RRs for the 25g/day. Yes, these generally indicate an increased risk but often the additional relative risk isn't that high, comparatively speaking. And 25g/day approximates to three units of alcohol. So, one might anticipate that drinking just one or two units a day would have an even lower increase in relative risk.

So, there's some truth to the old adage of 'everything in moderation'. And, as noted above, any potential benefits of alcohol, if borne out, are also associated with moderate consumption.

This knowledge allows us to judge the sorts of risk we're willing to take. There is no known 'safe' dose as such when it comes to alcohol and cancer, but for those who can't bear to give up their favourite tipple, moderate or occasional consumption (say up to 1–2 units a day) might be a pragmatic approach. The key is to avoid exceeding it. Binge drinking is known to be more harmful than regularly drinking small amounts. A word of caution though; there is a synergistic relationship with other carcinogens, which means that alcohol in combination with other cancer-causing agents – e.g., smoking – increases the risk further.

Some of you may be curious to know the answer to the question as to whether we know how or why alcohol causes cancer. So, here's our current understanding.

5.4.2 Fourteen Reasons Why Cancer Loves Alcohol

1) Alcohol can cause direct damage to cells it comes in contact with and, hence, it is no surprise that the risk is highest for cancers of the mouth, throat, and oesophagus. Repeated damage and the need for continuous repair lead to the mutation of genes.

2) Oxidative stress: Alcohol causes oxidative damage[78] to cells and their genes. The body has a limited capacity to repair this damage and once it is overwhelmed, the repair processes start to fail and cumulative damage leads to formation of cancers over time.

3) Inflammation: Alcohol causes chronic inflammatory processes in multiple organs, eventually leading to DNA damage and mutations which are pre-cancerous in nature.

4) Malnutrition: People who consume alcohol get energy, 7 kcal per gram of alcohol, and hence loose the desire to eat. This leads to malnutrition, as alcohol does not have any nutritional value on its own.

5) Poor dietary habits: Alcohol consumption is associated with poor dietary habits. The diet of people consuming alcohol often lacks the antioxidant and beneficial compounds which could offset the damaging effects of environmental carcinogens, including alcohol.

6) Long-term alcohol use affects the naturally occurring bacteria in the gut, known as the *gut microbiome*. The technical term for this is *dysbiosis*, meaning defective or abnormally altered bacteria in the gut. Alcohol also weakens the barrier in the gut between the bacteria and bloodstream. This leads to increased exposure of the body to bacterial products, and is associated with increased risk of liver and colorectal cancers, to name a few.

---

[78] By producing reactive oxygen containing compounds which we talked about in previous sections.

7) Alcohol acts as a solvent for easier penetration of dietary or environmental carcinogens, especially those found in cigarette smoke.

8) Alcohol induces expression of many enzymes, such as cytochrome P4502E1 (CYP2E1), especially in the human oesophagus, and in a dose-dependent manner too. This means the more alcohol consumed, the more the production of this enzyme. The CYP2E1 activity yields substantial quantities of reactive oxygen species that can cause damage to DNA.

9) One of the major metabolites of alcohol is a toxic chemical known as 'acetaldehyde'. This is a genotoxic carcinogen, promoting cancer by damaging DNA and affecting gene transcription processes involved with cellular growth and differentiation. Alcohol doesn't have to wait until it reaches the liver before being converted into acetaldehyde. It is converted in saliva, resulting in salivary acetaldehyde levels that are 10 to 100 times higher than in the blood, a factor in the development of mouth, throat, and food canal (upper aero-digestive tract) cancers. Genetics certainly plays a role in alcohol-related cancer risk. The amounts of acetaldehyde present in various tissues not only depend on the quantity of ethanol consumed but also the individual's ability to metabolise it. Some people have variations in enzymes (such as alcohol dehydrogenase or aldehyde hydrogenase), making them more vulnerable than others. In such individuals, acetaldehyde levels following alcohol consumption can be elevated and prolonged, increasing the cancer risk. This is common in certain races, such as Native Americans, Australian Aboriginals, and Far East Asians. Due to the slower breakdown of acetaldehyde, they can suffer from hot flushes, especially on the face, known as the 'Asian glow'. The phenomenon is known to affect 30–50% of Chinese, Japanese, and Koreans. It also makes them feel very sick, gives them a splitting headache and a racing heart (palpitations). This is nature's way of discouraging them from consuming alcohol.

10) Alcohol also affects hormone metabolism, resulting in increased levels of circulatory oestrogen, for example, increasing the risk of breast cancer.

11) Alcohol affects DNA repair mechanisms and disables the body's capacity to fix DNA damage, hence increasing the chances of pre-cancerous mutations.

12) Alcohol reduces levels of vitamin A (especially its metabolite, retinoic acid) and helps set the stage for cell proliferation and possibly malignant transformation.

13) Alcohol also affects the immune surveillance of cancer cells. Due to alcohol, the capacity and efficacy of immune system to combat early cancerous lesions is impaired.

14) Alcohol causes changes in folate metabolism, which once again increases the risk of cancer formation.

Last, but not the least, as alcohol has all these multiple mechanisms of causing cell damage, it unsurprisingly also has a major impact on cancer treatment. If people consume high amounts of alcohol while receiving treatment for cancer, the efficacy of treatment can be compromised; not only because alcohol can interact with the enzyme systems involved in metabolism of chemotherapy, but also because it will cause more DNA damage in an already mutated cancer cell population, and may cause the emergence of new mutated treatment-resistant clones of existing cancer cells.

So how can we reduce the risk of alcohol-related cancers?

The answer depends on your relationship with this 'old friend' of the human race.

1. If you are not drinking alcohol and only benefiting from its other forms (antiseptics, disinfectants, and vinegar etc.), don't start now.

2. If you drink occasionally – once in a blue moon – try quitting altogether.

3. If you drink regularly, keep it as low as possible. Do not binge and have regular alcohol-free days. This will allow the body's DNA repair system to fix the damage done by alcohol and also have a much-needed rest.

4. If you find yourself hooked on it, seek professional advice. There are many effective remedies which can help you reduce the intake.

5. And there are many ways to offset the damage done by alcohol. Regular exercise, coffee, tea, healthy diet, fresh food, chillies, spices, fruits, nuts, and vegetables, to name a few.

6. Last but not least, don't combine alcohol with other cancer risk factors such as smoking, as alcohol can augment their cancerous effects and they can worsen its damage, too.

5.5 Tobacco, Smoke and Smoking

5.5.1 History of Smoking

In the beginning there was lightning.

Then came fire. Then smoke. Then man, who found both, and became obsessed with them. But they did more than just cook with fire. Humans have been playing with fire and smoke since antiquity and across all cultures.

Archaeological evidence suggests that around 7,000 years ago people were making fire offerings to deities and burning stuff like clarified butter, fish offal, incense sticks, cannabis, and generally whatever was flammable or combustible. They found all kinds of excuses to do it. It was done for the purposes of fumigation, religious ceremonies, cleansing rituals, and as a ritualistic practice by shamans and priests to invoke their spirituality. Initially, this smoke was passively inhaled from the environment, but as soon as the mind-altering qualities of certain substances became evident people started to inhale it directly.

Cannabis was discovered and smoked in India and hence the name *Cannabis indica* for the plant producing the drug. If you visit the Indian subcontinent, especially the regions around the river Indus in present-day Pakistan, you will find that the cannabis plant is ubiquitous as a local weed and is considered a nuisance by gardeners.

From India, the practice of smoking cannabis was taken by Indian and Arab traders to East Africa, especially Ethiopia. From here it tracked all the way down to sub-Saharan Africa and became quite popular, for obvious reasons.

Smoking is one of the best ways to get a drug to the brain within a minute, second only to injecting it into a vein. Hence, it was the preferred mode of taking mind-altering drugs before the invention of needle and syringe.

Today, people smoke tobacco, cannabis, opium, and heroin using cigars, bidis (beedi, a thin cigarette or mini cigar wrapped in a tendu leaf), hookahs, and bongs.

Smoking tobacco takes the lead and there are about 1,000,000,000 (one billion) users worldwide, mostly in developing countries, making it the commonest recreational drug in use. It is highly addictive and the trend for smoking tobacco seems to be rising, especially in the developing countries, despite the fact that it causes over 5,000,000 deaths a year and eventually kills approximately half of long-term smokers.

Smoking tobacco in pipes was used as a ritual and social activity by Native Americans. The credit for introducing it to Europe goes to Jean Nicot, a Frenchman who brought it over to France in 1560 and had the dubious honour of getting its active ingredient, 'nicotine', named after him. From France, the fashion spread to England, as it usually does and has done for centuries. Historical record mentions the sighting of English sailors emitting smoke from their nostrils in the major port of Bristol around this time.

Originally, tobacco was used as a form of medicine, as was the case with most of the drugs used for recreational purposes. It took a long time for people to realise that it caused cancer, heart attacks, birth defects, erectile dysfunction, COPD (chronic obstructive pulmonary disease), and a myriad of other diseases.

Thanks to the efforts of English, French, and Portuguese traders, the practice of smoking was carried across the world.

The first ever *smoking ban* was initiated by the Ottoman Emperor (Khalifa) Murad IV (1623–1640), who considered it a threat to public health and morality. However, this did not prove effective and today the Turks are considered to be one of the nations associated with a strong smoking culture. In fact, legend has it that the very first cigarette was devised by a Turkish solider during the Crimean War (1853–56) when he ran out of clay pipes and decided to wrap his tobacco in a piece of paper and light it up.

The credit for initiating the first ever *smoking cessation campaign* goes to His Holiness, patriarch of Moscow and all Rus (Russia), Bishop Joasaphus the First (1634–1640), who forbad tobacco use and sentenced men and women who flouted the ban to have their nostrils slit and then whipped them until the skin came off their backs.

The results were not long-lived and today Russia tops the table of countries smoking tobacco, with Indonesia coming second, Laos third, Ukraine fourth, Belarus fifth, Greece sixth, Jordan seventh, and China eighth. The trend has been declining in other countries. For example, in the United States of America the smoking rate has dropped from 42% in 1965 to 20.8% in 2006.

5.5.2   Smoking, Cancer, and Carcinogens

Human lungs are able to cope with occasional incidents of smoke inhalation such as a forest fire, a barbecue party, a bonfire night, or sitting next to a fireplace. Our lungs are gifted with a limited capacity to deal with these situations and even repair the damage incurred.

But diligently sucking in pure smoke, one cigarette after another, is a totally different ballgame and its consequences are beyond scope of the body's capacity to neutralise the damage.

Don't get me wrong, human lungs have a lot of capacity to cope with challenges of smoke and other environmental particles like dust, pollen, and spores. Billions of these undesirables are filtered out by our respiratory system.

We have an excellent filtration system from the nasal passages all the way to the tiny air chambers that make the lungs. The nasal hair traps any dust or other particles in air. The lining of the airways has special cells that produce a sticky mucus which filters out any tiny particles, be it dust or smoke. These cells also have brush-like bristles called *cilia* (millions of them altogether) on their surface which continuously move in a sweeping motion away from the lung, effectively removing the mucus and its trapped particles upwards to the throat, where it is unconsciously swallowed and falls into the stomach acid to be destroyed and dissolved.

We are only aware of this phenomenon when there is an excess production of this mucus in conditions of infection or inflammation, and it's coughed up as phlegm.

Lungs are also capacious, even though they don't look very roomy. There is about 1,000 square feet of breathing surface folded in them and if the airways were to be stretched out they would be more than 1,000miles long.

Their extra capacity and resilience are their undoing when it comes to smoking. Lungs have a capacity to breath in six litres of air but normally we only breathe in half a litre. The extra space is for times of stress and exertion, when we require more oxygen in the body; for example, making a run to climb the nearest tree when being chased by a lion. But as lions are becoming increasingly rare, we do not have the need to breathe all six litres. Instead, we can sit against the nearest tree and smoke for decades, taking advantage of the extra lung capacity before it is damaged enough for us to notice. And by the time we notice, it's too late for the lungs to recover.

On a positive note, there is now evidence emerging to suggest that if we stop punishing our lungs in time, they have a capacity not only to recover but also regain some of the loss caused by smoking. After 20 years of stopping smoking, the excess risk of lung cancer is reduced by 75%.

Not all life-long smokers end up with a smoking-related disease. Only five out of six do. So, it's a gamble. Smoking is like taking a six-chamber revolver with only five bullets, spinning the barrel, and then putting it up to your head and pressing the trigger. So, the philosophical among you may think we can't just blame the cigarette. There is an element of bad luck to it, too.

Secondly, every free and fair society gives its members freedom of choice. This includes a free will to smoke, inhale, inject, ingest, or insert whatever they might please. The fact that human body has limitations whereas human choice does not is the main problem. To strike a balance between the two it's important that humans are provided an opportunity to make well-informed decisions in life.

And this is the spirit of our discussion on smoking and its effects on human health.

The main ingredient of cigarette smoke, nicotine, by itself may not induce cancer, but its metabolic products (for example NNK, nitrosamine ketone) are carcinogenic. However, nicotine by itself is known to inhibit the natural cell death known as apoptosis, thereby accelerating the lifespan of existing cancer cells.

The process of cancer development with cigarette smoking is multifactorial. For example, the polycyclic aromatic hydrocarbons found in the tar component of cigarette are produced by thermal decomposition (a process known as *pyrolysis*; *pyro*, 'fire' and *lysis*, 'separating', in Greek) of organic matter, and these are emitted into the smoke.

Some of these chemicals are toxic by nature and others become toxic and carcinogenic after being metabolised by the liver. These chemicals are not water soluble, and the body needs to dissolve them in water to enable it to excrete them through urine. To change them to water-soluble forms, the liver uses an enzyme system called *cytochrome P450* to add oxygen to them. Although this addition makes them water soluble, it also creates a higher volatile reactive chemical, an epoxide, and this can cause mutations by reacting with cell DNA.

An epoxide is a highly reactive three-atom triangular ring containing oxygen. The resulting DNA damage can lead to pre-cancerous lesions and, over time, further damage by cigarette smoke's chemicals such as benzopyrene, which permanently attaches to DNA and either kills or mutates the cell, can lead to a fully-fledged cancer.

Another pyrolysis product found abundantly in cigarette smoke is a well-known cancer-causing agent called 'acrolein'. If you have ever been around a lit cigarette, you would have felt it. It is the chemical giving cigarette smoke its acrid smell (hence the name, 'acrolein' – an acrid smelling oil; *oleum* in Latin) and causes irritation to the eyes, making them tearful. It is considered to be a major carcinogen.

Acrolein is 1,000 times more abundant than polycyclic aromatic hydrocarbons in smoke and reacts without metabolic activation by the liver. Scientists have tried to test it in animal models and assess its toxicity in forming cancer, but they have not been able to confirm its cancer-inducing potency because it kills the animals before they can live long enough to develop cancer.

Cigarette smoke also contains chemicals called *alkylating agents* which transfer an alkyl group from one molecule to another. These have a tendency to permanently bind to DNA, inducing mutations. Alkylating agents are so good at damaging cells that some of them have been modified for use as anti-cancer drugs.

In addition, nitrosamine compounds, which are notorious carcinogens, are also found in cigarette smoke. And here's a very little-known fact that tobacco companies would never want you to know. Cigarettes not only contain carcinogenic chemicals; they also come laden with radioactive carcinogens. These include lead-210 (Pb210) and polonium-210 (Po210). Tobacco growers use fertilisers with phosphates which can also contain uranium, radium, and radon.

The radioactive elements are mostly found in the cigarette tar, a sticky substance that deposits at places where the airways branch (bronchial tubules). Cigarette tar is resistant to the dissolving effect of lung fluids which are normally able to dissolve any impurities found in inhaled air and remove them from the lung in the form of mucus. As the tar sticks around for a long time, the radioactive compounds undergo slow decay, releasing radioactivity which damages nearby cells and their DNA resulting in cancerous mutations.

For a comparison, if you are living near a nuclear power station you will be exposed to radioactivity in the range of 0.001 mSv per year. The 'mSv' stands for 'millisievert', a measure of radiation dose to the human body. However, when smoking 30 cigarettes a day (one and a half packs), you are exposed to radiation in the range of 60–160 mSv per year. Needless to say, that is a lot of radiation going to straight to the lungs, sticking to the airways and releasing over time.

Second-hand smoke, also known as 'environmental tobacco smoke' (ETS), or passive smoking, is also a serious risk factor for health. Smoke lingers in the air hours after extinguishing the cigarette. Among non-smokers exposed to second-hand smoke, the risk of heart disease is 25 to 30% higher compared to those who have not been exposed to it, and similarly the risk of lung cancer is 20 to 30% higher. It approximately accounts for 38,000 deaths per year.

5.5.3   Why Is It Difficult to Quit Smoking?

The reason why people smoke is not just because it's associated with glamour (remember the Marlboro Man and James Dean) but because it is laden with chemicals which get you easily hooked.

If you stand next to a pile of burning dry leaves, you will not be able to tolerate it for long and might end up choking. However, on the contrary, smokers take a small pile of dried leaves wrapped in paper, light it up and suck in the smoke as if their lives depend on it. This is all made possible by additives, often specific to the brand of cigarette maker. Unsurprisingly, smoking addiction is often a 'brand addiction 'and people who prefer a particular brand tend to smoke more of them than they would another brand. Many of these additives have additional toxic chemicals and metabolites harmful to human health. In my research on cigarette additives, I've uncovered 619 chemicals so far (YES, OVER SIX HUNDRED!), and there could be more, which only the cigarette manufacturers know of.

Nicotine is highly addictive, but it is not the only addictive chemical in cigarette smoke. It also contains acetaldehyde, and during its metabolism it forms a compound known as *harmane*[79].

Harmane, in combination with nicotine, causes addiction by increasing the levels of dopamine in the brain. This is the same chemical associated with almost all types of addictions, from caffeine and cocaine to alcohol and heroin. It also plays an important role in addictive behaviours, such as gambling. Studies have shown that nicotine in cigarette smoke can cause more addiction than cannabis, caffeine, alcohol, LSD, and cocaine. However, its withdrawal effects are not as strong as these drugs.

Addiction to cigarettes occurs approximately five months after starting smoking. It takes a total of 10 seconds for nicotine to reach the brain. One usually needs three months off cigarette smoking to quit the addiction. Quitting is often associated with a risk of depression, as is the case with quitting most psychoactive drugs.

5.5.4   E-Cigarettes

There has been a lot of commotion and fuss[80] about electronic cigarettes and their benefits versus dangers. Experts seem to be polarised in opinion, but the fact of that matter is that it is too early to say what the long-term toxic effects of electronic cigarettes will be.

Remember, it took centuries before the harmful effects of cigarette smoking became evident. Hopefully, it will not take so long with electronic cigarettes, as serious studies and research have already started.

The positive aspect of electronic cigarettes is that they don't contain any tar, ash, or carbon monoxide. The latter is a toxic compound similar in structure to carbon dioxide, but containing only one oxygen atom. It binds to the haemoglobin in blood resulting in an abnormal form called *carboxyhaemoglobin* which does not have the proper capacity to carry oxygen. So, despite normal haemoglobin levels and oxygen in the air, the body's cells lack the delivery of oxygen.

---

[79] It belongs to a group of chemicals known as *MAO* (monoamineoxidase) *inhibitors*.

[80] I have been told it's better to say 'commotion and fuss' than 'hoo-ha', my preferred term for discussions regarding electronic cigarettes.

Further good news has come from the Royal College of Physicians in England, which says that the harmful effect of electronic cigarettes might only be 5% of the harmful effects from smoking, but this can also mean that, so far, we have only identified 5% of the dangers associated with it.

Although e-cigarettes have fewer toxicants compared to combustible tobacco, they are not without their risks. Use can cause severe lung illness and nicotine poisoning. The cytotoxicity (toxicity to the cell) of e-cigarettes varies from one type to another. Metal parts in contact with the e-liquid can contaminate the liquid with tiny, microscopic metal particles. This effect is not seen in conventional cigarette smoking. The heating element (nichrome wire) that touches the e-liquid can produce toxic compounds such as formaldehyde and other carbonyl compounds, all well-known carcinogens.

Vapours from an e-cigarette have fine and (mostly) ultra-fine particles including propylene glycol, glycine, nicotine, flavours, toxicants, carcinogens, heavy metals, and metal nanoparticles. Nanoparticles are tiny, about one millionth of a millimetre. Although e-cigarettes lack many of the toxins found in tobacco smoke, they have some chemicals which are not found in tobacco smoke and hence we do not know what their long-term toxic effects will be. There is a strong indication that e-cigarettes may have toxic effects during pregnancy on the baby.

E-cigarettes also have formaldehyde and acrolein, which are well-known carcinogens causing mutagenesis and DNA damage. They also contain nicotine, of course, although the amount is less than that in conventional combustible cigarettes.

Nicotine by itself is a nasty and toxic compound. Although it may not cause cancer, it promotes them by causing cells to divide rapidly, avoiding apoptosis (programmed cell death), developing new blood vessels (angiogenesis) and helping them in moving out of the main tumour and spread to other parts of the body (metastasis). Making new blood vessels also helps to bring more nutrition to a growing cancer and speeds up its growth. By these effects, nicotine can stimulate progression of cancers.

Nicotine can cause DNA damage, however, stimulating cell proliferation and decreasing tumour suppressor gene activity, especially for the tumour suppressor gene CHEK2 (Checkpoint kinase 2). This gene controls cell growth, repairs damaged DNA, and thus avoids mutations persisting, and works as a team with other tumour suppressor genes, especially TP53, the Guardian of the Genome, which we discussed earlier. If the DNA mutations cannot be fixed, CHEK2 forces the damaged cell to undergo programmed cell death (apoptosis). By suppressing CHEK2, nicotine opens the pathway for uninhibited cancer growth.

Mouse models have shown increased size, number, and metastasis of tumours when exposed to nicotine. Studies have also shown that use of nicotine products may reduce the effects of anti-cancer treatment. And there is mounting evidence coming to light now that e-cigarettes can be a risk factor for lung cancer.

Important constituents of e-cigarettes are two chemicals: glycerine and propylene glycol. These are added to make the smoke less irritant and 'smooth' to inhale. Long-term effects of glycerine and propylene glycol are not known. But we do know that heating propylene glycol could turn it into propylene oxide, which is a suspected carcinogen.

To cover the bitter taste of nicotine, flavourings are added. We do not know the long-term effects. These can include aldehydes and reactive oxygen species. Second-hand smoke particles found from e-cigarettes are smaller than the combustible tobacco cigarette molecules. Their mean size is 3 nm (nm stands for 'nanometre', or one billionth of a metre). Exposure to first or second-hand electronic cigarette smoke is not recommended in pregnancy due to its dangerous effect on the foetus, causing abnormalities in the development of a baby's lung, heart, brain, and immune system. Time will tell what the full spectrum of hazardous effects will be for adults.

5.6   Get High (but Not Stoned)

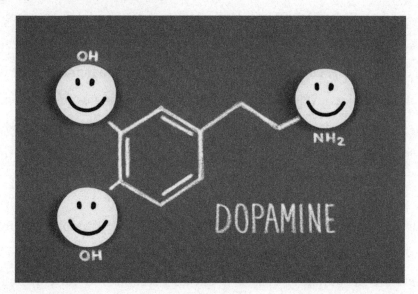

Here's a controversial statement: *Getting high's OK because we are meant to*. Let me explain. The reason why most drugs work is that our body already has receptors for them and the reason why we have receptors for them is that we have natural chemicals made in our body which bind to them.

Our bodies are made to enjoy getting high but not getting stoned. That's an extreme which is not good for us. Getting high is pleasurable but getting stoned may lead to fits, seizures, and a catatonic state which can cause death or disability. And the supply is meant to be indigenous, not off the street from a drug dealer.

The human body is a narcotics drug factory. Opiates (called *endorphins*, similar to heroin and opium), cannabinoids, dopamine, adrenaline and noradrenaline (the stuff released by amphetamines, Ecstasy, ICE, crack, and cocaine) are all made by our bodies.

Let's have a look at the three main types of these drugs.

(i) **Dopamine** is released in many organs, especially the brain. It is made to support normal functions of the body and its release is also the common thread running through all addictive stimuli: smoking, alcohol, cannabis, cocaine, amphetamine, and even love, sex, and gambling. Dopamine makes us happy and gets us hooked to things that make us happy. It is also involved in reward, motivation, memory, attention, pleasure, and even movements of the body.

Low levels of dopamine make you feel low by causing reduced enthusiasm and motivation. The body needs amino acids (two types, tyrosine and phenylalanine) to make dopamine. These are found in proteins. A diet low in protein causes low levels of dopamine and makes us unhappy. No wonder the sight of a sizzling steak[81] fills the human heart with joy. High intake of fats can also interfere with dopamine by lowering its levels. A rare but rich source of dopamine is a type of bean known as *Mucuna pruriens*, which contains high levels of a chemical called 'L-dopa' that changes to dopamine in the body. However, high doses can be harmful. Dopamine levels also increase with 10–30 minutes of exercise. When awake, our body is continuously consuming dopamine, so one way to preserve its supply in the brain is not to use it all the time, and a good night's sleep helps to conserve levels. Things that make you relax and be happy – like sunlight, music, and meditation – also help increase levels in the body.

Ironically, all the drugs of abuse which are used to get a so-called 'dopamine high 'do not contain dopamine. They work by releasing the dopamine already stored in our body. We feel the intense 'Highs' because almost all the stored dopamine is released in one go, depleting the stores in our body. What follows is a *prolonged come down* (*lowest of the lows*, if you may) as the body goes into a deep depression, struggling to restore its dopamine reserves. This is what causes a comedown/crash/exhaustion, or the well-known hangover.

---

[81] Or, in case of vegans, the sight of soya milk sends them into throes of ecstasy.

Drugs don't bring happiness, they just release all the happiness we have stored up in our mind and body in one go, leaving us emotionally bankrupt. They are like an evil 'friend' who comes to you when you are feeling very low and throws you an awesome party that cheers you up, but by using all of your savings and credit cards, leaving you in debt and in an even deeper depression.

(ii) **Marijuana or cannabinoid** receptors are abundant in the body, too. They help with mood, memory, sleep, appetite, cognition, and pain. Cannabis-like chemicals made by our body are known as *endocannabinoids* (*endo* means 'internal' or 'inside the body'). These include virodhamine, oleamide and anandamide (from the word *ananda* in ancient Sanskrit, meaning 'joy', 'bliss' and 'delight'). Anandamide does what the name suggests and also helps in fertility by facilitating embryo implantation.

Faced with stress, the body releases anandamide to calm us down, more so in Caucasian males than African Americans and Asians. It's no surprise that the latter are known to supplement their anandamide levels with cannabis, a weed endemic to Afghanistan, Pakistan, Nepal, and India, but now grown all over the world. In acute stress the body produces high levels of anandamide to calm us down, but long-term anxiety lowers these levels. Levels of anandamide can also be boosted by eating dark chocolates and black truffles, or taking cold showers. Anandamide has shown to inhibit breast cancer cell proliferation in experimental cancer cell lines in the laboratory, giving rise to hope and rumours that cannabis can cure cancer. So far, the laboratory benefits in experimental cancer cells have not been translated to any notable success in real-life disease.

As cannabis and cancer is one of the hotly debated topics nowadays, let's look in detail on the evidence available.

One of the largest studies was conducted in Israel, involving 2,960 patients. It showed that cannabis or marijuana may improve a variety of cancer-related symptoms, including nausea and vomiting, sleep disorders, pain, anxiety, and depression. The researchers looked at cancer patients who used cannabis over a six-month period. Most had advanced stage cancer (51.2% had stage 4) and at six months about 25% had died. Of the 1,742 patients who survived to six months and finished the study, 60% achieved treatment success. This was defined as moderate or significant improvement in a patient's overall condition at six months, as well as not quitting treatment and not having any serious side effects. People who had previous experience with cannabis, a high level of pain, were younger, and lacked concerns regarding the possible negative effects of cannabis treatment benefited the most.

Israel has a relatively long experience with medical cannabis. Their ministry of health approved its use in 2007. The primary use is palliation (control) of symptoms. In one study[82], the trial population had a mean age of 59.5 years, and about half (43%) were older than 65 years. Most were either retired (31%) or did not work (46%), probably the ideal situation for someone regularly taking cannabis. There were slightly more women (54%) than men in the study. About one quarter (26%) had previous experience with the drug. The main types of cancers included those of the breast (20%), lung (13%), pancreas (8%), and colon (7%), as well as lymphoma (4%). Predominantly, four different cannabis strains were used and consumed in different forms: as an oil, through ingestion via capsules, cigarettes, or evaporators. Unfortunately, around half (45%) of the patients chose smoking as a delivery method. Dose of the drug was adjusted according to patient tolerance and requirement. At the start, patients reported an average of around 11 symptoms. Most commonly these were trouble sleeping, pain (with median intensity of eight out of 10 on a well-established scale), weakness, and fatigue. The symptoms which improved most were nausea and vomiting (91%), sleep disorder (87%), restlessness (87%), anxiety and depression (84%), pruritis/itching (82%), and headaches (81%). Cannabis also helped patients reduce the use of a variety of drugs for pain relief and their cancer-related condition. During the study period, 35% of participants reported a decrease in concomitant drug consumption (drugs taken alongside their cannabis) such as painkillers, steroids, and sleeping tablets.

Among the painkillers, opioids were the most prevalent drug used by participants at the study start. Notably, at six months, 36% of those patients had stopped taking opioids and about 10% had reduced the dose. A further 51% continued to take the same dose and only around 1% increased the dose. Most common side effects of medicinal cannabis at six months were dizziness (8%), dry mouth (7%), increased appetite (3%), sleepiness (3%), and psychoactive effect (2%). The most common reasons for stopping treatment were lack of ongoing need (28%), no therapeutic effect (22%), and side effects (19%).

So, it can be reasonably concluded that cannabis has benefits in controlling the symptoms in many but not all cancer patients. But most importantly, contrary to the myths and urban legends, cannabis was not effective in treating or curing any type of cancer.

Hopefully, in the future more research will be done by independent sources and the benefits of cannabis in treatment of cancer can be fully and neutrally determined.

(iii) We are also good at naturally producing **opioid** narcotics, known as *endorphins*. Heroin, opium, and other opiates (fentanyl, oxycodone etc.) cause their effects by binding to endorphin receptors. Some of the

---

[82] Numbers and percentages have been rounded (e.g., 43.1% is rounded to 43%).

endorphins that our internal narcotics factory produces include alpha endorphins, beta endorphins, gamma endorphins, enkephalins, dynorphins, adrenorphin, amidorphin, leumorphin, endomorphins, opiorphins, spinorphin, hemorphins, codeine, and morphine. That's quite a list! Even the infamous Cuban drug lord, Pablo Escobar's laboratories produced less variety than you and me. When it comes to making drugs, we are all 'living legends'. Endorphins are very important in our daily life. They control motivation, emotion, attachment behaviour, response to pain, stress, and control of appetite. You can increase their production by doing exercise and incorporating spices and chillies in your diet.

5.7　Coffee (Caffeine) & Khat

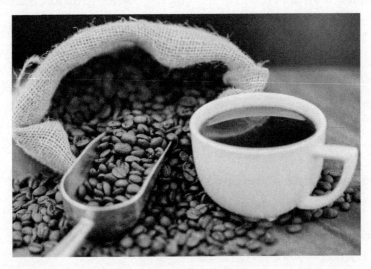

Coffee and cancer is a hotly debated topic, full of controversies and confusion. There are many opinions – literally, hundreds of millions on the internet – with conflicting views. But we are not going to be bogged down by them. Instead, we'll walk the path of scientific evidence, separating fact from fiction.

But, first, we'll start with a story: the legend of a man, his goats, and a very special berry bush.

The year is around 850 AD, and somewhere on the Ethiopian highland plains a simple goat herder called Kaldi (also known as Khalid) is about to stumble on one of the greatest discoveries of all time.

Kaldi was a keen and clever young man. He loved his goats and others knew him to be a passionate and conscientious herder. As dusk fell at the end of each day, an exhausted but contented Kaldi would settle beside the glowing warmth of his fire, draw his cloak tightly about his shoulders against the chill, and look forward to a good night's sleep. His herd settled and the ensuing darkness would be filled with little more than the occasional bleat and rustle of grass.

One night, however, his goats had a different idea. They refused to settle and bleated all night long with zeal, keeping a despairing Kaldi awake. The next day, bleary-eyed, Kaldi encountered another problem.

His goats seemed almost delirious, showing no signs of settling. After another sleepless night, Kaldi grew suspicious. He watched his herd closely, noticing that they seemed to enjoy eating berries from a particular type of bush. It was after feeding on these berries that they pepped up, and became hard for him to control. Over the ensuing days he saw they were very keen to revisit the same grazing grounds and the same bushes. All attempts to keep them away by calling out and waving his stick failed miserably. They simply ignored him. And they never seemed to tire of those berries. Fearful that he might fall asleep, only to wake and find that his goats had wandered off, Kaldi supposed that if you can't beat them, join them. And so he did.

Kaldi tried the berries and found a bitter-tasting bean at the centre. He dried the beans under the sun and tried again, but they still tasted awful. At a loss, he took the berries to an abbot at the local monastery and explained his problem. The abbot, a wise man, crushed the beans and brewed them in water. It made a dark concoction with a nice fragrance, and when drank gave him the same rush and freshness which the goats had been exhibiting for weeks. The abbot saw the potential; such a brew would help him stay awake during endless hours of prayer. Soon, many of the priests were converted drinkers, too.

Kaldi and the abbot had just discovered the stimulant and mildly addictive effects of coffee and, as news spread, the brew gained in popularity across Ethiopia. Of course, neither Kaldi nor the abbot knew that the beans contained caffeine, or that such a drug even existed. It wasn't isolated until 1819, when the German chemist Friedlieb Ferdinand Runge extracted a relatively pure form of caffeine he called *kaffebase*.

From Ethiopia, drinking coffee spread across the Red Sea to Yemen and soon made its way to Arabia, where the beverage was refined by roasting the beans and boiling the crushed roast to create a stronger brew. At the time, Arabia was going through a new religious revolution, much akin to the Christian Gnostic and Jewish Kabbalistic movements, and the Muslims were developing their own spiritual orders known as the 'Sufis'. The Sufi mystic orders were quick to incorporate this new drink, which they called *qahwa* (sometimes pronounced affectionately as 'gahwa') into their daily soul-searching sessions. Its stimulant and addictive qualities made it an ideal companion for long nights of devotional prayers and meditation. Coffee rapidly became associated with the Arabian Peninsula. A certain variety with a chocolatey taste made the port of Mocha in Yemen famous, becoming synonymous with it. The finer and more expensive beans are still called 'arabica' while the cheaper type, known as 'robusta', is often used in making instant coffee.

The Arabs introduced coffee to Turkish and Persian lands. Coffee houses, called *qahvey khaneh*, sprang up and proved popular, with coffee consumption being accompanied by music, performances, games of chess, and debate. They became known as 'schools of the wise'. From here it crossed over to Europe, although along its journey coffee encountered the occasional dissenting voice. In 1623, in Constantinople (nowadays Istanbul), Murad IV claimed the Ottoman throne and set about banning coffee. The penalty for a first offence was simply a beating, but repeat offenders risked being sewn into a leather bag and thrown into the Bosporus.

Unlike Ethiopia and Arabia, where coffee was generally welcomed by the monastic and mystic sects of Christianity and Islam, in Europe it was often treated with suspicion, as most things foreign were then, and sometimes are even now. The Church decreed it to be 'the drink of the infidels', banning the practice of drinking coffee, driving it underground where it sold like a potent and illegal drug. It was not until 1600 that it was legalised, and the credit goes to the most important religious figure of the time, His Holiness Ippolito Aldobrandini, also known as Pope Clement VIII.

Pope Clement VIII was a force to be reckoned with. He had little pity or patience for his opponents. When the Italian Dominican friar, philosopher, mathematician, poet, and scientist Giordano Bruno came up with revolutionary ideas, including the concept that stars were distant suns surrounded by their own planets, Pope Clement VIII was appalled by such heresy and had him burned at the stake in Rome.

When His Holiness tried a cup of coffee and enjoyed its effect, he proclaimed that it would be a pity to let the infidels have the exclusive use of this 'Satanic drink'. With his reputation, needless to say not a single word of opposition was heard throughout Christendom. It is alleged he became such a coffee aficionado that he blessed the bean, baptising the brew which had hitherto been called a 'Muslim drink'. Soon the blessed bean was being brewed and served all over Europe.

In Oxford, England, coffee houses called 'penny universities' were established where, for a one-penny admission fee, you could buy coffee and have intellectual discussion in an alcohol-free environment. Later on, you could visit the local alehouse for less intelligent talk and other entertainments!

Partly thanks to Pope Clement VIII, today the top nine consumers[83] of this blessed bean are the European nations. Namely, Finland, Norway, Iceland, Denmark, Netherlands, Sweden, Switzerland, Belgium, and Luxembourg. Number 10 is Canada. Coffee, I have been told, is not only the world's most widely consumed psychoactive drug but is also the second most traded commodity after petroleum. And everyone claims to own it too; Ethiopian coffee, Arabic coffee, Turkish coffee, Italian, Brazilian, Guatemalan, Ecuadorian, Jamaican, and the list goes on. There are about 70 nations producing coffee beans, with Brazil at number one. Coffee, it can be said, is going from strength to strength. There are dozens of varieties with new ones being developed all the time.

---

[83] In pounds of coffee per person per year.

The latest and the most expensive, known as 'kopi luwak' or 'civet coffee', sells at a price more than 100 times the ordinary brands. The story of kopi luwak is very similar to the discovery of coffee, but with a repulsive twist. When coffee farming was brought to Southeast Asian countries, like Indonesia, it quickly became very popular among humans and other creatures of God, including a small mammal known as a 'civet'. Civets love to raid the coffee farms and eat the berries. Unlike the Ethiopian goats, the East Asian civets proved to be connoisseurs of coffee, selectively eating only the best and the ripest berries, leaving the sub-standard beans for the farmers to harvest.

One day, a very frugal and frustrated farmer noticed that although the civets were able to eat the coffee berries, their digestive system was unable to digest the central beans, the source of coffee. The beans were passed intact and slightly roasted (from hours of exposure to the low body heat of the animal's stomach and intestines). More importantly, the beans were still sealed in a fine membrane which had kept them untouched by the surrounding 'unmentionable' products of the civet's digestive process. With great inquisitiveness and greater indignity, and not wanting to waste the results of his hard work, the farmer washed and dried the beans and ground them into a fine powder, brewing the first cup of what was to become the most expensive coffee in the world.

Professional coffee tasters testify that the civet coffee has a certain smoothness which is lacking in other coffee types. It is also thought to be milder in taste. Needless to say, drinking kopi luwak is an acquired taste which takes a lot of courage, not to mention parting with a lot of cash for something dug out of a small South Asian mammal's droppings. Having said that, it is proving both popular and lucrative. There are huge farms teeming with civets being force-fed coffee berries to produce the "caviar of the coffee world", and sales are rising every year. The price reported in 2019 was around $700 per kilogram.

Kaldi and his goats must have turned in their graves at hearing this news.

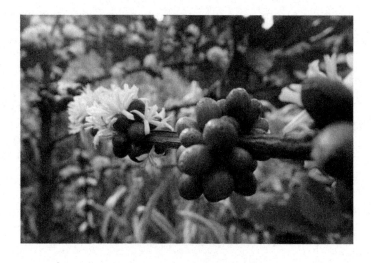

Berries on a coffee plant in Indonesia.

Ever wondered how caffeine creates that buzz, keeping us awake and alert and helping us to concentrate? Well, that drowsiness we feel as the day wears on is partly due to the build-up of a chemical called *adenosine* in the synapses of our brain. Synapses are the junctions between our nerve cells. Adenosine binds and activates receptors that lead to a range of responses that we feel as drowsiness. Caffeine competes to block this, and therefore promotes wakefulness. This also stimulates some of the brain's centres, increasing our breathing rate, reducing our heart rate, and constricting our blood vessels.

Caffeine is able to do this because it is soluble in both water and lipids (fats), allowing it to cross the blood-brain barrier, and structurally is very similar to adenosine. But this isn't the only way caffeine works. It also affects the release and binding of dopamine in certain parts of the brain. Dopamine, you will recall, is a hormone and neurotransmitter released by every addictive drug. In our brains it has a role in influencing various functions, including motor (muscle) control, motivation, arousal, and reward.

If, like me, you have ever overindulged, you may have experienced some of the less desirable effects of coffee. As well as insomnia (sleeplessness), you might have felt mild anxiety, a little bit jittery or restless, excited even. Your tummy might get upset. Your face might get a little flushed, and you might perspire (sweat) more than usual, or your friends might think you look a little bit 'clammy'.

So, is coffee safe to drink? Well, the US Food and Drug Administration categorises caffeine as *Generally Recognised As Safe* (GRAS) at levels of up 0.02% as a food additive to, for example, colas, and the World Health Organisation (WHO) includes caffeine citrate in its Model List of Essential Medicines, its use being to treat *apnoea* (where you temporarily stop breathing, especially during sleep) in neonates (newborns). It may improve athletic performance, both aerobic and anaerobic, enhancing power and endurance. However, in children, high doses of caffeine (greater than 400 mg) are generally not recommended as it might cause harm, particularly in those with existing psychiatric or heart conditions.

During pregnancy it is often recommended that caffeine intake is avoided or limited, but this is largely due to the fact that caffeine may be metabolised more slowly, increasing the exposure to its effects.

In terms of general health benefits, coffee has many. For example, it reduces the risk of obesity, of type 2 diabetes (non-insulin dependent), mental health issues such as anxiety, dementia, cognitive impairment, hypertension, heart disease, Parkinson's disease and, yes, even cancer. No surprise it has also been associated with longevity and preserving youth. Coffee is one of those magic beverages which continue to amaze scientists and doctors with its beneficial effects.

The highlights regarding these are as follows:

Indirect Effects

1) Coffee contains chlorogenic acid, a strong antioxidant, neutralising any cell-damaging chemicals and molecules. Chlorogenic acid improves insulin sensitivity, making the body more responsive to the effects of this hormone. This reduces the absorption of glucose from the intestine, which is good news because cancer cells love to feed on glucose.

2) Coffee consumption reduces insulin levels, especially among overweight women. Because insulin and its related chemicals act as growth stimulants for cancer cells, the less insulin circulating, the better.

3) Coffee increases a protein in the blood known as *sex hormone binding globulin* or SHBG. SHBG does exactly as its name suggests – it binds sex hormones, like the female hormone oestrogen (oestradiol), reducing its levels. These hormones are implicated in the growth and development of many cancers, especially those of breast and uterus. Therefore, reducing the level of SHBG is potentially beneficial.

4) Further good news is that not only does coffee help bind these cancer-promoting hormones, but it also helps break them down in the liver. Coffee intake increases the levels of liver enzymes (in this case enzyme systems called *CYP1A2* and *CYP3A4*) which break down oestradiol and inactivate it.

5) Coffee, whether caffeinated of decaffeinated, lowers the levels of chemicals in the blood which can increase body fat levels. One of these chemicals is called *C-peptide*. On the other hand, coffee increases blood levels of another substance, called *adiponectin*. This is an enzyme that regulates glucose and fat in the body. This is helpful because increased body fat is known to increase the risk of cancer.

6) The same is true with diabetes. Uncontrolled diabetes is known to promote cancer growth and coffee consumption decreases the chances of getting diabetes.

Direct Effects

7) Research has also shown direct anti-cancer effects of coffee. Coffee discourages development of new blood vessels among cancer cells. Cancer cells use these blood vessels not only to get nourishment from the body but also as an escape route for spreading to other organs and tissues, where they form new colonies (a process known as *metastasis*). Fewer blood vessels mean less nutrition and fewer escape routes for cancer cells.

8) And I saved the best for last. Coffee kills cancer, and does so very kindly. It has been shown to cause programmed cell death (apoptosis) in damaged cells, including cancer cells. This stops damaged pre-cancerous cells from developing into a full-blown cancer.

And more evidence of the beneficial effects of coffee continue to emerge every day. But there is a catch. The way coffee is processed can alter the levels of beneficial chemicals. This is best illustrated by similar studies done in different countries, looking at the effects of coffee consumption on cancer prevention, but each using a different method of making coffee.

Sweden has high levels of coffee consumption (in fact one of the highest in the world, with an average coffee consumption of 8.2 kg per person in 2008). A study carried out there, and published in the *Breast Cancer Research Journal* in 2011, looked at a large population and found that there was a decrease in overall breast cancer risk with increased coffee consumption. The reduction in risk was statistically significant for a certain type of breast cancer known as *oestrogen receptor (ER) negative breast cancer* (in this type of breast cancer, cells are not sensitive to oestrogen hormone stimulation for growth, and this kind of cancer tends to be more difficult to treat compared to ER positive breast cancer, which responds to anti-oestrogen therapy). The maximum benefit was seen in women who drank more than five cups of coffee per day (57% less likely to get ER negative tumours). The benefit was also noticed to be more significant among post-menopausal women.

However, similar studies from Germany did not show such a significant benefit. Notably, Germans tend to use filtered coffee, whereas Scandinavians are keener on boiled coffee. It is possible that the differences in results could be down to the chemical differences between filtered and boiled coffee. The benefits of decaffeinated coffee in this regard are not established yet. In Sweden, the use of decaffeinated coffee is negligible, less than 1%, so their study was unable to answer this question.

A combined analysis (meta-analysis[84]) of 37 published studies on the effects of coffee concluded that in post-menopausal women the risk of breast cancer decreased by 2% for every two extra cups of coffee per day consumed, and 1% for every 200 mg per day increment in caffeine intake. Similar results were reported in Canada in 2013. The researchers found a significant reduction in risk with the highest category of coffee consumption (five or more cups per day). Multiple, large, observational studies (including a total of 850,000 patients) have shown a protective association for caffeinated coffee, but not for decaffeinated coffee. The protective effects of caffeinated coffee seem to be more significant in women compared to men. Consuming coffee also reduced the risk of endometrial cancer (cancer of the womb). There is an approximately 7% reduced risk of endometrial cancer per cup of coffee consumed per day. And good news for consumers of decaffeinated coffee, this benefit is also found with it, reducing the risk of endometrial cancer by approximately 8% for every cup consumed.

---

[84]A meta- analysis is a statistical analysis which combines the results from many scientific studies addressing the same question.

Finally, there is strong evidence that coffee helps repair damage to liver cells and reduces the risk of developing liver cancer. And studies have also shown that coffee consumption tends to reduce the risk of pancreatic cancer.

Not bad for a bean from a berry discovered by a herd of bleating goats. But a word of caution. Today, Yemen, the hub of coffee production for centuries, is nowhere to be seen among the list of top producers. The port of Mocha is no longer filled with ships of chocolate-flavoured coffee beans. And ever since the discovery of coffee, goats have not contributed significantly to human health in terms of beating cancer. But that's not to say they haven't been busy. The latest, and probably the least beneficial goat-based discovery, is a leafy shrub called 'khat'.

Yemenis are now into growing khat (or 'qat'; botanical name, *Catha edulis*), whose leaves produce an alkaloid stimulant called 'cathionine', similar to cocaine produced by coca leaves grown in South America. Its effects on the brain are like that of amphetamines and ephedrine but slightly milder. The leaves are chewed to release the stimulant chemicals, giving the brain a bigger buzz than caffeine. The tell-tale sign of eating khat is a bulging cheek on one side of the face, filled with a wad of leaves slowly releasing the brain-stimulating alkaloids to be absorbed by the blood vessels in the mouth. Once again, history is repeating itself, because the stimulant effects of the leaves were first discovered by goat herders in Ethiopia and Somalia. Just like coffee, khat became very popular in the eastern Horn of Africa before crossing the Red Sea to Yemen, as coffee did many centuries before.

But the similarity ends here. Unlike coffee beans, the leaves of *Catha edulis* have a very short shelf-life, a few days at best. The stimulant effects reduce quickly as the leaves and their chemical components rot away. Attempts at synthesising the stimulant chemicals resulted in the production of a compound known as 'mephedrine' or M-GAT, subsequently introduced onto the international drug scene as 'meow meow'. This lab-made derivative of khat proved to be unpredictable and dangerous. I have personally managed streams of young victims brought into the hospital with seizures and hallucinations after consuming this drug. Khat and meow meow are already banned in most countries around the world. So, thankfully, it is very unlikely that khat or its inspired synthetic products will ever become as popular as coffee.

5.8   Fantastic Tea

The first time you have tea with a Balti[85], you are a stranger, the second time you take tea, you are an honoured guest. The third time you share a cup of tea you become family.

(Ancient Balti saying)

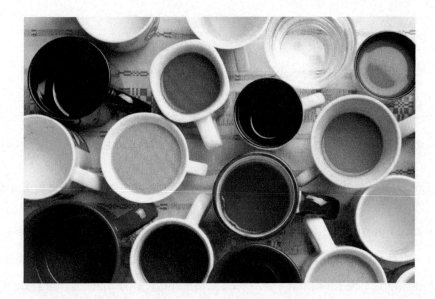

Shennong was a legend, literally. The mythological Chinese ruler from 2737 BC was also known as the 'Divine Farmer' and the 'Medicine King'.

He is considered the father of Chinese medicine and agriculture. He taught the Chinese how to irrigate and cultivate. A genius inventor, among other things he introduced acupuncture and the first Chinese calendar.

But his most famous discovery happened by chance.

Legend has it that Shennong used to boil water before using it (which is a sensible method of sterilising it). One day, while travelling in the countryside, a dead leaf from a wild tea bush fell into the boiling water, going unnoticed by his royal servants. As a result, Shennong was presented the first cup of tea in human history.

It didn't take him long to realise the medicinal value[86] of the brew and soon he had incorporated it into his medical practice and also used it as an antidote.

---

[85] Balti people are an ethnic group of Tibetan descent who are native to the Baltistan region of northern Pakistan, known for their peaceful nature, friendliness, longevity, and a low incidence of cancer.
[86] It helps control pain and reduces fever.

Ironically, the great Medicine King died due to a lack of tea. Shennong often experimented on himself and during one such experiment he consumed a yellow flower from a wild weed which caused his intestines to burst just before he could take a sip from his cup of 'antidote tea' which would have neutralised the poison.

In Chinese language *tu* means a bitter herb.

In the Min dialect of Chinese language, it is called *te* and the Dutch who bought their tea from the regions of China where the Min dialect was spoken introduced it to Western Europe as 'Tea'.

The Portuguese, Russians, Turks, Persians, Arabs, and other nations bought their tea from the Mandarin-speaking Chinese who called it *cha* and that is what it's known as to the rest of the world[87].

Camellia sinensis, the evergreen shrub whose leaves are brewed as tea, is native to China and East Asia.

It was used for medicinal purposes for centuries, but the recreational use was made popular by European colonists who discovered its potential as a trade commodity and established commercial tea plantations around the globe. Although trade bloomed, there was a huge untapped market that proved difficult to break into: the Indian subcontinent (present-day Pakistan, India, Nepal, Bangladesh, and Sri Lanka).

Although there was a tradition of drinking tea in the mountainous regions of Pakistan (local green, pink, and salted butter versions of imported Chinese tea), the rest of the region (including Assam, which had its own variety of indigenous tea) only used tea as a medicine in traditional therapies. The reason was simple – hot weather! Nobody with an ounce of common sense wanted to drink a piping hot drink in the blazing heat of the subcontinent. But tea is an addictive drink, and the British knew that once people got hooked, it would quickly develop into a culture of tea drinking. The biggest obstacle was to get people hooked on it in the first place.

An innovative and merciless marketing campaign to promote tea began, involving a three-pronged approach:

1. In the blazing Indian summer, passengers travelling on the railroads found there was no water to drink either on the trains or the platforms. For the thirsty and dehydrated travellers[88], the only choice was hot tea, served *free* of cost.

---

[87] With the exceptions of the Arabs, who call it *shai* as they do not have a word which sounds like 'ch' in their language.
[88] My great grandfather was a target of this campaign for many years while travelling across the country, and used to tell the story for many years.

2. Tea was also sold *for free* by vendors on bicycles with tanks of tea, in all major towns and cities.

3. In contrast to the popular native drinks such as lassi (made from yogurt) and sattu (made mostly from ground barley flour, and sometimes ground chickpea/millet/almonds or cashew nuts, mixed with cane juice and water, served chilled), tea was promoted as an urban intellectual drink favoured by the British elite. It was even suggested that the secret of the European scientific and industrial revolutions was due to their consumption of tea, which stimulated the brain, whereas the traditional drinks had a sedating effect on it.

The campaign was successful; slowly and steadily the populace was converted to tea. As a result, today this region is the largest consumer of tea with 30% of the world production consumed within India.

Tea is the most popular and commonly consumed beverage in the world, equalling the combined consumption of coffee, alcohol, and soft drinks. And in case you are wondering, the Indian railway has started offering water again, but this time neither the water nor the tea is free.

Tea and Its Anti-Cancer Effects

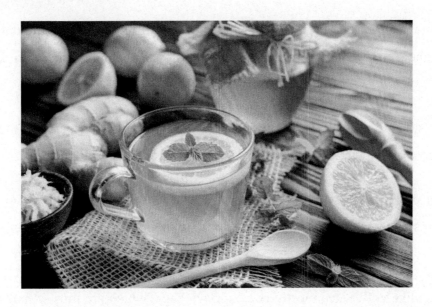

The two major types of tea, green and black, actually originate from the same plant, *Camellia sinensis*, discovered in China thousands of years ago. Processing the leaves yields different results; fermenting them makes black tea, unfermented being used for green.

Tea contains chemicals known as 'catechins' which have many benefits for human health. Green tea has more catechins than black because during fermentation some catechins are changed to other chemicals.

Catechins and other beneficial chemicals in tea help reduce weight, decrease the levels of insulin in the body, reduce inflammation, discourage growth of new blood vessels in tumours, and also help the body in killing cancer cells by apoptosis.

The anti-cancer effects are quite stunning in the laboratory environment and animal models, especially in rats, but when subjected to human trials the results are inconclusive at best and sometimes even controversial.

For example, some studies done in Japan have shown that green tea can delay the average age of onset of cancer by 7.3 years. Others have shown some benefit in bowel and prostate cancer, but none have been very convincing.

Ironically, studies from other countries have reported an increase in the risk of oesophageal (food pipe) cancer with increased consumption of tea. I suspect the reason for this is probably due to the damage and irritation done by drinking very hot tea (more than 65 degrees centigrade) and not the chemicals in tea.

In my opinion there are four important factors which can mask or neutralise the beneficial effects of tea:

1. The types of tea, especially green and black, have a big difference in the amount of chemicals they contain and hence the benefit is difficult to study unless a person is strictly drinking one particular type.

2. Addition of sugar to tea would mitigate many beneficial effects as it increases the levels of glucose, insulin, and other growth factors in the body which fuel cancer growth.

3. Addition of milk, more commonly done to tea than coffee, would also be counterproductive, as milk contains many growth-promoting chemicals that would neutralise the anti-growth effects of tea.

4. Tea bags. Unlike coffee, tea mostly comes in tea bags, which are mostly made of filter paper or food-grade plastic. They also contain a plastic known as 'polypropylene'[89] to seal them. At a brewing temperature of 95 degrees centigrade, a single plastic teabag releases approximately 11.6 billion microplastics and 3.1 billion nanoplastics into a single cup. We still don't know the long-term effects of these chemicals, but there is a good chance that they might interact with the chemicals released by the tea leaves.

---

[89] A thermoplastic polymer that can be sealed by heat rather than gluing.

So, a proper study of the potential anti-cancer effects of tea need to compare three major groups of people – those who drink black tea vs green tea vs no tea – and then each group should be subdivided into those who use sugar/milk/teabags.

Speaking of teabags, it's easy to avoid them. Just tear them open, pour the tea leaves into the cup/kettle, and brew it to your heart's delight. Use a tea strainer, if you have one, to filter out the leaves. There is the risk of getting those nasty little bits of soggy tea leaves with the last few sips but it's better than ingesting 14.7 *billion* bits of invisible plastic.

The curative and preventive potential of tea may not have been utilised by us yet, but it has already saved millions of human lives. Recently, too. And here's how it happened.

In early 2019, India and Pakistan were at the brink of a nuclear war.

It all started when Adil Ahmad Dar, a Kashmiri teenager, was stopped, beaten, and publicly humiliated by Indian security forces while returning from school for no apparent reason. The experience deeply traumatised the boy who ended up leaving his home and joining a local militant separatist group that had been fighting for independence for decades.

On 14th February, 2019, when other lads were wrapping gifts for their valentines, this angry young man packed 80 kilograms of high explosive, probably stolen from a construction site, in a car and drove it into a bus carrying security personnel, killing 40 and injuring many more.

The militant group with cross-border ties eagerly took credit for it.

An angry Indian government laid the blame squarely on Pakistan (which condemned the attack and denied any involvement), even before any investigations were conducted and, under political pressure from hardliners, decided to launch a 'pre-emptive strike' across the border.

On 26th February, Indian Air Force jets crossed into Pakistan, dropping bombs on a suspected militant camp to thwart any future attacks.

Heavy cross-border artillery fire ensued between the two countries, killing and seriously wounding soldiers and civilians on both sides. The next day, Pakistani Air Force jets bombed Indian targets in the disputed Jammu and Kashmir territory that both countries lay claim to. Indian aircraft tried to intercept them and in the ensuing fight one was shot down over Pakistan, the pilot captured by the Pakistani military.

Warmongers on each side of the border demanded revenge.

Both nations mobilised their armies, navies, and air forces, and nuclear weapons were deployed with missiles targeting major cities in both countries. International defence experts estimated that even a limited nuclear war would result in the loss of 125 million lives and five million tons of radioactive soot would be released into the stratosphere, plunging the whole world into an ice age-like nuclear winter for many years to come.

At this point, a leaked video of the captured pilot, Abhinandan ('Abhi' for short) made its way to the internet. It showed what could only be described as the friendliest interrogation ever undertaken by two warring sides. Abhi, sat with a cup of tea in his hands, sipping audibly, was praising the gentlemanly attitude of his captors, declining to answer any technical questions about his mission, and looking more like an honoured guest than an enemy combatant.

But the catchphrase of the video, which went viral, was when his interrogator asked him,

"I hope you like the tea."

"The tea is fantastic," replied Abhi enthusiastically.

It made everyone who watched the video break into a smile.

The two nuclear-armed hostile nations were bound together in the love and appreciation of a British brew from their common colonial past. Hospitality prevailed over hostility. Voices of reason overtook those calling for a bloody revenge.

On 1st March, Pakistan returned the captured pilot, dressed not in his military uniform but a spanking new tailor-made suit (a gift from the captors) to his home country. Calls were made for de-escalation, missiles were rolled back into their silos, and once again peace prevailed.

So, three cheers for Shennong, the legendary Chinese king who discovered this life-saving brew.

Let's put on the kettle and have a cuppa.

5.9   Aspirin (A Wonder Drug?)

Aspirin has been around for at least 2,400 years in one form or another. The precursor to aspirin was found in the leaves from the willow tree and used as a traditional medicine for treating fever and pain.

In 1853, Charles Frederick Gerhardt made synthetic aspirin by treating sodium salicylate with acetyl chloride. In 1899, Bayer, the German pharmaceutical company, improved on the formula and named it 'aspirin'. At present, every year people consume between 50 to 120 billion aspirin tablets for a multitude of maladies. The chemical name for aspirin is 'acetyl salicylic acid' (ASA). It is a painkiller (a non-steroidal anti-inflammatory drug) found to be beneficial in many other diseases; for example, reducing the risk of death after a heart attack, ischaemic stroke, and blood clots.

You have got to love the drug. It comes from a natural source, is dirt cheap, and works like a charm. And when it comes to cancer prevention, it is a magic drug.

Evidence suggests that aspirin not only prolongs colorectal cancer survival but can also activate T-cell-mediated anti-tumour immunity, and it synergises with immunotherapy through inhibiting production of a chemical called *prostaglandin E*.

Studies have shown that treatment with daily aspirin for five years (at least 75 mg) or longer reduce the subsequent risk of colorectal cancer. Several lines of evidence suggest that aspirin might also reduce the risk of other cancers, particularly of the gastrointestinal tract.

A study published in the medical journal *Lancet* in December 2010 looked at eight different trials of aspirin originally designed for prevention of vascular events such as heart attacks and strokes. These trials had allocated patients to receive either aspirin or a placebo for many years. The trials established the benefit of aspirin in reducing vascular events and saving patient lives. However, the risk of developing cancer was also found to be affected.

The benefits in reducing the risk of cancer by use of aspirin are not evident immediately. Detailed analysis of data showed that the benefit is seen after five years for oesophageal, pancreatic, brain, and lung cancer, but was more delayed for stomach, colorectal, and prostate cancer. For lung and oesophageal cancer, the benefit was evident after 20 years of using the drug.

The benefit does not increase by taking more than 75 mg of aspirin per day but does reduce if the dose is dropped below this level. The benefit is also greater in older patients.

Thank God for aspirin. The lifetime risk of developing cancer in the developing world is up to 50%, and little progress has been made in the use of drugs for prevention of the disease.

So, how does aspirin work its magic?

Aspirin reduces the incidence and growth rate, or both, in several cancers in animal models. This is mediated by reduced production of inflammatory chemicals in the body[90]. The beneficial effect is evident after a delay of several years, probably by reducing pre-cancerous lesions (known as *adenomas*; these can develop into adenocarcinomas over the years).

The implications are especially important for colon cancer, which is rising by 1.8% annually, and in rectal cancer, which has incidences rising by 1.4% on average each year for those in the UK[91]. People are getting this cancer at an earlier age, and it is being argued that they should be screened earlier in life too. Public Health England has already lowered the age of screening to 50.

As if news was not good enough for aspirin as a heroic drug, saving lives, further hope was given by a study done by Dr Allard, the lead investigator and a urologic-oncology fellow at Brigham and Women's Hospital and Massachusetts General Hospital in Boston[92], USA. He reported that aspirin slows the rate of disease progression for prostate cancer and also reduces the risk of dying from the disease. The risk of developing lethal prostate cancer was 25% lower in men who took aspirin on a regular basis. Men *with* prostate cancer who took aspirin regularly had a 39% lower risk of dying from the disease.

Until now, the usual recommendation for prostate cancer patients is to have active treatment, along with rest, exercise, less stress, more leafy green vegetables and fruit, and less red meat. With mounting evidence, it is possible in future that they would also be prescribed regular aspirin. In a round-up of 71 studies involving 520,000 people, researchers at Cardiff University discovered that the number of patients alive would be 20 to 30% greater if they had regularly taken low-dose aspirin[93]. The spread of cancer to other parts of the body was also substantially reduced in patients using aspirin. Hence, now aspirin has an important role in tertiary prevention (preventing an existing disease from worsening) of cancer too.

The side effects of aspirin, especially the risk of internal bleeding, have always been a concern but the data so far has shown the incidence of serious bleeding to be very small.

---

[90] Inhibition of the cyclo-oxygenase (COX) enzymes and reduced production of prostaglandins and other inflammatory mediators.

[91] This is the percentage rise in the cancer rate; for example, if there are 42,000 new cases of colorectal cancer in UK in a year, a 1.8% rise would mean an additional 756 cases in the next year.

[92] The findings were presented at the Genitourinary Cancer Symposium in 2016 in San Francisco.

[93] Peter Elwood, honorary professor at Cardiff University, who directed the study said, "The use of low-dose aspirin as a preventative for heart disease, stroke and cancer is well established, but evidence is now emerging that the drug may have a valuable role as an additional treatment for cancer too. Evidence from further studies are urgently required. All patients should consult their GPs before starting new medications".

5.10   Vitamins: The Jekyll and Hyde of Cancer Prevention

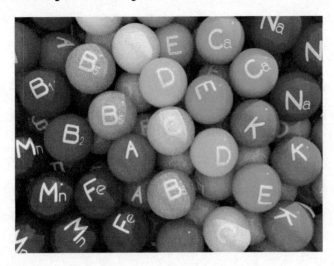

Can vitamins prevent and even cure cancer?

This question has intrigued and divided the medical community for decades. And the answer to this question is one of the best-kept secrets of our time. So, lets answer this question by revealing the secret and find out why it has been hidden for so long.

A vitamin is an essential nutrient needed by the body in small quantities for proper functioning and health. There are many classes of vitamins such as A, B, C, D, E, and K. Vitamin B comprises a number of vitamins, including B9 (also known as 'folic acid') and B12.

Vitamins are found all around us; nature is full of them. For example, eggs, milk, bananas, strawberries, fish, and cheese contain them; even coffee, too. The best sources of vitamins are fresh fruits and vegetables, preserved, packaged, and delivered to us by Mother Nature herself.

A diet rich in fruits and vegetables helps your body function properly and it also reduces the risk of many cancers. For example, prostate, breast, bladder, brain, bowel, stomach, and lung cancer, to name a few.

However, natural vitamins have an alter ego – namely, man-made synthetic vitamins, also known as 'vitamin supplements'. These commercial products come in all colours, shapes, and forms as tablets, capsules, and syrups. These synthetic vitamins are big business, and when I say big business, trust me I mean big business, both in the number of people using them and the billions of packs sold.

For example, in America almost half of the population use these vitamins, spending more than 140 billion dollars every year.

But there is a stark difference between these two types (natural versus synthetic) of vitamins, which the health agencies, manufacturers, and even doctors don't talk about, and this is the deadly secret that I want to share with you. So here it is.

Natural vitamins, the ones from vegetables and fruits, eggs, and cheese, reduce risk of cancers and there is scientific evidence to back it up. But synthetic vitamins can <u>increase</u> the risk of cancer.

Yes, you heard me right, synthetic vitamins can increase the chances of me and you getting cancer. Shocking, isn't it? The health authorities are letting them be sold openly over the counter without any warning. But where's the evidence, I hear you ask. So, let's look for it together. In fact, I will classify it for you in three categories. As an oncologist I see the world divided into three groups:

1. People with low risk of cancer.

2. People at higher risk of cancer (like smokers, for example).

3. People who already have cancer.

What happens when these three groups are given synthetic vitamins?

1) <u>People with low risk of cancer.</u> In 2006, two Norwegian trials, Norvit ('Norwegian Vitamin Trial') and WenBit ('Western Norway Vitamin B International Trial') were looking at benefits of vitamins in heart disease. The results were a double shock for everyone, since not only did synthetic vitamins fail to show a benefit for heart disease, there was an increased risk of cancer and cancer deaths in Norwegian patients given vitamins for heart disease. In 2009, another trial looked specifically at the benefits of synthetic supplements and vitamins in reducing the risk of cancer. Previous studies had shown that use of natural vitamin E and selenium reduces the risk of prostate cancer, so they decided to try synthetic vitamin E and selenium to see the effects. Some 33,533 men were recruited. The outcome was nothing short of disappointing. Patients taking vitamin E had more incidences of prostate cancer. The difference was statistically significant with a 17% increased relative risk.

2) <u>People at high risk of cancer.</u> In 1994, a study involving a high-risk group of male smokers recruited more than 29,000 patients, in which half were given vitamin E and beta-carotene for five to eight years, and half were not. The results showed that there were more deaths from lung cancer among smokers who used synthetic vitamins.
In1996, 18,313 smokers or ex-smokers were recruited to another trial. They were divided into groups and given vitamin A plus beta-carotene or a placebo. Guess what happened? There was a greater risk

of lung cancer with synthetic vitamin use and more deaths from lung cancer. The trial was stopped after only 21 months. Yet more trials were done, as people thought we should be able to cure cancer with vitamins or, at least, reduce risk. In 2007, researchers decided to give a folic acid supplement to reduce bowel cancer, but people who received synthetic folic acid had a higher risk of multiple polyps in the bowel (18.9% with folic acid compared to 4.3% without[94]). Polyps are precancerous lesions which can become cancers over time. There was an additional shock for the investigators. An increased incidence of prostate cancer (10.5% vs 6.3%[95]) occurred in those getting the synthetic folic acid.

3) <u>Patients with existing cancer.</u> So, maybe vitamins help in patients who already have cancer? Unfortunately, not. A trial published in 2009 looked at breast cancer patients who were taking vitamin supplements such as vitamin A, C, E, and carotenoids. They were found to be more at risk of their breast cancer coming back after it had been successfully treated, and had a higher risk of treatment failure and death.

All quite surprising and shocking, isn't it?

We get vitamins naturally from fruits and vegetables, and they reduce cancer risk. Studies have shown it to be a statistically significant reduction in risk. But then you have these synthetic vitamins, the alter ego, which increase the risk of cancer. What's the reason? Why on earth is this happening?

To answer this question, we have to go back to the definition of vitamins. I said that a vitamin is an essential nutrient needed by the body in *small quantities for proper functioning and health.*

The quantity or amount may be crucial here.

When you ingest natural vitamins, they are in small amounts, and they are released slowly in the body. We only absorb what we need; the rest is left unabsorbed. However, when we take synthetic vitamins, larger amounts are released from the products. This happens very fast, and the body takes more than it needs. So, where does this extra amount go? Remember our earlier discussion about cancer? I told you that normal cells develop normally, but cancer cells develop abnormally and grow in large numbers. Because they grow faster, cancer cells steal food, water, and nutrition, and that includes vitamins. So, if you have a cancer cell born in the body (and we have many of them born every day and usually our amazing body kills them all) feeding them with high-dose vitamins helps them to grow, making it more difficult for the body's defence system to overcome and kill them. Our body has a limited capacity to fight

---

[94] The findings were statistically significant, p value 0.008 (just in case you are a statistician and wondering how significant it was).

[95] Once again statistically significant, and not a chance finding (p value 0.02).

cancer and we reduce it further by feeding the cancer. No wonder the incidence of cancer increases as the use of synthetic vitamins increases.

In 2000, the global nutritional supplements and vitamin industry was worth around $20 billion dollars, and the lifetime risk of cancer was 33% in UK. In 2020, the industry was worth more than $140 billion dollars and the lifetime risk of getting cancer has risen to 50% in the UK.

About half of US citizens use synthetic vitamins and around 48% get at least one cancer in their lifetime. I am not suggesting that the rise of cancer can be totally attributed to an increased use of synthetic vitamins, but clinical trials have shown a strong association and therefore I believe we need to regulate their use.

So, the million-dollar question is should we take vitamins or not? And the answer is both yes and no.

Vitamins should be used only when required, like antibiotics (you don't take them every day).

So, check you vitamin levels, and if they are low take vitamin supplements. Recheck the levels, and when they normalise stop taking the supplements and go back to natural sources of vitamins, such as fruits and vegetables.

Don't waste your time, your money (and life) buying man-made vitamins otherwise.

Last but not least, we need to create awareness about the dangers of unregulated vitamin use. I believe that vitamins should be prescription only and come with a warning of their benefits and harms.

No one else will do it for us. It's a big industry, like alcohol and tobacco, providing employment and generating tax revenue. No wonder there has been such a massive oversight from the health authorities, despite evidence from clinical trials showing their harms and shortcomings.

If their use goes unchecked, we will end up with a worsening health crisis. Before you know it, we could even end up taking these chemicals without our knowledge and choice. Let me give you an example.

On 19th September, 2021, the BBC reported plans by the British government to add folic acid (yes, the very same folic acid which has shown in trials to increase the risk of pre-cancerous bowel polyps and prostate cancer) to flour (yes, the very same flour which is used to make bread, cakes, nans, chapatis, and all other sorts of staple food) in the UK.

This "mandatory fortification" of flour with folic acid for a population of 60 million would be done to reduce the risk of folic acid deficiency in pregnant women, which affects around 1,000 pregnancies a year in UK. It would help reduce the incidence of spine defects at birth per year (currently about 200 per year). The reason is good, but the rationale is poor.

Instead of identifying the 1,000 high-risk women and giving them folic acid supplements, the government would feed 60 million people folic acid every day, more than half of whom have a zero risk of giving birth to babies with any kind of health problems – because they are men – and many millions more who are either too young or too old to bear children. But 100% of them could be at an increased risk of bowel cancer and half at an increased risk of prostate cancer. The UK is not alone in this folly, as some 80 countries, including Australia, are already adding it to their flour.

And in case you think we are safe for now, the BBC reported that the UK government has already been adding two types of vitamins, B1 and B3, along with iron and calcium since the Second World War.

INFECTIONS
THAT MAY LEAD
TO CANCER

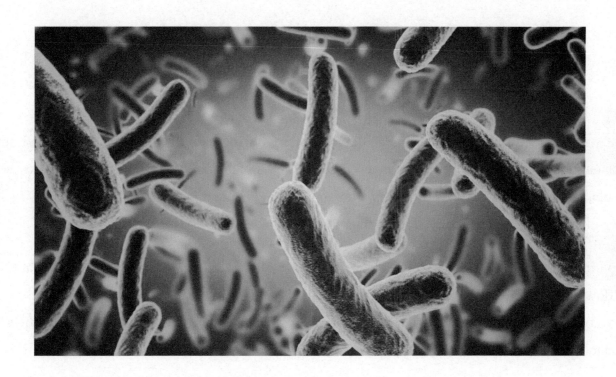

PART 6: INFECTIONS THAT MAY LEAD TO CANCER

6　Infection and Cancer

In Part 5, we saw how several types of infection, e.g., by the human papilloma virus (HPV), can give rise to cancer. There are others too, and it is an area that is probably less well understood by the general public, despite being a major cause of the disease, and so this section will hopefully address this.

6.1　Bacteria and Viruses

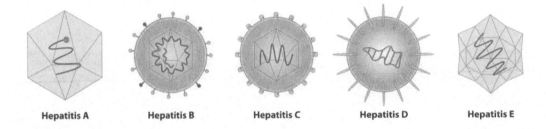

Hepatitis A　　Hepatitis B　　Hepatitis C　　Hepatitis D　　Hepatitis E

Here's some food for thought. Our world is dominated by microorganisms: bacteria, viruses, and fungi. Even our body is more microbes than human cells. We are normally not aware of them until they cause us trouble, like infections. They usually keep a low profile, and being microscopically small helps. Let me give you an idea of how tiny they are in comparison to us.

If a virus was the size of a tennis ball and bacteria the size of a beach ball, you would be so tall that if you lay down your head would be in Edinburgh, the capital of Scotland, with your feet touching the port of Calais on the northern coast of France. Now, imagine how many tennis balls can fill the distance between Scotland and France and you have an idea how numerous the microbes can be.

Having trillions upon trillions of microbes in and around us means we are always at risk of getting an infection. Fortunately, most of these bugs are not interested in hurting us. Indeed, many help provide us with nutrients by digesting food that we cannot break down.

But there are exceptions, as not all of these bugs live by the principles of good will and coexistence. When given a chance, such as when our body's defences are compromised (low immunity states), they attack – a process known as 'infection'.

Infections are an important preventable cause of cancer worldwide. It is estimated that approximately 13% of all cancers are due to infections. In numbers, this is estimated to be 2.2 million cases every year. Overall, the trend seems to be decreasing as more and more infections are becoming treatable and preventable. The percentage of cancers attributed to infections worldwide used to be much higher: 18% in 2002, 16% in 2008, and 15% in 2012.

Not all infections lead to cancers and those which do make it happen over a long period of time. For example, gastric cancer caused by *Helicobacter pylori* (*H. pylori*) infection, and cancers caused by human papilloma virus (HPV) infections, can take decades to develop from the start of infection (See section 5.1 on sex for more on HPV).

The pathogenesis (development process) of cancer due to infection is usually due to recurrent and repeated damage to the cells. In an attempt to repair this, the cells undergo division and during this process DNA damage can occur over time, having an accumulative effect. If this damage is to tumour promoter genes and tumour suppresser genes involved in DNA repair, the cells start to grow and form a tumour. Long-term, they can accumulate further damage to other important genes, leading to features of an aggressive cancer, with the capability of spreading to other parts of the body.

Some cancers can be caused by more than one infectious risk factor. For example, lymphoma is a type of blood cancer which can occur due to four infectious pathogens. The first is HTLV-1 (causing adult T-cell leukaemia or lymphoma); the second is Epstein-Barr virus (causing Hodgkin and Burkitt lymphoma); the third is hepatitis C virus (non-Hodgkin's lymphoma) and the fourth is a bacterium, *Helicobacter pylori* (gastric lymphoma).

Geographically, more than a third of the infection-related cancer cases occur in China. Of these, most are caused by *Helicobacter pylori* and *hepatitis B* virus.

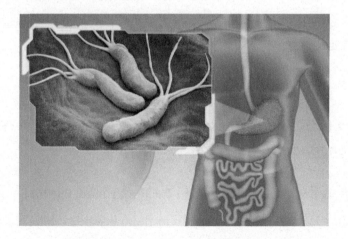

H. pylori bacteria in the human stomach.

Generally, more than 90% of infection-related cancers are caused by just four types of infectious agents (the *Famous Four*), namely, the *Helicobacter pylori* bacterium, the human papilloma virus, the hepatitis B virus, and the hepatitis C virus.

Although the human immunodeficiency virus (HIV) has been implicated in cases of different types of cancers, due to its ability to suppress the immune system and hence allow cancer cells to develop and mature, there is suspicion now that it can directly cause the squamous cell carcinoma of the conjunctiva (a membrane that covers the eyeball and lines the eyelids). Co-infection of HIV and other viruses increases the risk of cancers. For example, HIV with Epstein-Barr virus increases the chances of non-Hodgkin and Hodgkin's lymphoma. HIV and human herpes virus (HHV-8) causes Kaposi's sarcoma. HIV and human papilloma virus (HPV) significantly increase the risk of cervical and anal cancer.

Infection with the typhoid-causing bacterium, *Salmonella typhi*, can also cause gall bladder cancer as a long-term complication of the disease.

The Merkel cell virus can cause Merkel cell carcinoma of the skin. Merkel cells are oval-shaped cells in the skin which detect light-touch sensation. They are especially abundant in the fingertips, lips, and face, and this is the reason why these areas are very sensitive to touch.

6.2   Parasitic Infections

Depending on where you live, parasitic infections may or may not be relevant to your daily lives. There are large regions, however, where parasitic infections are not just a hazard but are widespread. Here are some key culprits.

1. Plasmodium Falciparum (Causing Malaria)

The malarial parasite, *Plasmodium falciparum*, has been identified as a cause of Burkitt lymphoma. How it did so was an enigma until recently, when it was discovered that the malaria-causing parasite also activates an enzyme in the human cells which causes DNA breaks and mutations, leading to a lymphoma over the long term (years).

2. Clonorchis Sinensis (Thankfully, Also Known as The 'Chinese Liver Fluke' Which Is So Much Easier to Pronounce)

Rediscovered in 1874 by James McConnell, when he found it in the body of a 20-year-old Chinese carpenter who had died unexpectedly, the Chinese liver fluke has been detected in corpses dating back to 278 BC, indicating that this particular parasite has been plaguing the human race for thousands of years. Its life cycle involves freshwater snails, freshwater fish, and mammals such as humans, dogs, cats, rats, pigs, badgers, weasels, camels, and water buffalos.

The Chinese liver fluke has an interesting life cycle. Eggs from this parasitic flatworm are eaten by freshwater snails. Inside the snail's body, the eggs dissolve and larvae emerge. The larvae then bore out of the snail's body and hang upside down in the water, waiting for any fish to pass by. When fish come into contact with the larvae, the larvae attach to their scales, make a hole in the fish's skin, and lodge in its muscles. When this fish is caught and consumed by the final host, including humans, the larvae infect them. Usually, the risk is highest with raw or undercooked fish. However, the larvae have a cyst around them, protecting them from low-intensity heat and cooking. Once consumed, the cyst is dissolved by the acid produced in the stomach. The liberated larvae then penetrate through the gut wall, entering the host's bile duct. Here, they feed on the bile produced by the liver and start to grow. The lifespan of this liver fluke is an impressive 30 years, and it is capable of laying 4,000 eggs per day. The eggs are released in the faeces, and when sewage mixes with fresh water they have the opportunity to find their initial host, the freshwater snail, and start the whole lifecycle again, spreading to more and more target hosts.

The Chinese liver fluke is most commonly found in Asia and Russia. It causes inflammation of the bile ducts and liver, often resulting in scarring of the liver (liver cirrhosis). Over a period of time, repeated infection and damage to the liver and bile cells can lead to liver cancer (hepatocellular carcinoma) and bile duct cancer (cholangiocarcinoma).

Its treatment is quite simple, using anti-parasitic drugs (albendazole, levamisole, and mebendazole) which are mass-produced and readily available. The infection can be cured easily.

3. *Opisthorchis Viverrini (Also Known as The Southeast Asian Liver Fluke, Thank God for That)*

The life cycle of the Southeast Asian liver fluke once again involves freshwater snails, from where it spreads to fish. Once this fish is consumed raw or undercooked by mammals such as humans, dogs, cats, or rats, it infects their liver and bile tract. Like its Chinese cousin, it is very fond of the biliary ducts and feeds on the bile produced by the liver. Most commonly, it is found in Thailand, Vietnam, and Cambodia. Continuous and repeated damage by this infection can eventually lead to bile duct cancer, known as cholangiocarcinoma. Infection can be treated effectively by the use of anti-parasitic medication.

4. *Schistosoma Haematobium (the Urinary Bladder Fluke or More Simply Called 'aaa')*

This parasite is mostly found in Africa and the Middle East. It has been plaguing the human race for at least 5,000 years. It causes infection of the urinary bladder causing blood in urine, a condition the ancient

Egyptians recorded as *aaa*[96]. Incredibly, Egyptian mummies from 1,250 BC have yielded parasitic eggs belonging to this fluke.

Most of the Egyptian papyri on medicine mention *aaa*. The ancient Egyptians had recognised that the bladder fluke came from infested waters in the Nile Valley and the cycle was continued due to infected patients urinating and polluting the river. They advised people to avoid polluted waters and asked the farmers and fishermen, who were in regular contact with the river, to wear penile sheaths made of linen like a primitive condom. Regretfully, these preventive measures did not work, and the bladder fluke continued to make the Egyptians go "aaa!".

By the 18th century, the infection was so common that French physicians accompanying Napoleon's campaign in 1798 were bewildered by the symptoms among the Egyptian men, and after much 'research ' and 'brainstorming 'documented their conclusions with the following words, "Egypt is the only country in the world where men menstruate."

By the 1920s, 70% of the Egyptian male population was infected with this disease, known to the West as *bilharzia*[97], although I prefer the ancient name, *aaa*. Since then, the Egyptian government has made several attempts to eliminate the parasite, especially by killing the river snails. Infection rates fell to 50% by the 1950s.

At this time, an injectable drug became available to treat the infection and a mass campaign was started to treat Egyptian men suffering from the disease. This worked well for treating *aaa* but due to the practice of re-using glass syringes, millions of Egyptian men were inadvertently infected with hepatitis B and C viruses. Fortunately, in the early 1980s, an oral drug called 'praziquantel'[98] became available. It killed the parasite with a single dose. By 1988, the Egyptian government was providing the drug for free.

But rates of bladder infections persisted, as did cases of bladder cancer. Then one man, a petroleum engineer turned actor and comedian, turned the tide by launching a health campaign with support from the government. Mohamed Reda, beloved of Egyptian TV, cinema, and theatre, starred in adverts, dressed up as a farmer, asking the infected Egyptians to do two things:

---

[96] I salute the ancient Egyptians for their knowledge and common sense, especially when it came to naming diseases. *Aaa* explains not just the disease but also the pain and agony associated with passing blood in urine. Compared to it, schistosoma haematobium sounds like a bowel problem complicated by piles.

[97] It may sound Arabic but it's not. This name was actually given to 'honour' Theodor Maximilian BILHARZ (1825–1862), a German physician who worked as the chief of medical services and medical school at Cairo, Egypt. Bilharz discovered the worm while performing an autopsy on a patient.

[98] In case you are thinking it won the Nobel Prize, I had the same thought but sadly it didn't. The 'prazi' in its name comes from the German *pyrazin*, a blend of pyridin and azine, and 'quantel' from **qu**inoline *ant*i h*el*minthic.

1. Take your medication.

2. "Turn your back to the canal."

And the message had the desired effect. By 1993 the prevalence of bilharzia bladder infection had fallen to less than 7%. It took a comedian to end the agony that Egyptians suffered for 5,000 years! A happy ending? Well, not quite. Despite the low number of bladder infections, the rate of bladder cancer started to rise again among Egyptians. This time the culprit was not a snail-riding waterborne parasite but something that the French had introduced to the country during Napoleon's campaign – smoking. It is estimated that Egyptians consume around 20 billion cigarettes a year, importing all the tobacco from abroad, which is a big drain on the national reserves.

If only Mohamed Reda, the Egyptian heartthrob comedian, was around to tell the Egyptians, "Turn your back to the cigarette." Sadly, he passed away in 1995.

Back to the bladder fluke, which is found in fresh water and its first host is the freshwater snail. After growing from eggs to larvae, the parasite emerges from the snail and swims around, looking for its next host, usually humans. It attaches to the skin by suckers and starts to bore into the body. Once inside, the first symptoms of itching develop – but by then it is too late. It enters the blood vessels and goes to the heart and liver, and then spreads out to other organs, especially the urinary bladder.

There are few things which are quite unique to this parasite. Firstly, it is permanently paired as a male and female (a very romantic arrangement known as a 'copula') and the loving couple very rarely separate, except for a very brief time when the female needs to lay between 500 and 1,000 eggs per day. Secondly, our immune system can detect this pathogen and attack it. To save itself, it coats its body with human proteins (known as *antigens*) to deceive the immune system. Its favourite abode is the urinary bladder, where it lives in the wall. From here it releases its eggs, and they penetrate the bladder mucosa (lining) by releasing toxic chemicals, causing necrosis (death of the tissue). The eggs are released into the urine and make their way to freshwater reservoirs to infect more snails and carry on their lifecycle. The usual lifespan of the fluke is 3–4 years.

The trapped eggs in the bladder wall can cause inflammation and infection. Repeated injury to the wall eventually leads to formation of bladder cancer, usually of a certain type known as a *squamous cell carcinoma* (in contrast to transitional cell carcinomas caused by other bladder toxins, such as smoking and arsenic).

PART 7

FOOD
AND DIET

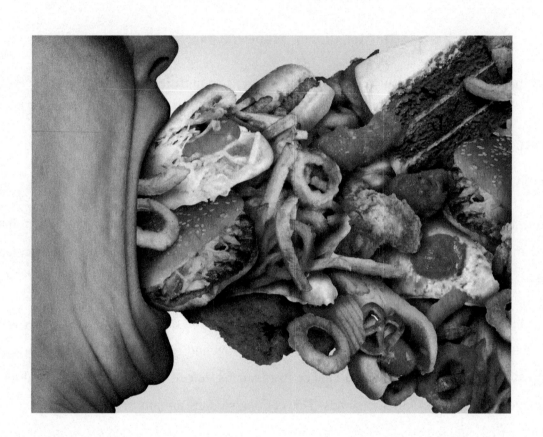

PART 7: FOOD & DIET

7 Food & Diet

One man's food is another man's poison.

From the poem *De Rerum Natura* ('On the Nature of Things') by Titus Lucretius Carus, 99–55 BC.

Too much food is any man's poison.

Dr Mohammad Muneeb Khan

It is estimated that 35% of cancers can be attributed to dietary and nutritional factors.

7.1 Most of Us Eat Too Much

The human body is not designed to overeat.

We are healthiest and functionally best when remaining slightly under-filled and hungry. When there is a dearth of food and nutrition, the basic elements required for the growth and production of new cells are in limited supply.

At such moments, the body does a remarkable thing. It starts to ration the growth process. Only perfectly healthy cells with no damage to their genes are allowed to grow and reproduce. Any cell with damaged genes is stopped from growing and given a chance to repair its defect. If a cell is unable to do so, it is killed by activation of a group of killer enzymes. This cellular suicide, apoptosis (programmed cell death), we learnt about earlier, and the circuit of enzymes invoked in this process is called *apoptotic* or *cell death pathways*.

This is our body's essential control mechanism to stop cancer from developing. Remember, cancer starts with genetic damage in a normal cell. If that cell divides and goes on to accumulate further damage to its genes, eventually it becomes a full-blown malignant cell, shutting off all of its regulatory systems and becoming an immortal menace called *cancer*.

Fasting and activation of cell death mechanisms nips this process of cancer formation in the bud.

On the other hand, when humans are overfed, the body's regulatory pathways for stopping defective cells from reproducing are suppressed and cancers develop with relative ease. One such pathway is the mTOR[99], especially active when a human is well fed. The mTOR pathway system encourages cell growth and proliferation, and discourages normal cell death. Together, these are a recipe for cancer growth and progression. Fasting (and certain drugs) inhibit the mTOR pathway.

So, why do we overeat?

The reasons are many but let us start with the basic one.

First and foremost, the human body is designed to survive and flourish on fewer calories than what we generally consume. If you desire two slices of bread, the body is probably perfectly able to function on one, and in fact prefers to do so by cutting down on unnecessary growth. Sort of an 'economy mode', like in a car or a washing machine.

Now the question arises, why? And the answer is that for thousands of years we have always struggled to find enough food. So, the body is well adapted to this situation of food scarcity.

However, severe deficiency of food can cause malnutrition and death, of course. So, our body evolved a system where *occasionally*, when food was surplus, we would be tricked into eating more, and that extra bit of nutrition could be stored as fat to be used in times of famine. In fact, very much like camels, who thrive in the desert on little water and vegetation but whenever given the occasional opportunity to overeat and drink, do so, and store the food as body fat in their hump. Our bodies do the same except that it creates the hump at the front! And, just like camels, once we have the 'hump' it's difficult to lose it.

The mechanism of tricking us into overeating is simple. The stomach does not tell the brain when it is full. We get filled up long before our mind feels the sensation of fullness (16–20 minutes estimated by one study[100]).

---

[99] MTOR stands for *mammalian target of rapamycin*, referring to an enzyme found in mammalian cells which becomes attached to a chemical called *rapamycin*, found in certain bacteria. These bacteria in turn are found on a far-flung island in the Pacific known as 'Rapa Nui'. The island was settled by Polynesians hundreds of years ago. They became obsessed with making big stone statues with massive heads. In the process they cut down all the trees on the island and destroyed its environment. Eventually, they could not survive and had to leave the island, leaving behind their obsessively crafted statues forever. Today, we call this island 'Easter Island' and its stone heads are a big tourist attraction. Cancer has a very similar story. It destroys the organ which feeds it and consumes all the resources before moving on to other parts of the body. It's ironic that rapamycin, the chemical which helped discover an important cancer-control mechanism of human cells, was found on this island which suffered a fate similar to cancer at our hands.

[100] That is why, every so often when you find yourself seeking a second helping, by the time (15–20 minutes later) you have prepared it, you realise that you are not hungry anymore.

However, having extra food was meant to be a rarity for most if not all humans. Ironically, in the modern world the majority of us eat excess food most of the time. But our stomachs and minds are still running on primitive reflexes rooted in historical conditions[101]. So, every day, at every mealtime, we end up overeating, inhibiting our body's anti-cancer mechanisms.

That is the reason why you often hear that, "The increase in cancer incidence is associated with modern lifestyle and is more common in the developed world."

We are like a camel which was designed for the sparsity of a desert but ended up living in the confines of an oasis.

Cancer is a disease of prosperity. The second most important reason is the type of food we eat. Yes, you heard it right. Our food makes us overeat. Especially the commonly used refined sugar, sucrose. This contains the notorious sweet-tasting chemical 'glucose', which stimulates our appetite and makes us feel hungry, even when we have had a full meal. Once again, having tons of refined sugar available in our diet is down to the modern-day lifestyle. Historically, sweet substances were a luxury, only consumed on special occasions, like celebrations such as a wedding, or at Christmas. Nowadays, every mealtime is party time, with cookies, candies, and super sweet drinks (one popular brand of fizzy cola is known to have 42, let me say it again, FORTY-TWO cubes of sugar in a 300 ml can).

And that's the tip of the iceberg; just the sugar we're aware of. There is a lot of hidden sweetness in the food we presume not to be sweet. For example, cereals and bread. Some of this sugar is natural and other is added to make it more appetising.

Now, if that wasn't bad enough, here's the really, *really* bad news. Cancer cells LOVE glucose[102]. And there's worse news – glucose encourages the body to secrete chemicals, acting as a stimulus for cancer growth[103].

---

[101] Interestingly, this phenomenon was recognised and documented more than one thousand years ago in a book recording the sayings of the prophet of Islam. It is stated that "Mohammad (may peace be upon him) advised his followers not to eat to their fill and stop eating when they were still feeling a bit hungry as this would ward off diseases."

[102] Cancer cells prefer to feed on glucose as it provides quick and abundant energy for them to grow and divide. In fact, they consume it at such an alarming rate that normal body cells are left starving.

[103] Glucose causes release of insulin from the pancreas. This acts on the liver and tells the liver to produce a chemical called IGF (insulin-like growth factor), which helps all cells grow. Cancer cells, however, are loaded with receptors for IGF and benefit from this growth stimulus more than other cells of the body.

For centuries, we had a sensible diet, then somewhere, somehow, we lost the plot. To understand how, when, and why it happened, we need to go back 1,000 years to meet one of the most influential and least appreciated experts of all time.

7.2   Ibn Sina (Physician Extraordinaire) and the First Calorie-Controlled Diet

The year is 997 AD and King Nuh II is suffering from an advanced and serious illness of unknown cause, and taking his last breaths. King Nuh II is no ordinary king. He rules the Samanid Empire (present-day Afghanistan, Pakistan, Iran, Turkmenistan, Uzbekistan, Kyrgyzstan, and Kazakhstan and many other 'stans'[104]) which not only is a vast realm but also controls the bulk of trade between Asia and Europe. Mostly unheard of today, Nuh II was known all over the world 1,000 years ago as the sovereign of the biggest economic power in the world. Coins issued in his name, both silver and gold, were the internationally acceptable and most desirable currency of the time, very much like the dollar is today, and hence his name was as familiar as Benjamin Franklin's is to us. Even today, archaeologists continue to find hoards of Samanid silver and gold coins in the name of Nuh II as far away as England and Sweden. So, it was a matter of grave concern – global concern in fact – that the king was about to die.

When the best physicians of his time had given up, someone suggested that Nuh II should seek advice from a 17-year-old medical student named Abu Ali Sina (known to the West as Avicenna, a Latin corruption of his Arabic patronym, Ibn Sina).

The king was desperate, clutching at straws and had nothing to lose, so he sent for the lad. The boy took a detailed history, carried out a clinical examination and prescribed some medication which worked like a charm and spared the king's life. A miracle of global fame indeed. In his gratitude, the king offered Ibn Sina any reward that he wanted and, much to everyone's shock, instead of asking for gold, silver, and other fortunes, Ibn Sina asked for something that no teenager has or will likely ever ask for *again*.

Free access to the royal library.

This must have impressed and pleased King Nuh II immensely (even royalty loves a bargain) because Ibn Sina was appointed to the post of chief royal physician. Who wouldn't want life-saving treatment for free?

---

[104] The word/suffix 'stan' comes from an ancient Indo-European language and means a place/land where you stand or live. In fact, the English word 'stand' comes from 'stan'. Just like England means the land where the English live, Afghanistan means the land where Afghans live. Interestingly, in many parts of Asia England is still referred to as 'Englistan'.

172

This was the first and probably the last time in human history that the state entrusted a teenager with … well, anything.

Born in 980 AD, in a small village near the historical city of Bukhara in present-day Uzbekistan, Abu Ali Sina was a child prodigy. By the age of 10 he had memorised the whole Quran and also became an expert on classical literature. Next, he turned his attention to mathematics, jurisprudence, philosophy, metaphysics, astronomy, and other sciences, mastering all fields, including contemporary and historical works of Greek scholars such as Aristotle, Ptolemy, Euclid, and Porphyry … and all by the age of 16.

At this point he began studying medicine and by the age of 18 he was a fully qualified and popular doctor, something that usually took up to 14 years for other medical students to achieve.

After saving the king's life and gaining unlimited access, Ibn Sina made good use of the royal library. He read and then embarked on writing books on different subjects, including medicine, meteorology, mathematics, music, chemistry, education, and philosophy. He correctly identified that sound travels in waves (he called them 'invisible ripples') and if these waves are disrupted the sound would not reach us. He also recorded that light travels faster than sound.

Of the 450 books he wrote, only 240 survive today and among them 40 are on medicine, including a five-volume medical encyclopaedia named *Al-Qanun Fi't-Tibb*, or 'The Laws of Medicine', translated in Europe as *The Canon of Medicine*.

'The Cannon', as it was popularly referred to, became the most famous medical textbook ever written. It was the standard medical textbook until 1715, and is still being taught in traditional medical schools in Asia and Africa.

Ibn Sina was not only a genius but also way ahead of his time. He did pioneering work on cancer and its treatment. To his credit, he correctly identified that cancer spreads to other parts of the body and does so by using veins as a channel, not arteries. He recommended surgery as a potentially curative treatment and emphasised the importance of wide excisions around the cancer. For inoperable tumours he used cauterisation (damaging the tumours with heat) to control them, very much like modern-day laser therapy or radiation treatment. He also used herbal extracts from a plant to treat cancer, which is the first recorded use of chemotherapy. In addition, Ibn Sina acknowledged the futility of treating advanced cancers, and suggested palliative care by providing symptomatic relief to patients. He established hospitals aiming to separate the ill from the healthy, and provide them with 24-hour care and treatment.

He revolutionised the art of surgery by introducing antiseptics, painkillers, and anaesthetics. His patients would receive pain control before surgery. During operations, they would inhale anaesthetics from a sponge saturated with a mixture of drugs. These sponges were preprepared with the correct dosage of the drugs and then stored, making them available to be used at short notice. Ibn Sina waited until his patients were in a deep sleep before operating on them. This was the first recorded use of inhalation anaesthesia in history, and the practice did not return until centuries later. His compassion for the patients did not stop with the surgery. He also made sure they were pain-free afterwards, and only stopped their medication when they had recovered from the effects of their operation.

Compare this to the surgical practice of the famous English surgeon, Thomas Hollyer, in 1658, and you will have an idea of how ahead of his time Ibn Sina was. Hollyer operated on the famous diarist and historian Samuel Pepys to remove a bladder stone. 'Anaesthesia' involved four people holding Pepys down, no antiseptics were used, and an instrument was passed through Pepys' penis into the bladder to hold the stone in place. Then a cut was made between his scrotum and anus to deliver the stone, while Pepys lay fully awake and in excruciating pain. Pepys was bed-bound for weeks after the operation and was so traumatised by the experience that for the rest of his life he marked the day as an anniversary with special prayers, begging God that the disease did not return. It wasn't until 1846 that anaesthesia was established as a medical practice in England.

As if Ibn Sina hadn't achieved enough, he was also the first known child psychologist and educationalist. He recognised that the process of learning for a child began from the moment of birth and not at the age of six as it was believed by many experts at the time. He identified the first year of life as the most important time for development of personality, discovered the effects of breastfeeding on protecting the baby from diseases, advised teachers to customise their teaching methods according to a child's individual capabilities and talents, and emphasised the concept of reward and punishment, without any physical punishments, to modify a child's behaviour.

One thousand years ago, Ibn Sina also established the field of elderly medicine, recognising the different nutritional and medicinal requirements of elderly people. In the modern era, it only became recognised as a separate speciality in 1909, when Dr Ignatz Leo Nascher coined the term 'geriatrics' for it, and Dr Nascher was given the title of the 'father of geriatrics'.

No other physician has single-handedly contributed more to medicine and been less appreciated than Ibn Sina. One of the many, least recognised contributions is that he gave us the concept of calories in food.

He described food as having a dual quality: an outer temperature and an inner, concealed heat, or energy, which it releases in the human body. For example, green tea is hot on the outside but 'cold' in nature as it has few calories. In contrast, ice cream (which was present in times of Ibn Sina, but did not come in the hundreds of fancy flavours we have today, for example the crab-flavoured ice cream popular in Hokkaido, Japan) is cold on the outside but considered 'hot-natured' because it contains more calories.

Similarly, fruits, vegetables, and diluted soups are considered a 'cold' diet because they carry fewer calories. Rationalising calorie intake, he recommended high-calorie diets for children, malnourished patients, and in cold weather. In contrast, he advised low-calorie diets for adults, those who were less active, and patients suffering from diabetes, kidney disease, and cancer. He was so obsessed with the effects of diet on human health that he dedicated a whole section in his medical books to preparing various dishes, describing in detail the advantages and disadvantages of using different ingredients. His specialty was the rice dish known as 'pilau rice' and he is considered to be the father of modern pilau. An endorsement by the most famous physician in the world did well for pilau, and it soon became one of the most popular dishes in in Asia, Africa, and Europe[105], especially Spain, where it is known as 'paella'.

Ibn Sina's recommendations for maintaining a balanced diet depended on a person's age, health, physical activity, and weather (climate) and were followed internationally for almost 800 years.

But then things changed for the worse ….

7.3   The Scientific Revolution & The High-Calorie Diet

By the 1800s, Europe had moved from the Renaissance[106] and the Age of Enlightenment[107] to the Scientific Revolution[108].

Great strides were made in the field of science and technology during this time but there was also a drive to redefine what had already been known. And the work of Ibn Sina, especially *The Cannon of Medicine*, was no exception.

---

[105] In Armenia it's called *pilaf*; Azerbaijan, *plov*; France, *pilaf*; Greece, *pilafi*; Brazil, *arroz pilau*; Caribbean, *pilau*; Indonesia, *nasi kebuli* ('rice from Kabul'), and the list goes on and on across the globe.
[106] 14th,15th, and 16th century.
[107] 17th and 18th century.
[108] The rest of the world was moving at its own pace. The Indian subcontinent, for example, had moved from the Era of Pilau Rice (10th to 16th century) to the Golden Age of Biryani (16th century onwards) which we continue to live in.

In Europe, the French and Germans were competing to discover, or should we say rediscover, the concept of calories in food.

Nicolas Clement, the famous French physicist and chemist, was calculating the maximum amount of energy that could be obtained by burning a kilogram of coal. In the process he defined the term 'calorie' as a unit of heat.

Julius Robert von Mayer, the German physician, chemist, and physicist (of 'energy can be neither created nor destroyed' fame) was keenly studying thermodynamics and the chemical processes of generating energy in a living creature. That is, before he found out that the credit for his work was being given to an English scientist called James Prescott Joule. On learning this he took a career break, attempted suicide, and spent some time in a mental institution before resuming his scientific pursuits.

Pierre Antoine Favre, a physician, and Johann T. Silbermann, a physicist, were studying thermochemical reactions and measuring the heat released in calories.

Enter Wilbur Olin Atwater, an American chemist, who established the United States Agricultural Experiment Station. Wilbur was born in Johnsburg, New York, the son of a Methodist minister, and was a keen student who preferred to stay in school, giving up a once-in-a-lifetime historical opportunity to participate in the American Civil War.

In 1869, he got his doctorate in agricultural chemistry and went to Germany for his post-doctoral studies. While working with German physiologist and dietician Carl von Voit, he became aware of the work being done by the above-mentioned famous European scientists, Favre and Silbermann. On his return to the US, he was appointed as a professor of chemistry and using his position and resources created the first agricultural research station in America. In his laboratory, Wilbur made a special chamber, 7 foot long, 4 foot wide and 6 foot high, known as a 'respirator calorimeter'. With it, he studied human subjects, meticulously calculating how much heat was being generated in the human body by different kinds of food. Everything recordable was recorded: input of food and water, output of faces, urine, carbon dioxide etc.

The basic principle underpinning his work was the first law of thermodynamics, as described by Julius von Meyer, 'energy can neither be created nor destroyed'. Energy was measured in units called 'food calories'.

Based on this principle, Wilbur calculated the calories found in thousands of food items, including alcohol, which he published in his 1896 book, *The Chemical Composition of American Food*. But interpreting his data, Wilbur made a monumental mistake, the price of which we are still paying.

He wrongly concluded that food with high calories such as meat, sugar, and alcohol was superior to low-calorie food, such as fruits, nuts, and vegetables. The logic was simple but toxic. Why eat large amounts of fruits and vegetables when we could get the same, or more, calories from smaller amounts of meat, sugar, and alcohol?

Ibn Sina's ancient philosophy of a balanced diet was unceremoniously chucked out of the window and replaced by the new scientific experiment-based concept of a 'high-calorie diet'.

Ironically, getting rid of so-called 'inferior, low-calorie fruits, nuts, and vegetables' also resulted in losing the benefits of vitamins and minerals, which are essential for human health. In his naivety, Wilbur Atwater had thrown out the baby with the bathwater.

The concept and curse of high-calorie food being good gave birth to the modern diet, the menace of which has stayed with us since. High calorie became such a rage that even fruits, grains, and vegetables were selectively bred to have a higher calorie content, especially being rich in sugar.

The World Health Organisation recommends no more than five teaspoons of sugar a day, but most people knowingly or unknowingly consume between 20–40 teaspoons a day. The public also started preferring sugar-enriched processed foods, such as conserves made out of fruit rather than the fruit itself. Thanks to Wilbur Olin Atwater's interpretations, the modern human has achieved something that was considered impossible for any species: we are overfed and malnourished at the same time!

It wasn't until the end of last century that we rediscovered the ancient wisdom of a balanced diet, and recommendations were made to reincorporate the 'inferior' low-calorie 'five-a-day fruits and vegetables' in our diet. It took us a thousand years since Ibn Sina to reinvent this wheel.

7.4   The Debate Regarding Vegetarianism and Veganism

Vegetarianism (a diet based on plants with or without eggs and dairy) and veganism (a practice of abstaining from use of any animal products), is an acquired human behaviour. By nature, we are omnivorous, meaning we eat both vegetables and meat. Historically, it was not possible to be a vegetarian in most geographic areas of the globe. For example, in Northern Europe, Sahara desert, Central Asia, Arabian Peninsula, and most other parts of the world, it was not possible to have access to fruits and vegetables all year round, especially in the winter months. Hence, people had to consume meat, which became a staple of the human diet. However, with the modern lifestyle and year-long availability of fruits and vegetables in almost all parts of the world, it is now possible to have an almost purely vegetarian diet. Previously, this was just a luxury enjoyed by those living in tropical climates, like in some parts of India. In the Indian peninsula's northern areas, where the winters are harsh, you see a trend of consuming meat, even among religious communities such as Buddhists and Hindus, religions which are usually associated with a vegetarian diet. It comes as a surprise to most that Buddha, who belonged to northeast India, was himself not a vegetarian and ate meat[109].

There are dangers associated with vegetarianism. Such a diet is usually low in proteins, vitamin B12, calcium, iron, and zinc. Proteins can be consumed as soya milk, tofu, grains, beans, seeds, and nuts. Vitamin B12 is usually difficult to find with a vegetarian diet. Fortified soya products and breakfast cereals can partly compensate for the deficiency. Calcium can be gained from vegetables such as spinach, kale, broccoli, almonds, or dairy products. Iron is found in lentils, chickpeas, beans, spinach, bran flakes, and dried fruits. Zinc, which is important for the immune system, can be found in pumpkin seeds, as well as beans and nuts.

Another drawback with vegetarian diets is that people compensate for the lack of calories by consuming more carbohydrates. A high-carbohydrate diet helps to gain weight and undo most of the benefits of eating fruits and vegetables.

An alternative to a vegetarian diet is a plant-based diet which includes some lean meat but mostly comprises of whole grains, vegetables, fruits, and legumes. A mostly (but not exclusively) plant-based diet is consistent with what human beings have been consuming traditionally for thousands of years, and this is the kind of diet which our body is most adapted to. Meat has always been a luxury, or a supplement, to the normal human diet, unlike today when it is considered to be an essential daily ingredient.

It is important that we should consume as little refined sugar as possible. Everything in moderation is also helpful. Which brings us to our next discussion, diet and dieting.

It is a well-established fact that the incidences of cancer rise significantly with an unhealthy diet and increased weight. Diets are dime a dozen when it comes to weight loss. We will talk about those which have got backing by scientific evidence and are most relevant to cancer prevention.

---

[109] There is, however, evidence to suggest that Buddha forbade his followers from eating human flesh (aka cannibalism). Thank God for that.

So, let's start with the well-known diets that can help with preventing cancer. We won't go in a lot of detail as there is a lot of information available on them including entire books and documentaries.

7.5   The Mediterranean Diet

The Mediterranean diet has been shown to reduce the risk of cardiovascular disease and cancer. A Mediterranean diet is high in cereals, fruit, and vegetables, and low in red meat. It is linked to a lower incidence of cardiovascular disease, diabetes, cancer, and mortality.

A study, performed in the UK which included 23,902 healthy people who were followed for 12 to 17 years, showed that people who had a Mediterranean diet (or closely adhered to it) had a six to 16% lower risk of future heart disease and death than those with poor adherence. The researchers estimated that 12.5% of cardiovascular (heart disease, including high blood pressure) deaths could be potentially avoided by having a Mediterranean diet.

The Mediterranean diet is based on a combination of foods rich, mainly, in antioxidants and anti-inflammatory nutrients. It depends on a high intake of vegetables, legumes, fresh fruit, non-refined cereals, nuts, and olive oil (especially extra virgin olive oil – from the first mechanical pressing[110] and which has an acidity rate lower than 0.8%). The diet also contains some fish and dairy, but a low intake of red meats. Alcohol consumption is in moderation, usually in form of wine taken with meals.

The constituents of a Mediterranean diet are associated with a lower risk of epithelial cancers, digestive tract, breast, female genital, urinary tract, liver, bowel, pancreas, lung, and nasopharyngeal cancers.

7.6   Low Carbohydrate (Ketogenic) Diets

Some experts have proposed that a ketogenic diet is helpful in controlling cancer growth because cancer cells are less efficient at metabolising ketone bodies. There are many variations of low carb, ketogenic diets.

The basic concept of a ketogenic diet is having high fat, moderate protein, and low levels of carbohydrates. By doing so, we force the body to burn fats for energy instead of carbohydrates. The whole body's metabolism switches from burning glucose to breaking down fats. This helps in weight loss and reducing the levels of insulin in the body. An additional advantage is that the brain also switches from using glucose to consuming fatty acids and ketone bodies (breakdown products of fat produced by the liver), helping to

---

[110] Extra virgin olive oil is the oil obtained from the first press of olives.

reduce the frequency of seizures in epileptic children. The benefit seen in adults is less evident. However, the ketogenic diet comes at a cost. It can cause increase in cholesterol levels, and constipation. Increased incidences of renal stones and slowing of growth in children have also been observed.

Another famous diet is the Atkins diet, devised by Robert Atkins, which has been used to achieve weight loss all over the world. There is scientific evidence which has demonstrated that the benefits of increased ketone levels in the body are associated with anti-tumour and anti-angiogenic (reduced blood vessel formation by tumours) effects. The benefit has especially been demonstrated in brain tumours, prostate, colon, pancreas, and lung cancers. There is limited evidence for benefit in breast, stomach, and liver cancer, too.

7.7   Intermittent Fasting and Time-Restricted Eating

One of the most effective methods of generating ketones in the body is by fasting. Recently, a lot of interest has grown in studying the effects of intermittent fasting and restricted feeding, and their benefit on preventing and controlling cancer.

The 5:2 (Feast and Fast) Diet

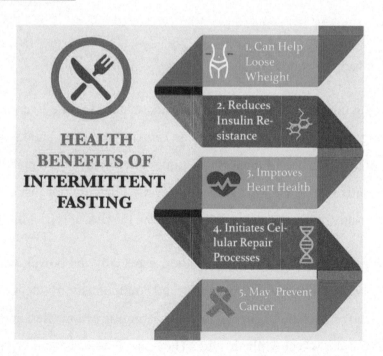

The 5:2 diet is an intermittent fasting diet which has two fasting days, followed by five feasting (eating) days. The two days can be spread out over the week; for example, a Monday and a Thursday[111].

---

[111] The earliest documented record of the 5:2 diet comes from the biography of Prophet Mohammad, who used to fast on Mondays and Thursdays regularly.

Studies carried out in South Australia showed that the 5:2 diet is effective, especially for people with diabetes. The 5:2 diet is a suitable alternative to a daily diet effective for body weight loss and blood glucose control, especially in type 2 diabetics. It results in the same weight loss and improvements to blood glucose as people who are moderately restricting their energy intake on a daily basis.

The 16/8 Diet

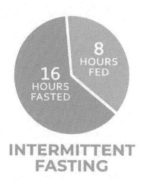

A 16/8 diet is a diet in which the participant eats daily, but only within a set time window. So, instead of eating meals across a 12 to 14-hour period, they eat only during an eight-hour period and fast for the remaining hours of each day, hence the name, the '16/8 diet'.

* * *

So, the question is, what happens when we fast?

When our body is running normally, it is drawing on glucose stored in the liver and muscles for energy, but once we start fasting it goes into a state known as *ketosis*. The liver breaks down fat and produces ketones, which can be used by the body for energy. Ketones have many beneficial properties. They reduce appetite and reduce oxidative stress and inflammation levels. They are not just used for energy but also have a lot of additional positive effects. Such a diet can reduce the risk of type 2 diabetes and heart disease.

This fasting break also provides some rest to our bodies, especially the bowel, which can be exposed to the harmful effects of food products if eating regularly and continuously. Evidence from scientific studies has shown that people who restrict their time window for eating stay more alert and are less susceptible to falling asleep at work or at the wheel while driving. They also tend to have a brighter mind. Intermittent fasting has also shown to cause weight loss, improve brain function, and perhaps even reverse diabetes, especially in the early stage of disease.

A study published in the *Journal of Proteomics* in April 2020 showed that intermittent fasting from dawn to sunset (around 14 hours a day) for 30 consecutive days in healthy subjects (as done in the month of

Ramadan by Muslims) results in the human body producing proteins (the technical term for body proteins in blood is *serum proteome*) which are protective against cancer.

The interesting thing about the study was that the intermittent fasting was done without calorie restriction, meaning that the participants could eat as much as they wanted between sunset and dawn (i.e., overnight). Also, the benefit was independent of any weight loss during the fasting period.

Intermittent fasting from dawn to sunset for 30 days upregulated (increased) proteins protective against obesity, diabetes, and metabolic syndrome. In addition, it induced key regulatory proteins of DNA repair and the immune system. Researchers also found an increased production of proteins that are thought to be protective against Alzheimer's disease and neuropsychiatric disorders. Overall, key regulatory proteins of glucose and lipid metabolism, insulin signalling, circadian clock, DNA repair, cytoskeletal re-modelling, immune system, and cognitive function were produced more than normal in healthy subjects.

The findings suggest that fasting from dawn to sunset for 30 consecutive days can be preventative and a possible an adjunct to therapy in cancer, metabolic syndrome, and several cognitive and neuropsychiatric diseases.

The anti-cancer proteins found in abundance after fasting are those which are deficient in several cancers[112].

7.8   How to Avoid Overeating

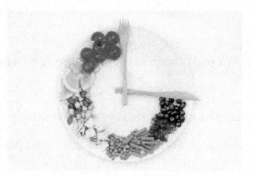

So, how do we avoid overeating?

---

[112] For example, LATS1 (an abbreviation for *large tumour suppressor kinase 1*) is an enzyme protein which, as the name suggests, suppresses tumour growth and when absent makes the body vulnerable to carcinogens and tumour production. It has also shown to have an inhibitory effect on the proliferation, progression, and invasion of several tumours, like hepatocellular carcinoma, cervical cancer, and non-small cell lung cancer. In the fasting subjects, the researchers found an average ninefold increase in the LATS1 level at the end of the fourth week during 30-day intermittent fasting, compared with the level before fasting began.

The simple method is to stop eating when you are still feeling a bit hungry. Never eat to your fill. Second, is to avoid sugar in your food, especially glucose-rich, refined sugar (which increases our desire to eat). Third, and very important, is to create a scarcity of food every now and then to stimulate the body's anti-cancer mechanisms. This has been traditionally done by fasting (see above).

7.9 Obesity

For thousands of years, mankind has fought a war against hunger and finally triumphed. Ironically, today, this victory has transformed into a war against obesity. Obesity is a major concern not only of the developed countries but also the developing world. For example, on the Polynesian island country of Nauru, more than 94% of the population is overweight and the rates of obesity are more than 71%.

Being overweight is defined as having a body mass index (ratio between weight and height, calculated by dividing the weight in kilograms by the height in metres) of between 25 and 29.9. People with a body mass index (BMI) of 30 or over are considered obese. In 2016, Britain had the dubious honour of being the most overweight nation in Western Europe with obesity rates rising at a higher level than in the United States.

At present, around 62% of the population is considered to be overweight or obese in the United Kingdom. In January 2016, Cancer Research UK reported that the increasing epidemic of obesity is going to fuel a surge in cancers. The report, 'Tipping The Scales: Why Preventing Obesity Makes Economic Sense', predicts that almost three in four adults will be overweight or obese by the year 2035. The cost of managing (treatment and social services) obesity-related disease would be an extra £2.51 billion per year to the National Health Service (NHS).

Predictions about 2035 say that more men than women will be overweight or obese, 76% compared to 69%. Another alarming prediction is that the poorest people in society would be affected most by obesity. The reason is that junk food is cheaper compared to a natural, healthy diet, and more people with a lower social-economic background consume junk food due to the high cost of fresh food.

In 2013, a staggering 257,200 new cases of type 2 diabetes were reported due to being overweight or obese in the UK. Over the next 20 years, rising levels of obesity may lead to around an additional 4.62 million cases of type 2 diabetes, 1.63 million cases of coronary heart disease, and 670,000 new cases of cancer.

Obesity puts us at increased risk of developing breast, colon, rectal, oesophageal, kidney, and pancreatic cancers. In 2017, the *British Journal of Cancer* reported that obesity is due to overtake smoking as a top cause of cancer in women. Cancer Research UK has suggested that obesity would become the leading preventable cause of cancer in women. The crossover is expected by 2043.

It is well known that increased body mass index is associated with many diseases, including cancer. Researchers in America did a meta-analysis (combined analysis) of seven studies from the Consortium on Health and Ageing, a network of cohorts (similar groups) in Europe and the United States. Data was analysed from 43,419 individuals from Denmark, Germany, Greece, and the Netherlands, along with Northern Ireland, Spain, and Norway. The mean age at study entry ranged from 54 to 67 years and the prevalence of obesity was from 11 to 42%.

During a follow-up period of 12 years there were 1,656 cases of obesity-related cancer. Across all studies, higher body mass index (BMI) was associated with a significantly increased risk of obesity-related cancers. Similar associations were seen for waist/hip ratio and waist circumference.

When it comes to fat in the human body, the three most important factors (just like buying a house) are *location, location, location.* Excess body fat, especially around the waistline, appears to be as important as body mass index is in increasing the risk of a range of cancers known to be associated with obesity. It also increases the risk of heart disease.

While increases in BMI raise the risk of developing a group of 10 obesity-related cancers by 11%, similar increases in waist circumference and waist-to-hip ratio raise the risk by 13 and 15%, respectively. Fat, in and around internal organs like the liver and stomach (known as *visceral fat*), especially fat deposits inside the liver, increases the risk of diabetes.

Needless to say, having fat in both locations is the worst possible combination.

The obesity pandemic is spreading fast. The Centers for Disease Control and Prevention (CDC) reported in 1985 that the prevalence of obesity was less than 10% in America, but by 2016 was above 20% in three states and above 25% in the rest. Obesity will soon pose a bigger risk than smoking. The reason why obesity is overtaking smoking as the commonest cause of cancer is not that smoking is becoming less dangerous but that fewer people are smoking. Added to which there is an increased incidence of obesity. The annual decline in prevalence of smoking is predicted to be around 4%, leading to 22% of the population being smokers by 2025. Unfortunately, being overweight or obese is projected to increase by similar amounts over the same timeframe. Based on these projections, the crossover point for women would be in 2043. The male population is likely to have this crossover much later because they continue to smoke more compared to women. The decline in smoking is an accumulative effect of public awareness programmes, taxation, removing tobacco marketing, and a ban on smoking in indoor public places. Maybe, similar measures need to be taken for junk food to combat the scourge of obesity.

Together, smoking and obesity/being overweight could cause more than 95,000 UK cancer cases in 2035 alone, compared with around 75,000 cases in 2015.

On a positive note, these dire predictions hide an obvious fact – most of these cancers can be prevented! For overweight people, intentional weight loss can reduce the risk of cancer death by 40–50%.

7.10   Sugars (Sucrose and Other Carbohydrates)

Technically, the term 'sugar' refers to sweet-tasting soluble carbohydrates which are used in different kinds of foods. Commonly, it refers to the white granulated sugar we are accustomed to, known as 'sucrose', which is composed of two types of carbohydrate: glucose and fructose.

Humans first came across sugar in plants, fruits, and honey. Honey is mostly composed of fructose with small amounts of glucose. Some plants have high concentrations of sucrose, such as sugar cane and sugar beet, and these are used to extract sugar for our use. The word 'sugar' comes from the Sanskrit word *śarkarā*, meaning 'ground or candied sugar', and is also found in the Persian language as *shakar* and Arabic *sukkar*. In 12th century French, the word *sucre* was used, later changing to the English word, 'sugar'.

Before sugar was produced commercially, honey was the most common sweetener used. The production of sugar started in the Indian sub-continent and spread from there to other parts of the world. Traditionally it was used as a medicine in Indian traditional folk medicine, *ayurveda*.

Alexander the Great of Macedonia, and his admiral, Nearchus, knew of sugar during their campaigns in India in 325 BC. However, this was the unrefined version. Sugar cane juice was a local delicacy, but once refined into granulated crystals it became easier to store, transport, and export. Crystallised sugar was discovered around the 5th century in India. Soon, it became the rage all over Asia. Indian sailors and travelling Buddhist monks from China took it to far-flung places. Historical documents confirm that the Chinese sent at least two missions to India in the year 647 CE to obtain the technology for sugar refining. The credit for introducing refined sugar to the rest of Asia and Europe goes to the Arabs. They became obsessed with sugar crystallisation and refinement. Legend has it that one of the Abbasid caliphs even made a mosque out of sugar so the devotees could pray and satisfy their sweet tooth at the same time. During the Crusades, the Europeans brought sugar back from the Holy Land and called it 'sweet salt'.

European Crusade chronicler William of Tyre, writing in the late 12th century, described sugar as very necessary for the use and health of mankind. However, today we know that nothing could be further from the truth. Excessive consumption of sugar has been implicated in the onset of obesity, diabetes, cardiovascular disease, dementia, and tooth decay.

Our modern obsession with producing sugar came with the discovery of the Americas. The sugar cane harvest became a major economic driving force in the New World. However, sugar remained expensive and did not come into common culinary use until the early 19th century. This was due to the rise of beet sugar in Germany, and later in France under Napoleon. Beet sugar was first produced in Germany in 1747, when Andreas Sigismund Marggraf discovered sugar in beets and devised a method using alcohol to extract it. His student, Franz Karl Achard, devised an economical industrial method to extract sugar in the late 18th century. The production of sugar from cane was fuelled by cheap labour as a result of slavery in the New World. After slavery was abolished, indentured labourers from the Indian sub-continent were hired to fill the gap. Hence the modern mix of Africans and Indians in the Caribbean, Americas, South-East Asia, Pacific Islands, East Africa, and Natal is as a result of an increased global demand for sugar.

In 2016, the combined world production of sugar cane and sugar beet, mostly for the purposes of refined sugar production, was about two billion tons. In the modern world, per capita consumption of sugar is highest in the United States, followed by Germany and the Netherlands. Globally, the average person consumes about 24 kg of sugar each year. In developed countries this is up to 33.1 kg, equivalent to over 260 food calories per day.

One hundred grams of granulated sugar (sucrose) contains 387 kcal and comprises 99.98% carbohydrates with 0% fat or protein. Some common sugary, carbonated drinks contain between 10 and 15 cubes of sugar per serving. Scientific research has shown that excessive consumption of sugar-sweetened beverages increases the risk of developing type 2 diabetes and metabolic syndrome, including weight gain and obesity, in both adults and children. Through its effects on type 2 diabetes and obesity, sugar is also contributing to the increased incidences of cancer all over the world.

Claims have been made regarding a possible relationship between sugar and Alzheimer's disease, but the evidence is inconclusive at best at present.

Sugar is also implicated in hyperactivity in children, tooth decay, and nutritional displacement due to 'empty' calories which discourage the consumption of food that contain essential nutrients. This usually occurs when sugar makes up more than 25% of daily energy intake. Displacement may occur at lower levels of consumption, too. The World Health Organisation (WHO) recommends that adults and children reduce their intake of free sugars to less than 10% and try to reduce it below 5% of their total energy intake.

In ancient tradition, sugar was used as an antidepressant. Its effects on mood are very evident among children who have a sugar rush after consuming it. However, the benefits of relieving depression and elevating the mood are short-lived, leading to an addictive behaviour in which more and more sugar is consumed for mood elation.

Seeking glucose to alleviate depression seems to be an instinctive behaviour for humans. It is the reason we tend to eat more when depressed (comfort eating) and raid the fridge late at night when unable to sleep. Probably, the mechanism is to feed and fatten our body in anticipation of tough times ahead, when we might be facing challenging circumstances with limited food supply. Historically, the biggest cause of depression could have been scarcity of food like during a drought, indicating an impending famine.

In the modern world this is probably the most unlikely cause of depression. Ironically, we have a primitive mechanism of combating depression (comfort eating) for new and unusual causes of low mood, which fail to benefit from overeating except for the short-term mood elation due to a sugar rush.

Research has suggested that sugar may fuel tumour growth in the body because cancer cells love to use it as a growth fuel. According to Johan Thevelein, a Belgian molecular biologist, the hyperactive sugar consumption of cancerous cells leads to a vicious cycle of continuous stimulation of cancer development and growth.

The 'Sugar Epidemic', as I like to call it, started in the last century. In the 1970s, due to a food crisis, America started growing more corn. The excess corn was converted into high-fructose corn syrup. This is 20 to 70% cheaper than cane sugar. High-fructose corn syrup makes a good preservative, often preferred by the food industry. It is added to soda drinks, processed meat, candy, chocolate, tinned fruit, and many other products. Between 1970 and 1990, the consumption of high-fructose corn syrup increased by 1000%. It is even added to bread. During the same period the rates of obesity in the United States increased from 15% to 39.8%.

Sugars, especially high-fructose corn syrup, are associated with increased obesity. Some 32% of all US adults are overweight, whereas 39.8% are obese. Obesity increases the risk of stroke by 64%, heart disease by 50%, and type 2 diabetes 20-fold. And it is associated with an increased risk of cancer too, as noted above.

Food sources containing fructose-containing sugars and high-calorie carbohydrates have a harmful effect on fasting insulin levels. A review published in the *British Medical Journal* in 2018 indicated that the levels of fasting insulin were higher with such a diet. High insulin levels are a major driver of cancer cell growth and proliferation.

Increased sugar intake leads to obesity, and it seems that the developed world is now exporting their epidemic of obesity to the developing and underdeveloped countries. Due to the low cost of junk food, it is very tempting for poorer communities to adopt an unhealthy diet.

The number of obese people is rising all over the world. In Brazil there are one million new cases of obesity every year. Since the 1970s, obesity has tripled globally. One of the main culprits is high sugar-containing food, especially soda drinks. A very popular brand is associated with the spread of obesity. As the consumption of that particular drink increases in any country, so do the levels of obesity and obesity-related problems, like type 2 diabetes and cancer. The high-sugar soda drinks can contain anywhere between 10 to 15 lumps (one lump has four grams of sugar so this is equal to 60 grams) of sugar per serving. You might be thinking your daily exercise regime will burn all this energy off.

The fact is, there is only a certain level of exercise we can do in a given day. The number of dry calories found in some colas would require a nine-to-five exercise regime to burn the amount of energy consumed.

Some manufacturers have started to substitute sugar with artificial sweeteners, but these are not good either as they change the normal flora of our gut and cause multiple health problems. Talking about the rapid rise of obesity, let's take China as a case study.

High-calorie colas spread from the USA, entering the Chinese market in the 1970s. Now they control half of the soda market in China. In 1975, the rate of obesity and being overweight was 10%, but since it has risen to 32% (2016).

The soft-drink companies have been financing direct and indirect interventions to formulate the health guidelines in China. The current Chinese health guidelines do not focus on reducing the sugar content of sodas and, in fact, are focusing more on increased physical activity, despite the overwhelming evidence that *both* exercise and calorie reduction are essential for weight loss and good health.

Another case study is that of Mexico. After Mexico joined the NAFTA (North American Free Trade Agreement) with the United States and Canada in 1993, its market was flooded with cheap, low-nutrient food products from the US and Canada. High-fructose corn syrup importation increased by around 1,200%. From 1983, when the obesity percentage was 34.5% in Mexico, the cases of overweight and obese people increased, and by 2018 Mexico had a 75.2% obese and overweight population. The leading cause of death in Mexico at present is diabetes mellitus, which is related to being overweight and obese. In Mexico, the high-calorie cola companies are having a field day. Their biggest consumers are children, who drink it instead of water in schools. Even babies get the calorie cola in their bottles. Ironically, in return, Mexico exports billions of dollars-worth of fruit and nuts to the United States.

Food and beverages containing high amounts of fructose sugar are associated with an increased risk of pancreatic cancer. There is approximately a 22% increase in the risk of pancreatic cancer per 25 grams of fructose consumed per day.

In the human body there is a special chemical produced which inactivates free radicals that can damage human cells and DNA. This chemical is known as *glutathione peroxidase*. Fructose inhibits it. Last, but not least, cancer cells consume fructose, especially when they are living in a low-oxygen environment, and use it to generate energy via a special metabolic pathway (known as a *non-oxidative pentose phosphate pathway*) for the purposes of cell proliferation.

The impact of high sugar and carbohydrate diet on cancer can be easily seen among indigenous societies which have abandoned their traditional diets and adopted the modern lifestyle. The rates of cancers among the Ojibwa tribe in northwestern Canada and the Canadian Inuit of the Artic region rose sharply as they moved away from traditional to imported food rich in grains and sugar. In the 1950s, cancer was a rare phenomenon among the Aboriginal Canadians; by 1972 it was around 10%, and shot up to 30% within ten years. Even the type of cancers changed from the traditional head and neck cancers to lung, breast, and bowel cancers, typical of the white European population in Canada.

7.11   Milk & Dairy

Scientists have closely studied the influence of milk and dairy diets on human health, especially with regard to cancer, and data has shown that consumption of milk and dairy products significantly influences our risk of developing the disease.

But before we get into this discussion, we need to know and understand our relationship with milk and dairy, and the reason why, out of all the creatures on this planet, we are the only ones who consume milk from cradle to grave.

The relationship of milk and mankind goes back a long way. As mammals, we all begin our life by deriving nutrition from milk. At the time a baby starts to wean, its body's ability to digest milk, especially the sugar known as 'lactose', reduces as it moves on to other sources of nutrition. This is the case with almost all mammals, but humans are an exception.

Due to a certain genetic mutation occurring more than 10,000 years ago in man, some humans developed the ability to continue digesting milk, and especially its lactose component, even after the initial years of life. To digest lactose, the body produces an enzyme called *lactase*. Around the same time, human beings also started to domesticate animals for the production of milk.

However, this did not happen to all humans. Only a small percentage had this advantage. Even today, for example, among the Chinese population only one percent can digest milk after the first two years of life.

This ability is known as *lactose tolerance* as compared to lactose intolerance, the default human condition of not digesting milk as a grown-up.

The ability to digest milk gave those able to do so a survival advantage in an environment and time when other sources of food were not available. This includes areas of northern Europe, which have long winters with very little chance of growing any crops, and deserts like those of Arabia and the Sahara. The steppes of Central Asia and the Gobi desert in Mongolia were also advantageous to these lactose-tolerant humans.

In such harsh environments, those who could digest milk survived and reproduced more than those who couldn't. As a result, the inhabitants of these areas, including northern Europeans, Arabs, Turks, and Mongol tribesmen, have a very high percentage of people who can easily digest milk, and hence milk forms an important source of nutrition for these communities.

Nowhere is this difference starker than between Mongolia and China. Although Mongols and Chinese are neighbours, among the Mongol population the ability to digest milk (lactose tolerant) is 99%. On the other hand, among the Chinese, where milk is not a stable diet (try to remember when was the last time you were served a milk or dairy-containing dish in a Chinese restaurant), the incidence of lactose intolerance is 99%.

Due to the variety of food available in mainland China, the Chinese have never had to depend on milk and dairy products as the Mongols did in the Gobi desert. In fact, the dependence of Mongols on milk can be gauged by the fact that they even make alcohol out of it.

A quick glance at global cuisines and you realise most ethnic cuisines (African, Chinese, South Asian, Southeast Asian, Native American, Aboriginal, to name a few) do not have milk as a significant component. On the other hand, it forms an important ingredient of European, Middle Eastern, central Asian and northern Indian[113] cuisines, where peoples are blessed with the lactose tolerance mutation.

Despite this, over the centuries milk has become very fashionable and acceptable even among some lactose-intolerant racial groups.

---

[113] Majority of the northern Indians are descendants of Central Asian tribes: Aryans, Scythians, Kushans, Juan Juan (not to be confused with the music group who sang 'Life is short, wanna get stoned') and White Huns, to name a few.

It also helped that humans processed milk in different ways, and developed many milk-related dairy products such as yoghurt, cheese, cream, butter, and, more recently, ice cream, to cater for their dairy taste. One of the advantages of these processed milk products is that they have a lower content of lactose and hence can be consumed in reasonable amounts by the majority of the human race, who are lactose intolerant.

Lactose intolerance was first recognised by Hypocrites (470–360 BC) who described milk as a 'laxative'. Consuming milk and dairy products come at a cost, especially for the lactose intolerant. People who are unable to digest lactose end up accumulating it in their gut where the bacteria, which are normally found in our body, feed on the lactose and produce chemical compounds and gases, giving rise to reflux, indigestion, nausea, cramps, bloating, and diarrhoea.

Another interesting fact is that even in lactose-tolerant people, the production of the enzyme lactase varies and gradually decreases with age. It can also vary dramatically in conditions causing inflammation of the bowel, like a simple gut infection (gastroenteritis) or long-term chronic gut diseases, such as Crohn's disease or ulcerative colitis. This phenomenon of reduced lactase production, due to a cause other than the genetic ability of the body, is known as *secondary lactose intolerance*.

In the modern-day lifestyle, milk and dairy products have become a very important constituent. Not only do we have them available commercially all over the world to both types of human population (lactose tolerant or intolerant), they are also being used in processed foods because milk and its sugar, lactose, is cheap to produce, smooth in flavour, and sweet in taste, making it a desirable, cheap component of many food products.

Hence, whether we like or tolerate it, or not, milk and dairy have become an integral part of human diet.

There are pros and cons to having milk and dairy products in the human diet.

In the traditional Western diet, which is now becoming the norm for most parts of the world, milk intake has been highly recommended. These recommendations are based on studies showing that milk consumption increases longitudinal growth and height in children, compared to those children who do not consume milk, despite having an adequate overall nutrition. This is because milk contains substantial amounts of essential amino acids which both directly and indirectly improve the growth of bones. The direct growth is due to availability of these amino acids for protein synthesis, along with ample amounts of calcium, with both being used for bone growth. The indirect effect is through increase in plasma concentration of a chemical hormone called *IGF-1* (*insulin-like growth factor 1*), which mediates the action of growth hormone.

Growing Tall at a Cost: Falls, Fractures, Clots, and Cancer ...

Ironically, the tall stature attained by increased growth also puts people at a higher risk of diseases such as hip fractures (an old English saying, 'The bigger they are, the harder the fall', comes to mind), pulmonary emboli (clots in the lungs), and certain cancers.

Studies have shown that countries with the highest intake of milk and calcium tend to have the highest rates of hip fractures at a later age. Among men, milk intake during adolescence has shown to be associated with a 9% greater relative risk of hip fractures later in life for every additional glass of milk consumed per day.

The risk of cancer with milk intake tends to be high for some kinds of cancers such as breast cancer, prostate cancer, and endometrial cancer of the womb. There is also suspicion that it might increase the risk of ovarian cancer but, more interestingly, consuming milk reduces the risk of colorectal cancer (see later).

The question arises as to why milk causes increased incidences of certain cancers. And the answer is as follows:

1) Milk has growth-promoting effects due to its content of amino acids and anabolic hormones, and especially the effect of the insulin growth factor IGF-1; all of these factors not only improve the growth and replication of normal cells but serve as a fodder for cancer growth.

2) The amino acid leucine, found in milk (which helps kids grow taller), activates the mTOR pathway cells, promoting replication of both normal and abnormal (cancer) cells and inhibits cell death of both normal and cancer cells.

3) Most milk found nowadays on the shelves of supermarkets is very different from traditional milk available to mankind over the centuries. To increase milk production, cows have been bred to produce higher levels of insulin-like growth factor (IGF-1). Also, commercial animals producing milk are pregnant for most of the time while they are milked; this greatly increases the level of hormones, such as progesterone and oestrogen. These hormones can act as a growth stimulus for cancer cells, especially endometrial and ovarian cancer cells.

However, it can be safely assumed that milk does not *cause* or start a new cancer but, instead, promotes the growth of cancer cells once they have already developed in the body. This means that for a person with the initial stages of cancer, consuming milk would give rise to clinically obvious disease much earlier compared to someone who does not consume milk.

A study conducted by scientists at Loma Linda University compared the effects of dairy products versus soya milk consumption in women. The study focused on the diets of more than 50,000 women in America over a period of eight years. There was no association between breast cancer and soya milk, but there was overwhelming evidence of a link between dairy intake and cancer.

The study concluded that women who had 2–3 cups of dairy milk daily, as per the current US dietary guideline, had a 70–80% increased risk of developing breast cancer (which means that if the actual risk of breast cancer is, say, 10%, drinking three cups of milk every day would increase it to 17–18%).

On the other hand, although a high consumption of dairy foods likely increases the risk of breast, prostate, and possibly endometrial cancer, it is associated with a reduced risk of colorectal cancer. The jury is still out on exactly why this is the case and further research is required. But I suspect the answer would be very simple.

Remember, in our earlier discussion about milk, the fact that most of the world population is lactose intolerant – something realised as long ago as the time of Hypocrites, when milk was recognised as having laxative qualities? This might be the key to milk's anti-colon cancer effects.

Even people who are able to digest milk tend to have a deficiency of this enzyme with advancing years, and eventually start suffering from the side effects of milk consumption. As mentioned earlier, when the milk sugar lactose cannot be digested by the human body and the normal bacteria found in the gut feed on it, they produce chemicals and gases, causing abdominal cramps, indigestion, flatulence, bloating, and often diarrhoea. The latter means that people who consume dairy products may have a faster gut motility and so whatever food they ingest does not stay in the gut for a long time. The shorter the transit time in the gut, the shorter the exposure time of the lining of the bowel to any potential carcinogens. However, people who have a milk-free or low-dairy diet will have a normal or longer transit time for food (and hence potential carcinogens) exposing their bowel to hazardous chemicals and cancer-causing toxins for longer. With the modern lifestyle, including low intake of fruits, vegetables, and water (the latter is substituted by sugary drinks, causing the water in the drinks to be absorbed quickly, along with the sugars, hence causing hard stools and constipation), the exposure time to carcinogens is much longer, as evident by a higher incidence of colon cancer in this population group.

So, should we drink milk?

The conclusion is that it would be safer for humans not to consume excessive amounts of milk and dairy products, especially those commercially produced on an industrial scale using techniques that increase the levels of hormones and insulin-like growth factors (such as the use of recombinant bovine somatotropin which causes significant elevation of levels of IGF-1 and residues of pesticides on commercially produced feeds, all of whom contribute to increased incidences of many cancers).

In addition, I would suggest that people who have suspicion of lactose intolerance should get tested for it (it is a simple test, analysing the breath for certain chemicals produced by breakdown of lactose by bacteria in the gut) and refrain from taking milk (or choose lactose-free milk and dairy products). This would prevent and cure most of the cases of bowel dysfunction, usually labelled as 'irritable bowel syndrome'.

The Menace of Milk Adulteration

The story of milk and cancer is incomplete without mention of milk adulteration and its effect on increasing the risk of developing cancers. In light of the increased demand of milk and dairy products, fake and adulterated milk has become quite common, especially in developing countries. There are three main approaches to milk scams:

1. Manipulating nature: To start with, cows are injected with a hormone called *oxytocin* for increased milk production. This hormone, also found naturally in the body, is known to have effects on cancer cell proliferation, especially in prostate cancer. Drinking milk from animals treated with oxytocin increases cancer growth.

2. Milk dilution: This is the more benign form of milk adulteration. It usually includes combining powdered milk with cooking oil and diluting it with water to make fake milk. There are commercial 'milk factories' using washing machines (old style top-loading designs from the sixties, as front-loading washing machines cannot be used for obvious reasons) to mix the three ingredients and make cheap, counterfeit milk, sold at the normal price of pure milk. Apparently, the counterfeit is quite convincingly milk-like and it's hard to tell the difference. The formula for this fake production (which I went to great trouble to find for you[114]) is mixing 2 kg of dry milk powder with one kg of cooking oil and 37 litres of water (please don't try this at home[115]). This doesn't increase the risk of cancer as long as the washing machine is detergent free.

3. Toxic processing of milk: The worst of all milk adulterations is the processing of milk using toxic chemicals, and has the biggest implication for cancer. Naturally produced milk has a lifespan of 1–

---

[114] I am grateful to the friends from the food industry who have provided me information in matters of milk and food adulteration, especially Mr Mohsin Bhatti. He is a world-leading expert on food adulteration and his work has been an important source for this section.

[115] On second thoughts, why not try it at home … as long as you are not selling it as pure milk. I would recommend a blender instead of a washing machine, take two tablespoons of dry milk and add it to 37 tablespoons of water, top it up with one tablespoon of cooking oil, and give them a whiz in the blender. Lo and behold, your fake adulterated synthetic milk is ready. Shake well before use.

2 hours before the bacteria start to break it down. To prolong its lifespan, formaldehyde (a toxic compound generally used to preserve dead bodies) is added to the milk to kill the bacteria. Formaldehyde is a well-established carcinogen causing damage to genes and inducing mutations that lead to cancer. There is clear link of formaldehyde with nasal sinus cancers, nasopharyngeal cancers, and leukaemias (a type of blood cancer), especially myeloid leukaemia. When formaldehyde is exposed to oxygen in the air it changes to formic acid, another cancer-causing chemical. Unfortunately, the use of formaldehyde is not just limited to preserving milk but has also been illegally used to prolong the shelf life of foods, vegetables, fish, and chicken.

The story of milk adulteration does not stop with the addition of formaldehyde. Once this milk has been preserved, the cream is extracted, and the leftover skimmed milk is fortified with industrial fat to make it thick again. However, animal fat does not mix with milk very well and requires potassium compounds to dissolve. Unfortunately, the cheapest source of such potassium is the fertiliser urea[116], which once again is hazardous to normal human cells.

Finally, to add insult to the injury, the adulterated milk which, after addition of animal fat becomes discoloured, is treated with caustic soda or washing powder chemicals to give it a brilliant white colour and a touch of froth.

7.12   Processed Foods & Cooking Methods

Before the invention of refrigerators and chemical processing, eating meat was a rare luxury because meat went off within a day or two and hence could only be consumed close to the time that the animal was killed.

And because one could not eat a whole cow in a day, you needed a group consensus before a butcher would pull out his knife.

But all this changed with chemical processing of food, especially meat.

Processed foods are designed to last for months and usually contain preservatives, not only in the form of their packing but also as added ingredients to enhance taste and texture. These salts and additives interact with the protein in the meat and can form toxic compounds which can damage cells in the gut. People

---

[116] That's the same stuff which is found in urine.

eating these meats, including smoked products, have been shown to have an increased risk of cancer, especially of the bowel.

Scientists in France have studied the link between people who eat more processed food and those who develop cancer and found that it is likely to increase the risk. At present, however, it is not clear whether the problem is in the preserving ingredients, the plastic packaging, or a combination of both, but evidence suggests that avoidance of processed food would reduce the risk.

Processed meats such as bacon and sausages increase the risk of cancer, especially breast cancer. The World Health Organisation reports that processed meat like hotdogs, ham, bacon, sausages, and others can cause cancer (classified as 'carcinogens'). This is because meat has been treated by salting, fermenting, curing, or smoking, which results in chemicals that can damage the DNA. A large new analysis of data of more than one million women by a team from Harvard University's T H Chan School of Public Health found that eating processed meats, such a sausages and bacon, increase the risk of developing cancer by around 9%.

It is possible that any kind of red meat, preserved or unpreserved, could be linked to an increased risk of colorectal cancers and there is some evidence to suggest that it also contributes to pancreatic and prostate cancer. However, the risk is higher with processed meat.

Consuming the equivalent of one hotdog or roughly two slices of bacon every day increases the relative risk of colorectal cancer by about 18%.

Another chemical of interest in cooking is acrylamide. This is an organic compound, one of more than 1,000 chemicals on the list of IARC's (International Agency for Research on Cancer) cancer-causing compounds. Acrylamide is a carcinogenic substance formed, albeit in very small quantities, during the browning of some foods when cooking at high temperatures, like bread, coffee, or French fries (chips).

When cooking between 140 to 165 degrees centigrade (280 to 330 Fahrenheit), this process happens naturally and is known as the 'Maillard reaction' (named after the French scientist Louis Camille Maillard, who described it in 1912). It is a chemical reaction between amino acids and reducing sugars without involving an enzyme, and adds flavour to the food. The amount of acrylamide produced in this process is very small and may not be significant enough to raise the risk of cancer significantly. However, its major source is cigarette smoking which has shown to increase levels of acrylamide in human blood.

7.13   Capsicum (Chillies)

Chillies are the biggest contribution to global cuisine made by Europe. Yes, you heard it right: *Europe!*

Europeans introduced chillies to the world. And no, it's got nothing to do with Chile the country. But the confusion was so widespread that the country had to change its name from 'Chilli' to Chile in 1900, so they are not confused with the fiery food. There is no consensus why Chile, the country, is called 'Chile', but it's either a corruption of *Tili*, the name of a Native American chief of the Picunche tribe who ruled there, or from the native South American Mapuche language, where *chilli* means 'where the land ends'.

As for the firebrand fruit, the name 'chilli' comes from the Central American Mexican language Nahuatl, spoken by the Nahua and Aztec people. The Native Americans discovered and began cultivating chillies, or Capsicum fruit, as it is formally referred to, around 7,500 BC, making it one of the oldest crops in the Americas. It is thought that initially it was used for medicinal purposes before it became an integral part of American diet. The Aztec used it as a painkiller, especially to treat toothache.

The *Codex Mendoza*, a record of Aztec lifestyle created by the Spanish after they conquered Mexico, has drawings of a parent exposing a teary-eyed child to the smoke from a pit of burning chillies. It is unclear whether this was done to treat a physical illness or as a punishment for naughty behaviour. In case of the latter, this would give chillies the distinction of being the first recorded behaviour-modifying medicine known to mankind. *Codex Mendoza* has since inspired many law-enforcing agencies and criminal gangs to use this method as an interrogation technique.

When Christopher Columbus and his Iberian crew came across chillies in the Caribbean, they called them 'peppers', confusing them with the 'black pepper' found in India. This was to be expected, since Columbus was looking for a new route to India[117] and had thought he had reached the west of India, hence the name 'West Indies' for the Caribbean islands, and 'Red Indians' for the Native Americans.

It wasn't until the 16th century that Europeans introduced Capsicum or 'chilli peppers' as they called them, to Asian cuisine. Until then, Asian food was spicy but not hot. Four hundred years later, Asians took revenge by introducing their food, laden with eye-watering amounts of chilli to Europe.

The phenomenon is known as 'karma'.

---

[117] Columbus was so sure of finding India across the Atlantic that he even took an Arabic-speaking sailor among his crew in case he ran into Arab traders on the way to India.

Today, millions of tons of chillies are produced all over the world. In 2016, the production of raw green chilli peppers alone amounted to 34.5 million tons.

Much of the production, almost 50%, comes from China[118]. Europe continues to benefit from this lucrative trade, being the fourth-largest producer of green chillies in the world. Mexico is second and Turkey the third-largest producer.

Why are chillies hot?

The Capsicum plant evolved to produce its fiery hot ingredient, *capsaicin*, to kill the fungus which attacks it. There was the added advantage of discouraging mammals from consuming it too. Capsaicin, however, is kind to birds as they lack the pain receptors that mammals have. This helps the plant, as birds don't chew the seeds, instead passing them whole in their droppings, helping to spread them. Chillies also contain carbohydrates, fibre, fat, vitamins (A, C and B6), minerals (potassium, iron, and magnesium), beta-carotene, and a famous fire extinguisher, water.

The hotness, or heat, of chillies is measured in units known as 'Scoville heat units' (SHU), named after American pharmacist Wilbur Scoville. In 1912, Scoville devised a simple test – take an extract of the chillies, dilute it in sugar water and see how much dilution is required to make the solution lose its fiery sting. If it requires 100 dilutions, the chilli is 100 SHU hot.

On this scale, the sweet bell pepper scores a big zero. Jalapeño scores up to 10,000 SHU, cayenne pepper 30,000–50,000 SHU, piri piri 50,000–100,000 SHU, habanero, scotch bonnet, and bird's eye, 100,000-350,000 SHU.

But these stand nowhere in comparison to certain, less familiar types.

For example, the British Infinity chilli scores 1.2 million SHU, Naga Viper 1.4 million SHU, and Dragon's Breath a numbing 2.4 million SHU.

The USA was lagging behind the UK with the Carolina Reaper at 2.2 million SHU but has taken the lead now with Pepper X, an eye-watering – or should I say gobsmacking – 3.18 million SHU.

It does somehow make you feel that the nuclear superpowers are diversifying their arsenal with stronger versions of Capsicum.

---

[118] Nowadays, what doesn't come from China?

Apart from using chillies as a punishment for misbehaving kids, the Mayans also used it as a chemical weapon in warfare by burning it to create a stinging smokescreen, as it caused pain and breathing difficulties for the enemy. Inspired by the Mayans, the active ingredients, *capasaicinoids*, are used in pepper sprays for personal defence and riot control. Capsaicin repellents are also used to deter pests, such as rabbits, squirrels, bears, dogs, insects, and even elephants. Add it to birdseed and it deters rodents from raiding it.

The US department of agriculture has approved it as a pesticide since 1962.

Chillies and spices have been used for centuries to add taste and flavour. But there is more to them than their fiery flavour and aroma. They act as natural non-toxic preservatives for food, and were essential in extending the shelf life of food before the more modern and toxic alternatives became available. Recent research has also shown that they possess antioxidant qualities, making them important anti-cancer agents.

The hot ingredient in chillies, capsaicin, also gives our brain a 'high' or euphoria due to the release of endorphins, which are morphine-like chemicals produced by the body.

The effect is not limited to humans as some animals, especially horses, also get a buzz by it, and its use as a performance-enhancing chemical has been banned in equestrian events. Four horses were disqualified from the 2008 Summer Olympics when they tested positive for capsaicin in their urine. Whether they have the same effect on human athletes is not known. However, looking at the dismal athletic performance of South Asian[119] athletes at the Olympics, I would place my bets on the horses.

Capsaicin is a well-known painkiller. Native Americans have used it for thousands of years and still do. Modern medicine has also rediscovered its analgesic potential and has made capsaicin creams, ointments, and skin patches to alleviate the nerve pain caused by shingles, HIV neuropathy, diabetic neuropathy, and arthritis.

The benefits don't stop there. Capsaicin has anti-inflammatory, antioxidant, and anti-cancer effects too.

Laboratory research has shown that capsaicin activates a receptor in the intestinal lining of mice, triggering a reaction that leads to a reduced risk of colorectal cancer. Researchers are quite hopeful that it has the same effect in humans.

---

[119] South Asia includes countries such as Pakistan, Bangladesh, India, Nepal, Bhutan, and Maldives, which are famous for their chilli-rich cuisine and poor performance at athletic events.

There is a receptor in our intestines, TRPV1 (transient receptor potential cation channel sub-family V member 1; it's a mouthful so I prefer the alternative name *capsaicin receptor* or, as I like to call it, the 'chilli receptor'). When TRPV1 activity increases, there is a reduction in the activity of another receptor known as the *epidermal growth factor receptor* (EGFR). The EGFR is a catalyst for normal cell production and turnover in the gut, usually turning over every four to six days. Increased activity of EGFR overproduces cells and increases the chance of developing tumours. The importance of the chilli receptor can be assessed by the fact that study of human bowel cancer cell samples has shown defective and mutated chilli receptors.

Chilli receptor activity is stimulated by capsaicin; hence chillies act as a *tumour suppressor* and keep our bowel free of cancer.

The benefit of chillies is not just limited to control of bowel cancer.

After compiling data from 4,729 studies, scientists have concluded that consuming chilli peppers helps you to live longer by reducing the risk of heart disease by 26%, cancer mortality by 23%, and overall/all-cause mortality by 25%.

Experiments on mice at the University of Wyoming also showed that adding capsaicin to their diet improved their ability to burn calories and prevented weight gain.

Mice infected with progressing human lung cancer cells had less growth and spread of cancer cells when fed on capsaicin compared to those who had a 'chilli-free diet'. The team who carried out this experiment at the Marshall University, Joan C. Edwards School of Medicine, in Huntington, West Virginia, are now planning to extend their study to human patients.

So, my recommendation for an anti-cancer diet is, 'Chillies and spice and everything nice'.

PART 8

THE
ENVIRONMENT

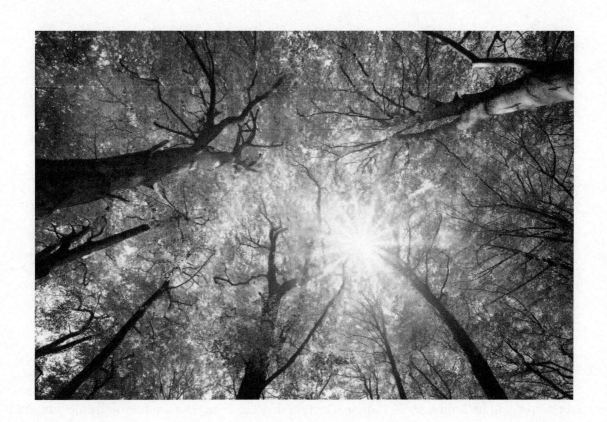

PART 8: THE ENVIRONMENT (OUR BEAUTIFUL BLUE PLANET)

8　　The Environment

Like me, you probably go about your daily lives with the sneaking suspicion that you are being exposed to toxic substances, whether it is the air you breathe or food you eat. Things you cannot see, hear, smell, touch, or taste, but somehow you know they are there. Perhaps this isn't so surprising, as we are endlessly being reminded about how we are polluting our beautiful blue planet. And it is true. But among these hazards are some not always of our making but part of our natural world. So, let's deal with these first.

8.1　　Radioactivity: We Live in a Radiant World

RADIOACTIVITY

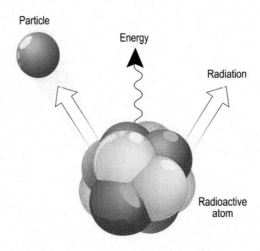

Everything around us, and including us, is radioactive to a degree; some emitting a miniscule amount of radiation, others considerably more. The reason for this is that the building blocks of our universe are atoms, and atoms of almost every element come in various forms, known as 'isotopes'[120].

Isotopes are either stable, which means they do not emit any radiation, or are unstable, which means they have a tendency to break down, emitting radiation in the process. The amount of radiation released from any object in the universe depends on the number of unstable atoms (isotopes) it contains, and how quickly

---

[120] From the Greek word *isos*, which means 'equal', and *topos* which means 'place', meaning that they are found in the same place in the periodic table.

they break down[121]. Depending on these two factors, a substance can be minimally or highly radioactive, or somewhere in-between.

For example, most lifeforms are composed of the element carbon. Carbon atoms exist as stable isotopes, such as ^{12}C (carbon-12) and ^{13}C (carbon-13), or the unstable isotope ^{14}C (carbon-14)[122], so the amount of radioactivity produced by a living creature would very much depend on how much unstable carbon-14 it has inside it[123].

In relation to human health, we measure the amount of radiation emitted by any substance in the form of the energy carried by that radiation. If this energy is small, it does not cause a significant hazard. If it is high enough, it may damage human cells, including the DNA, causing mutations and increasing the risk of cancer.

Radiation damages cells and DNA in various ways:

1. High-dose radiation kills cells and destroys their DNA. That is the reason why it is used to kill cancer cells, and for some types it can cure the cancer too.

2. Low-dose radiation causes irreparable damage to cells and DNA. The later results in mutations which can transform a normal cell to a cancer cell.

3. Very low-dose radiation causes repairable damage and hence is considered safe.

As you read this, you might be wondering about the aftermath of a nuclear explosion and the resulting radiation hazard, and the extent to which it gives rise to cancer. Although a man-made example, it might nevertheless help us get a handle on just what the risks from radiation are. Sadly, as a general rule, being bombed by a nuclear weapon is a fatal event for virtually anyone in the blast zone. This was clearly demonstrated in 1945 by the bombing of Japanese cities of Hiroshima and Nagasaki, killing up to 226,000 people. Even among the survivors, a large number suffered from radiation sickness and many died, although the exact number of fatalities was not recorded.

---

[121] How fast an unstable isotope breaks down, releasing radiation, is measured in terms of its half-life, which is the time taken for half of its atoms in a sample to decay.

[122] Actually, carbon has a total of 15 isotopes, but these three are the most common.

[123] The half-life of carbon-14 is 5,730 years. So, if you have 2 grams of radioactive carbon-14 in your body, after 5,730 years your body would only be left with 1 gram of radioactive carbon 14. In the real world, this does not apply to most human beings, except if they are Egyptian and were mummified 5,730 years ago. Measuring carbon-14 levels can help date the remains of a dead body and this method is known as 'carbon dating'.

After two years of exposure to the nuclear bombs' fallout radiation, the rates of cancers started to increase, peaking at around 6–8 years later. A significant increase was seen in blood cancers (leukaemias), followed by an increase in solid cancers. There is no reliable data to suggest what the effect was on pregnant females and the outcomes of their pregnancies. Similarly, we do not know how many women had miscarriages after being exposed to radiation.

As for the long-term consequences, seemingly good news came in 2015 from the Radiation Effects Research Foundation (RERF) in Hiroshima, which reported that children born to the atomic bomb survivors have not shown an increase in cancer or non-cancer deaths in relation to their parents' ionising radiation exposure. Dr Eric J. Grant of RERF said that researchers had found no association between maternal gonadal (ovarian) radiation exposure and risk of cancer deaths or non-cancer deaths among the offspring. However, this news has to be taken with a pinch of salt. As Dr David J. Branner, director for the Centre for Radiological Research at Columbia University Medical Centre in New York said, "Absence of evidence is not evidence of absence".

Radiation-induced germ line mutations have occurred in other species exposed to the fallout, although the mutation rates are low, and it is unlikely that human beings would have a fundamentally different response to such exposure. It was the longest study of its kind in the world, requiring the long-term cooperation of survivors and their children. The research was supported by the Japanese Ministry of Health, Labour and Welfare, and the US Department of Energy, and also had partial support of the US National Academy of Sciences.

Ironically, the authors who published this study in the medical journal *Lancet*, in 2015, did not recognise the contribution by the government of the United States in cooperation with the governments of the United Kingdom and Canada under the Manhattan Project, in the form of two nuclear bombs, 'Little Boy', dropped at Hiroshima on 6th August, 1945, and 'Fat Man' dropped at Nagasaki on 9th August, 1945.

So, despite these data, the question remains, how much radiation is safe?

The measure of radiation is expressed in terms of a unit called a 'sievert' (Sv), named after a Swedish medical physicist, Rolf Maximilian Sievert.

One sievert is equal to one joule of energy absorbed by a kilogram of human tissue[124]. One millisievert (mSv) is equal to 1,000th of this dose. One millionth of a sievert is called a 'microsievert' (μSv).

---

[124] Joule is a measure of energy named in honour of James Prescott Joule, an English physicist.

According to the Ionising Radiation Regulations 2017 (IRR17 by the HSE, or Health and Safety Executive, UK), a normal person is exposed to around 1 mSv dose of radiation per year to his or her whole body without any significant ill effects. For employees and trainees working with radiation (above the age of 18), the safe limit of radiation exposure to the whole body is up to 20 mSv. For the under 18s, who are working as an employee or trainee in areas where radioactivity is involved, the acceptable limit is 6 mSv.

Fortunately, the radiation emitted from most substances is much smaller than this amount.

So, let's see how radioactive our world really is.

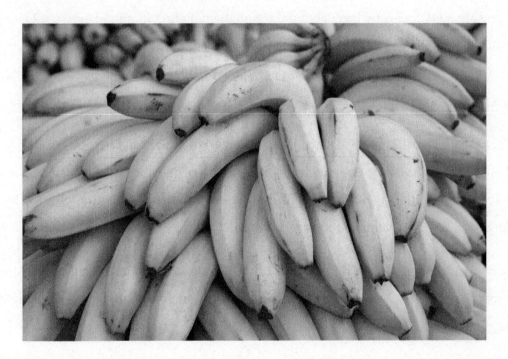

As we said earlier, all creatures great and small emit radiation. For example, an average human being would emit 0.05 mSv over a period of seven to eight hours from their body. An average banana (150 g or 5.3 oz in weight, in case you are wondering what an average for a banana is) would emit 0.1 mSv, twice as much as a human. The reason for this difference, despite the bigger size of a human being, is that the source of radiation in a human body is mostly the radioactive isotope carbon-14, but the major natural source of radioactivity in a banana (and most plant tissues) is an unstable isotope known as 'potassium-40' (^{40}K). As bananas and other plants have a higher concentration of potassium, the number of atoms that break down – releasing radiation – is higher compared to the number of atoms of carbon-14 (^{14}C) breaking down and releasing radioactivity in a human.

However, you do not have to stop eating bananas. Humans have developed a very effective system of keeping the dose and amount of potassium in their body fairy constant, due to a mechanism known as *homeostasis*. Homeostasis (*homeo*, 'same/similar' and *stasis*, 'stable') is maintaining a steady or stable state of internal physical and chemical conditions of the body despite changes in the environment. A simple example is our body temperature, which remains stable despite the cold or warm weather.

By this homeostatic system, any excess potassium absorbed from food is quickly compensated for by elimination of an equal amount. Radiation exposure due to eating a banana lasts only for a few hours after eating it because that is the time it takes for the normal potassium content of the body to be restored by the kidneys, which excretes the potassium in the urine.

Hence, eating or accompanying bananas is fairly safe. That is, unless you have a truck full of them – which is capable of causing a false alarm when passing through the radiation monitors used to detect the possible smuggling of nuclear material across borders or at ports. So, next time you are placed in charge of a truck or shipload of bananas crossing international borders, be aware that you might be stopped under suspicion of smuggling a nuclear weapon[125].

Measuring radiation emission from any substance can be hard to understand in terms of its relative hazard. To make it simple and interesting, let's measure it in terms of bananas[126]. We can call it the 'banana equivalent dose' (BED). One banana equivalent dose is the amount of radiation emitted by an average banana. So, let's measure life events in terms of bananas.

As an average human body emits 0.05 mSv over a period of seven to eight hours, eating an average banana, emitting 0.1 mSv of radiation, would be the same risk of radiation exposure as sleeping next to two people[127] in the same bed overnight.

Living within 50 miles of a coal-fuelled power plant for a year exposes us to 0.3 mSv (three bananas). Interestingly, living within 50 miles of a nuclear reactor power plant for one year would only expose you to 0.09 mSv, which is less than one banana. The reason for this dichotomy is that, thankfully, nuclear power plants employ rather strict radiation safety measures, such as thick concrete walls and lead shielding, reducing the amount of radiation leakage more effectively than those from a coal power plant.

Having an X-ray of your arm exposes you to 1 mSv, equivalent to 10 bananas.

Having a dental X-ray exposes you to 5 mSv, or 50 bananas.

---

[125] You have to be extra careful if your name starts with Mohammad and ends with Khan.

[126] I can't find the name of the genius who first coined this alternative measure, which has been around since the 1990s, but hats off to him/her.

[127] This is strictly in terms of radiation exposure and any additional risks to human health or morality cannot be measured in terms of banana equivalent doses.

If you keep safe and do not do anything risky, you are still exposed to background/general irradiation from the environment (remember we live in a radiant universe) and this is equal to 10 mSv a year, or the same as eating 100 bananas.

A flight from New York to Los Angeles exposes someone to 40 mSv, or 400 bananas. Interestingly, this is equal to the amount of extra radiation people living in Tokyo got from the Fukushima nuclear reactor accident. And you thought air travel was safe!

Having a chest X-ray involves 20 mSv, equivalent to 200 bananas.

Living in a stone, brick, or concrete building for one year exposes a person to 70 mSv or 700 banana equivalent doses.

A mammogram for detecting breast cancer involves 400 mSv, equal to consuming 4,000 bananas.

A computer tomography scan (CT scan) of the head would expose a person to 2 Sv, or 20,000 banana equivalent doses. A CT scan of the chest would expose one to 7 Sv, or 70,000 bananas (because a larger area of the body is exposed to the CT scan radiation, compared to the head). A whole-body CT scan would involve an exposure of around 10 Sv or a staggering 100,000 bananas.

Now, the question arises, how do we translate this exposure into a cancer risk factor? The answer is not straightforward, as it depends on your age, sex, and additional risk factors such as smoking or exposure to other carcinogens.

For example, the (lifetime) risk of developing cancer after a whole-body CT scan [128] is:

- *2.56% for a male and 4.78% for a female if the CT scan was done at birth.*

- *1.82% for a male and 3.38% for a female if the CT scan was done at the age of five years.*

- *The risk drops to 1.18% for a male and 2.06% for a female at the age of 15 years.*

- *At the age of 50 years the risk is 0.59% for a male and 0.74% for a female.*

- *For exposure at the age of 80 years the risk is 0.1% for a male and 0.21% for a female.*

The reason for this difference between different age groups and sexes is that although the energy released by radiation causes the same type of DNA damage, the risk of cancer depends on how fast the body cells

---

[128] Or being exposed to 100,000 bananas all at one time.

redivide and how long they continue to divide. With every cell division, the chances of accumulating further DNA damage increases. Cancer takes years to develop and the longer one lives after a DNA damaging event, more are the chances of developing cancer. Hence the risk is highest at birth because you've got longer to live with a mutation and declines over one's lifetime.

Let's now talk about a common source of environmental radioactivity – an invisible radioactive gas, radon.

8.1.1 Radioactive Radon

You may have heard of radon gas, but not given it much thought. Depending on where you live, you might want to look into it.

The year was 1984 and Stanley Watras, unknowingly, was destined for international fame. Mr. Watras worked as a construction engineer at Limerick Nuclear Power Plant, Pottstown, Pennsylvania, USA.

For several days, every time Mr. Watras went in or out of the still-under-construction nuclear power plant, he set off the radiation monitors. This was bizarre because the power plant was not yet fuelled and so it was impossible for Stanley to have picked up any radioactive material from the site. Despite being decontaminated and sent home 'clean' each evening, he would appear the next day only to trigger off the radiation monitors again. Suspicion grew that he might be bringing nuclear contamination from home. When an investigative team checked his house, they found amazingly high levels of radon gas (100,000 Bq/m^3)[129] in the basement. Typically, you would expect levels of 100 Bq/m^3 in an average dwelling.

To have an idea of how toxic the radiation levels were in his house, it is estimated that living in his home was equivalent to smoking 2,700 cigarettes (135 packs of 20 cigarettes per pack) a day. This meant he and his family had increased the risk of developing lung cancer by 13–14%.

Radon is a radioactive, colourless, odourless, and tasteless, naturally occurring noble gas. It is one of the densest substances that remains a gas under normal conditions and is considered to be a health hazard due to its radioactivity. So dense is radon that its breakdown products are all solid in nature (polonium, lead, and bismuth).

Radon's main source is from the breakdown of uranium. Uranium has been present since the earth was formed and its most common isotope has a very long half-life of 4.5 billion years (half-life is the time required for one half of the atoms to decay). Uranium breaks down into radium (the father of radon), which

---

[129] A becquerel (or Bq for short) is equal to one radioactive isotope breaking down and releasing its radiation in one second.

has a half-life of 1,620 years. Radium decays to form radon, which has a much, much, shorter half-life of 3.8 days. Radon then further breaks down to polonium (half-life three minutes), polonium decaying into lead (half-life 27 minutes), and this in turn forms bismuth (half-life 19.7 minutes).

Radon is often the single largest contributor to an individual's background radiation dose and is the most variable radiation source from one location to another.

According to a 2003 report of the US Environmental Protection Agency's (EPA) assessment of risks from radon in homes, evidence shows a clear link between lung cancer and high concentrations of radon, with 21,000 radon-induced US cancer deaths per year, second only to cigarette smoking.

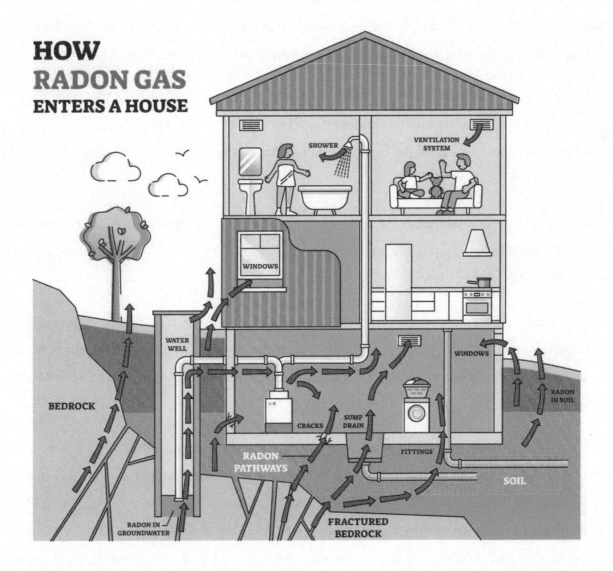

Radon is found in varying amounts all over the globe. The usual sources are regions with soils containing granite or shale, as these have a higher concentration of uranium. Every square mile of surface soil to a depth of 6 inches (2.6 km^2 to a depth of 15 cm) contains approximately 1 gram of radium.

Sand used in making concrete is the major source of radon in buildings. Radon gas from natural sources can accumulate in buildings, especially in confined areas such as attics and basements. It can also be found in caves, mines, some spring waters, and hot springs.

Fortunately, not only does it have a very short half-life but also its concentration decreases very quickly with increasing distance from where it is emitted. However, environmental factors like wind can affect its accumulation, and the concentration tends to be higher where there is less ventilation. As exposure to air reduces the concentration of radon, groundwater generally has higher concentrations of radon gas than surface water. Similarly, there will be more radon in saturated zones of soil.

Notorious areas in this regard are the towns of Boulder, Montana, USA, Misasa in Japan, and Bad Kreuznach in Germany, which have radium-rich springs that emit radon gas. In Merano and the village of Lurisia (Ligurian Alps in Italy), the activity of radon mineral water reaches 2,000 Bq per litre.

Radon exists in every US State and approximately 6% of American houses have elevated levels. The highest average radon concentrations are found in Iowa and in the Appalachians in southeastern Pennsylvania. Elsewhere, some of the highest readings have been recorded in Mallow, County Cork, Ireland.

Radon is also found in some petroleum sources. The products from the gas and oil industry often contain radium and its daughter products. A tell-tale sign is that radon decays to form solid isotopes, forming coatings on the inside of the pipework.

The effects of radon in food and drinking water are unknown. Following ingestion of radon dissolved in water, the biological half-life for removal of radon from the body ranges from 30 to 70 minutes. More than 90% of the absorbed radon is eliminated by breathing within 100 minutes. After 600 minutes (10 hours), only 1% of the absorbed amount remains in the body.

The health effects of high exposure to radon among miners was recognised as long ago as 1530 by Paracelsus, a Swiss physician and philosopher, who described a wasting disease of miners known as the *mala metallorum*[130]. Mineralogist Georg Agricola called it a 'mountain sickness' (*berauscht* in German) and recommended ventilation of mines to avoid it. In 1879 this wasting disease was finally identified as lung cancer by two other German researchers, Herting and Hesse, while investigating the health of miners from Schneeberg in Germany.

---

[130] A malady/malaise/disease related to metals.

Unsurprisingly, uranium mines usually have high concentrations of this gas. The first major studies with radon and health occurred in the context of uranium mining in the Joachimsthal region of Bohemia, and subsequently in the southwestern United States. Many uranium miners developed lung cancer and other pathologies as a result of high levels of exposure to radon in the mid-1950s. The increased incidence of lung cancer was particularly noticeable among Native American and Mormon miners because they usually have low rates of lung cancer. Over the decades, ventilation and other measures have been used to reduce radon levels in most affected mines that continue to operate. In recent years, the average annual exposure of uranium among miners has fallen to levels similar to the concentrations inhaled in some homes.

So, how does radon radiation cause cancer?

The isotope, radon-222, has been classified by the International Agency for Research and Cancer as being carcinogenic to humans. The primary route of exposure is inhalation. Two of radon's decay products, polonium-218 and 214, present a significant radiological hazard. If the gas is inhaled, the radon atoms decay in the airways of the lungs resulting in radioactive polonium, and ultimately lead atoms, attaching to the nearest tissue.

If dust or aerosol is inhaled then it carries radon decay products with it, and the deposition pattern in the respiratory tract depends on the behaviour of the particles in the lungs. If there is no co-existing lung pathology and the airways are healthy, particles get deposited higher up in the airways and are cleared by the body's mucociliary system (a combination of lung cells producing mucous, commonly known as *phlegm*, and brush-like cells which sweep it out of the lung). However, if the lungs are already damaged with exposure to dust and smoke – e.g., cigarette smoking – these particles are less effectively removed.

Radon atoms break down by emitting high-energy alpha radiation[131], with some associated gamma radiation, too, that can damage lung cells. It generates free radicals and causes DNA breakages and damage, leading to mutations that may eventually result in cancer.

The risk of lung cancer caused by smoking is much higher than the risk of lung cancer caused by indoor radon. In general, it is believed that exposure to radon and cigarette smoking are synergistic. They work as a team. This is because the decay products of radon often become attached to smoke and dust particles

---

[131] For the record, nuclear radiation is released from an atom in three common forms:

1. Alpha particles are the biggest and the heaviest, and comprise two protons and two neutrons. Due to their size and weight, they do not travel far and only damage nearby structures.
2. Beta particles are electrons which can travel farther than the big, chunky alpha particles.
3. Gamma rays are bursts of electromagnetic energy waves that can travel very far and penetrate through barriers. Their wavelength is shorter than X-rays.

and are then able to lodge in the lungs for a long period of time. There is also suspicion that radon exposure increases the risk of leukaemia.

Children are more prone to radon exposure because their respiratory rate is higher than that of adults, resulting in more gas exchange, and hence more radon is likely to be inhaled.

Health effects in children are similar to those of adults, predominantly including lung cancer and respiratory illnesses such as asthma, bronchitis, and pneumonia. There have been numerous studies assessing the link between radon exposure and childhood leukaemia, but the results are varied. DNA damage in cells has been noted in children exposed to high levels of radon and there is a significant increase in abnormal cells with chromosomal damage.

You might be surprised to learn that radon therapy has been used as a part of alternative medicine to treat arthritis and other conditions. 'Health mines' were established in the 20th and early 21st centuries in areas such as Basin and Montana, attracting people seeking relief from health problems such as arthritis through limited exposure to radioactive mine water.

Many places in the world offer radioactive water baths. For example, since 1906 it has been available in the Czech Republic in places like Jachymov. Radium-rich springs are also used in traditional Japanese medicine in Misasa, in the Tottori Prefecture.

Drinking therapy is applied in Badprambach, Germany. Inhalation therapy is carried out in Gasteiner-Heilstollen in Austria, in Kowari in Poland, and in Boulder in Montana, United States.

In the United States and Europe there are several radiation or radon spas where people sit (at their own risk) for minutes or hours in radon baths, sharing the belief that low doses of radiation will invigorate or energise them. The practice is controversial, at best because of the risk of high dose radiation to the body. Having said that, people do claim symptom relief from exposure to radon gas in air and water.

Nothing's an absolute evil in this world and so it is in the case with radon. As radon can damage cells, it has been produced commercially for use in radiation therapy to treat cancer. It is usually used in implantable seeds made of gold or glass. The gold seeds are produced by filling a long tube with radon pumped from a radium source. The tube is then divided into short sections by cutting. The gold layer keeps the radon within and filters out the alpha and beta radiations, while allowing the gamma rays to escape.

The gamma rays produced by radon and the first short-lived elements of its decay chain (lead, bismuth, polonium-214 and 218) are the main sources of radiation treatment. As radon and its first decay products are very short lived, the seed is left in place. After 12 half-lives (43 days), radioactivity is one 2,000th of its original levels, mostly due to lead (Pb^{210}) whose half-life is 22.3 years.

Since the recognition of radon as a carcinogen, you'll be glad to know that many steps have been taken to minimise its damage to human health.

In the USA, the Federal Radon Action Plan, known as 'FRAP', was created in 2010 and launched in 2011. The goal set forth by FRAP was to eliminate radon-induced cancer that can be prevented by expanding radon testing, mitigating higher levels of radon exposure, and developing radon-resistant construction.

FRAP was concluded in 2016 as a National Radon Action Plan (NRAP) took over, with the same aims plus the target of reducing radon risk in five million homes and saving 3,200 lives by 2020.

Iowa has the highest average radon concentration in the United States. Studies performed there have demonstrated a 50% increased lung cancer rate with prolonged radon exposure above the action level of the US Environmental Protection Agency (EPA).

Based on studies carried out by National Academy of Sciences in the United States, radon would thus be the second leading cause of lung cancer after smoking, and it accounts for 15,000 to 22,000 cancer deaths per year there alone. The EPA says that radon is the number one cause of lung cancer among non-smokers.

In the United Kingdom, residential radon exposure would be, after cigarette smoking, the second most frequent cause of lung cancer deaths according to models. Some 83.9% of deaths are attributed to smoking only, 1.0% to radon only, and 5.5% to a combination of radon and smoking.

The World Health Organisation has recommended a radon reference concentration of 100 Bq/m^3. The European Union recommends that action should be taken starting from concentrations of 4 Bq/m^3 for older dwellings and 200 Bq/m^3 for newer ones.

After publication of data from the combined 'North American and European Pooling Studies', Health Canada proposed a new guideline that lowers their action level from 800 to 200 Bq/m^3. The EPA strongly recommends action for any dwelling with a concentration higher than 148 Bq/m^3 and encourages action starting at 74 Bq/m^3. The EPA also recommends that all homes should be monitored for radon. If testing shows levels less than 160 Bq/m^3 then no action is necessary. For levels of 800 Bq/m^3 or higher, the homeowner should consider some type of procedure to decrease indoor radon levels. For instance, opening the windows once a day can cut the mean radon concentration by 75%. The EPA recommends homes be modified if an occupant's long-term exposure will be an average of 148 Bq/m^3 or more.

The EPA's radon risk level tables include comparisons to other risks encountered in life. They estimate that, nationally, 8% to 12% of dwellings are above their maximum safe levels.

For radon concentration in drinking water, the World Health Organisation issued guidelines in 1988 that remedial action should be considered when the radon activity exceeds 100 kBq/m^3, and remedial action should be considered without long delay if it exceeds 400 kBq/m^3.

So, how do we go about testing for radon gas in our homes?

Radon test kits are commercially available and come in several types. The short-term test kits used for screening purposes are inexpensive and in many cases are free. Discounted test kits can also be purchased online through some government programmes. The kit includes a device (collector) that the user hangs in the lowest liveable floor of their dwelling for 2–7 days. Charcoal canisters are another type of short-term radon test kit and are designed to be used for 2–4 days. The user then sends the collector to a laboratory for analysis. Both types of devices are passive, meaning they do not need power to function. The accuracy of the residential radon test depends on the lack of ventilation in the house when the sample is being obtained. Thus, the occupant will be instructed not to open windows during the test.

Long-term kits, collecting for three months to up to one year, are also available. An open land test kit can test radon emissions from land before construction begins.

What if you find your house has high levels of radon? What can you do about it?

Usually, the air pressure is lower inside a house than it is outside, and so a home acts as a vacuum, drawing radon gas in through cracks in the foundations or other openings, such as ventilation systems. Generally, the indoor radon concentration increases as ventilation rates decrease. In a well-ventilated home, the radon concentrations tend to align with outdoor values, typically 10 Bq/m^3, ranging from one to 100 Bq/m^3. Levels in indoor air can be lowered in several ways from sealing cracks in the floors and walls to increasing the ventilation rate of the building. More sophisticated methods include installing floor linings or slabs, crawl spaces, or basement ventilation systems, pumps, and positive pressure systems.

With the half-life of radon being 3.8 days, once the source is removed the hazard will be greatly reduced within approximately one month (seven half-lives).

Positive pressure ventilation systems can be combined with a heat exchanger to recover energy in the process of exchanging air with the outside. Simply exhausting basement air to the outside is not necessarily a viable solution, as this can draw radon gas into a dwelling. Homes built with a crawl space may benefit from a radon collector installed under a radon barrier or membrane (a sheet of plastic or laminated polyethylene film that covers the crawl space floor).

Water is another source of radon. If radon is present in a private well, installing either a point-of-use or point-of-entry solution may be necessary. Point-of-entry systems usually involve a granular, activated carbon filter or an aeration system, and both measures can help to remove radon before it enters the home's water distribution system.

So, despite natural radon gas posing a significant hazard to us in terms of cancer risk, there are ways to mitigate or remove the hazard.

8.1.2   Other Sources of Radiation

The last section might have got you wondering, or reminded you, about other sources of radiation that we encounter during our lives. Here's a quick overview.

Airport Scanners

Most airport body scanners use either radio waves or ionising radiation, but in both cases the doses are so small that they do not raise the risk of cancer significantly.

Mobile Phones

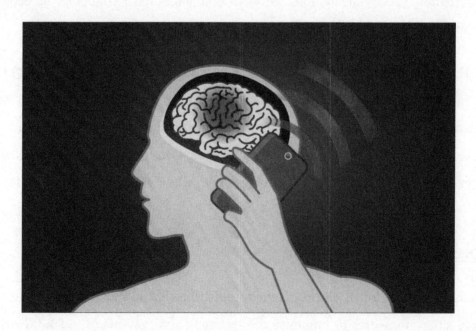

Mobile phones generate non-ionising radiation. So far, the large studies carried out to detect any link of mobile phone use and cancer have proved inconclusive. However, as mentioned earlier, the lapsed time between exposure to any kind of DNA-damaging factor and cancer development can be decades, and so it is still too early to determine whether mobile phone usage can significantly raise the risk of developing cancer. The general consensus is that the radiation given off by mobile phones is very weak and cannot directly cause cancer.

Nevertheless, most health authorities recommend avoiding heavy mobile phone use; for example, by using a hands-free set and keeping calls short. There is a significant lack of research into the effects of mobile phone use on children, and so the advice is that children under the age of 16 should only use mobile phones for essential calls. Looking at data for links to cancer with other causes of radiation, it would be sensible to conclude that the risk of cell damage by radiation from mobile phones would be higher at younger ages and among females.

Power Lines

Power lines are a source of non-ionising radiation. The radiation is a low-frequency electromagnetic radiation and does not have sufficient energy to damage cells or cause DNA mutation. Some studies have suggested a link between exposure to magnetic fields and small increase in the risk of childhood leukaemia, but the evidence for this is limited.

Computer Screens

Computer screens and monitors emit electromagnetic radiation at low levels that are considered safe according to international recommendations. Modern computers have conductor screens and the static field emitted is similar to background radiation from the rest of the universe.

The modern LED and plasma screens emit much lower radiation than the old cathode ray tube TV screens. For an average laptop screen, keeping it at a distance of around 12 inches (1 foot) substantially reduces the level of radiation reaching you. The bigger the screen, the further away you should sit from it to reduce the radiation dose. Keep moving back as you buy bigger screens until you have your back against the wall. You will then realise how pointless it is to buy a big screen when you have to move further away from it to be safe.

Microwave Ovens

Microwave ovens produce a lot of electromagnetic radiation, but in most countries the manufacturing standards specify safety measures to minimise the leakage from new ovens. If followed, according to these safety measures the amount of radiation leaking outside the oven is almost non-detectable. The leakage also drops as you move further away from the oven, so it is good practice to stay as far away as possible when a microwave is working. However, for some inexplicable reason, humans tend to stand next to a microwave and stare blankly at it, as if mesmerised by the device, while it is emitting electromagnetic radiation.

Cooking food in the microwave may not cause cancer, but it does affect the nutritional value of food, especially vegetables and fruit.

8.2   Rays of Sunshine (UV Radiation)

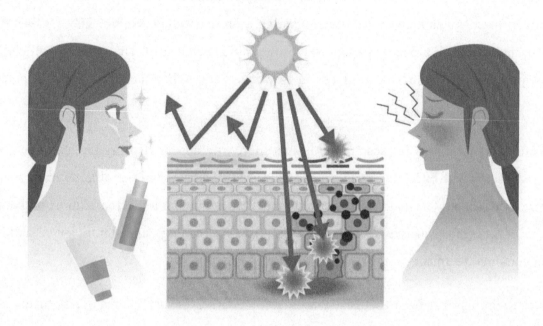

Earlier, in section 3.1, I mentioned how thousands of years ago man's migration to less sunny climes led, over time, to reduced skin pigmentation in order to maintain the ability to produce vitamin D – a useful evolutionary adaptation. But in recent times our fondness for lying in the sun has led to an explosion in the incidence of skin cancer, especially (but not exclusively) in the fairer-skinned.

The common types of skin cancer include basal cell carcinoma, squamous cell carcinoma, and melanoma.

Basal cell carcinoma (BCC) is the oxymoron[132] of cancers. It grows very slowly over years on easily visible parts of the body, usually sun-exposed areas such as the face, grows locally, does not spread to other parts of the body, at worse invades the underlying structures locally, and is very responsive to treatment with cure rates close to 100%.

---

[132] An oxymoron is a phrase in which two words with opposite meanings are brought together. For example, small crowd, fully empty, tragic comedy, liquid gas, original copies, clearly misunderstood, and the mother of all oxymorons … happily married.

Squamous cell carcinoma (SCC) is not as well behaved as BCC but does tend to be very responsive to treatment with high cure rates.

Melanoma, also known as *malignant melanoma*, abbreviated as *MM*, is a cancer of the pigment or melanin-producing cells, and is the bad boy of skin and all other cancers. It's a pretty ugly disease. It grows fast, is often diagnosed at an advanced stage, spreads far and wide, is refractory to treatment, and even when responding has a tendency to become resistant over time.

Skin comprises many types of cells, two of which are very common. The first are known as *keratinocytes*, forming part of the main skin structure and containing a protein called *keratin*. These, when damaged, mostly go through a natural process of apoptosis (programmed cell death). The other type of cell, called a *melanocyte*, produces the pigment that gives our skin its colour. When damaged, these cells tend to be preserved.

We will focus mainly on MM because not only is it more troublesome (to say the least) but because it shares the risk factor with BCC and SCC, so avoiding it also helps avoid the other two. Its incidence is increasing worldwide, but fortunately the mortality rates are beginning to decrease, most probably due to effective cancer prevention, increased early detection efforts (screening), and significant breakthroughs in advanced melanoma treatment.

There is overwhelming evidence to suggest that ultraviolet light exposure is a major risk factor and cause. The majority of melanomas develop on sun-exposed skin, particularly in areas that are more susceptible to sunburn. Individuals who have naturally dark skin or whose skin darkens easily on sun exposure have lower rates of melanoma.

Ultraviolet radiation is classified as a carcinogen for humans.

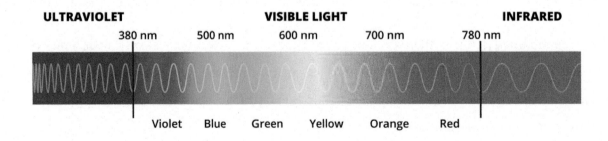

UV light is a component of natural sunlight comprising light of wavelengths from about 40 to 400 nm. While it is necessary for the production of vitamin D, a component – ultraviolet B radiation (UVB, wavelength 29 to 320 nm) – appears to be much more strongly associated with the development of melanoma, compared to ultraviolet A (UVA whose wavelength is from 320 to 400 nm). UVB radiation is most intense at the equator, whereas ultraviolet A intensity varies less across latitudes. The Earth's ozone layer does a good job in reducing the amount of UV reaching the planet's surface, and depletion of the ozone layer from pollution has led to greater levels of UV reaching us.

Melanocytes produce the pigment called *melanin* which has a protective function in the skin against light. So, whenever the ultraviolet radiation intensity increases, the melanocytes start to divide and increase in numbers. Recurrent damage by ultraviolet radiation puts them at risk of incomplete DNA repair and subsequent mutations may lead to the formation of a malignant melanoma.

In the United States, melanoma is the fifth leading cause of cancer in men and women. Overall, 96,480 new cases were diagnosed in 2019. The incidence varies greatly among different ethnic groups. For non-Hispanic whites it is 27 per 100,000, for the Hispanics five per 100,000, and among the blacks and Asians/Pacific Islanders one per 100,000. Historically, the incidence has been increasing. Between the early 1970s and 2000, the incidences of melanoma in Central Europe increased from three to four cases per 100,000 inhabitants per year to 10 to 15 cases per 100,000 inhabitants per year.

The incidence of melanoma is the highest in equatorial regions and decreases proportionately with distance from the equator. This corresponds to lower levels of ultraviolet exposure. The incidence of melanoma in Queensland, Australia, is the highest in the world at 72 per 100,000 per year. Melanoma is rare in children and adolescents and approximately 90% of these cases are in those who are 10 years or older.

Timing and pattern of sun exposure appears to be important for the development of all skin cancers, especially melanoma. Non-melanoma cancers are associated with cumulative sun exposure and occur most frequently in areas maximally exposed to the sun, such as the face, back of the hands, and forearms. In contrast, melanomas tend to be associated with intensity of the sun exposure. Intermittent sun exposure and sunburn can frequently occur in areas exposed to the sun only sporadically; for example, the back in men and legs in women.

Intermittent sun exposure may not be relevant for all body sites as, for example, melanomas of the head and neck are more frequent in patients with occupational sun exposure. Exposure in early life seems particularly important. Individuals who have had five or more severe sunburns during childhood or early adolescence have an estimated twofold greater risk of developing melanoma. Migrating from northern to more equatorial latitudes at a young age is also associated with an increased risk.

Unfortunately, people who have had other kinds of skin cancers, such as basal cell or squamous cell carcinomas, appear not only to have an increased risk of developing melanoma but also an increased risk of dying from it. However, evidence also suggests that a decrease in recreational sun exposure following the diagnosis of primary melanoma (use of preventive measures) can significantly diminish the chances of a second primary melanoma.

The extent of a person's skin pigmentation and their tanning ability also influence their risk of developing skin cancer, but they're not the only features. People who have red or blonde hair, blue or green eyes, a freckling tendency, and poor tanning ability, have a higher risk due to increased skin sensitivity. Having a light skin prototype, blue eye colour, red hair, and high freckle density is associated with a two to fourfold increase in risk. Skin moles (known as *naevi* in medical parlance) are usually an indicator of increased skin sensitivity.

People who have high numbers of naevi or have atypical naevi are at increased risk of melanoma and hence should be offered more sun protection, especially in childhood, when the risk of exposure to sun can lead to high incidences of melanoma later in life.

Race plays an important role. Although melanomas are very rare in black patients, if they do occur, they tend to be more aggressive and the 5-year survival rates are less for black people (69%), compared to white patients (93%). The melanomas in black people often occur in non-exposed areas. Age and social economic factors also tend to affect the prognosis, being poorer with more advanced disease and worse survival in people above the age of 50, especially white males and poor social economic groups. The reason could be that males over the age of 50, and belonging to a poor social economic group, are less self-aware of their skin changes.

Based on these factors we can establish general criteria for the high-risk category, e.g., who need screening for early detection of melanomas. Hence, white males above the age of 50, people with total naevus count above 50, one or more atypical or dysplastic naevi, family history of melanoma, significant childhood or adolescent sun exposure (including at least one blistering or painful sunburn under the age of 30 years), chronic outdoor activities without adequate sunscreen, indoor tanning bed use, immunosuppression (especially chronic use of medications that suppress the immune system), and red hair phenotype, would fall into a high-risk category.

The high-risk group would benefit from screening and education about self-awareness for detecting melanomas. Regular screening done by clinicians is also beneficial. The importance of intensive public and professional awareness has been demonstrated by multiple studies. Data from a large year-long population screening exercise in Germany, the 'Skin Cancer Research to provide Evidence for Effectiveness of Screening in Northern Germany' (SCREEN) project, showed that clinician-based skin examination was associated with a melanoma mortality reduction five years after the screening programme, although the mortality reduction did not persist in longer-term follow-ups. This is because screening is only as beneficial as the treatment options available. Detecting a disease earlier with limited curative options will not prolong life. Hence, detecting a melanoma very early when it can be surgically removed *completely*, followed by adequate education and awareness to reduce the risk factor for recurrent disease, could have an impact, but detecting it at a later stage may not make much of a difference.

A question I am often asked is how to identify and distinguish a potential melanoma from other skin marks (e.g., freckles and moles). Here's a quick guide to moles (section 8.2.1) and guide to diagnosis (section 8.2.2).

8.2.1 Moles (Naevi)

The term *naevus* is applied to a number of conditions caused by neoplasias and hyperplasias (proliferation) of melanin-producing cells (melanocytes), as well as a number of pigmentation disorders – both hypermelanotic (containing increased melanin, the pigment responsible for skin colour) and hypomelanotic (containing decreased melanin). They can be found in the superficial layer of skin, epidermis, where they're described as *junctional melanocytic naevi*, or in the deeper layer, the dermis, known as *interdermal melanocytic naevi*. Compound naevi occur in both the epidermis and dermis. For completeness, another type is called *atypical naevi* (also known as *dysplastic naevi*). This type has variable pigmentation and irregular borders.

Congenital Naevi - Congenital Melanocytic Naevi (CMN) are classically present at birth or within the first few months of life. One to two percent of newborn infants have congenital naevi. Large or giant CMN are rarer, occurring in approximately one in 20,000 births. For people with large CMN, the risk of developing melanoma is estimated to be 2 to 5% over a lifetime with most melanomas occurring in the first five years of life.

Atypical Naevi – Atypical naevi are not cancerous but benign in nature. They look like melanoma lesions due to their asymmetry, irregular borders, multiple colours, and size (diameter more than 5 mm). Although these are not cancerous, they act as a marker of an increased risk of melanoma, especially in individuals with numerous naevi and/or family history of melanoma.

An analysis of observational studies showed that the relative risk[133] of melanoma associated with atypical naevi was 1.5 for the presence of a single atypical naevus, and 6.36 for five atypical naevi, versus no atypical naevi, clearly suggesting that the more atypical naevi moles an individual has, the greater their risk of developing a melanoma.

FAMMM Syndrome and Atypical Mole Syndrome – Some inherited cases of melanoma occur in the setting of two syndromes: familial atypical multiple mole and melanoma (FAMMM) syndrome, and atypical mole syndrome (AMS). With FAMMM syndrome, the lifetime cumulative incidence of melanoma approaches a staggering 100%. In atypical mole syndrome (AMS), sometimes also known as *dysplastic naevus syndrome* (DNS), patients tend to have 50 to 100 or more naevi, at least one of which is 8 mm or larger in size, and at least one with atypical features, without personal or family history of melanoma.

Having a personal history of melanoma is associated with a higher risk of developing a second primary melanoma.

A Swedish study, which looked at cases from 1958 to 2010, found that patients with either familial or sporadic melanoma have a two to threefold increased risk of a subsequent melanoma and that the risk remains stable for patients with two or more previous melanomas. Similarly, a population-based study in the United States has shown that individuals with previous skin melanoma were more likely to develop a second skin melanoma or non-skin melanomas like oral melanoma and vaginal/exo-cervical melanoma. The risk was highest in the first year after diagnosis, two to 11% at five years, and tended to persist over time. However, having a safer lifestyle and preventative measures could reduce this risk.

In fact, about 10% of melanomas have a familial (inherited) aspect to them. There seems to be considerable genetic variability among such families, suggesting that multiple genes contribute to the risk. The causes are usually defects in both tumour suppressor and tumour promoter genes, also known as *oncogenes* (oncogenes are genes that in certain circumstances can transform a cell into a tumour cell – you can think of them as 'traitors' if you like).

An important culprit is a gene residing on chromosome 9b, the tumour suppressor gene CDKN2A[134]. Mutation of this is associated with multiple cases of melanoma in a family.

---

[133] Relative risk is the ratio of probability of an outcome (e.g., lung cancer) in a group exposed to a risk factor (e.g., smokers) to the probability of it happening in an unexposed group (e.g., non-smokers).
[134] Also called *P16INK4A* or *MTS1* (multiple tumour suppressor 1).

A second culprit is a gene found on chromosome 16q24. This is known as *melanocortin-1 receptor gene* (MC1R) and its variants associated with red hair and fair skin phenotype are known risk factors for melanoma.

The third is a BAP1 mutation with a propensity for uveal[135] and cutaneous (skin) melanomas, and other internal malignancies[136].

8.2.2 Identifying Melanomas

MELANOMA

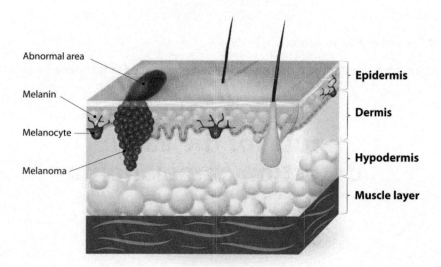

Most melanomas arise as a superficial indolent (painless) tumour which is confined to the upper layers of the skin (epidermis). They remain here for many years and tend to grow sideways (horizontal or radial growth). In this phase they are almost always curable by surgical excision alone.

Later on, it infiltrates deep into the skin (dermis) in what is known as the 'vertical growth phase' and finally becomes metastatic, spreading to other parts of the body. Melanomas occur in both sun-exposed and non-sun exposed areas. The non-sun exposed area melanomas are difficult to detect and less responsive to available treatment due to differences in tumour biology.

---

[135] Uvea is the pigmented part of the eye which gives the eye its colour. As melanoma occurs in pigment (melanin)-producing cells, it can develop in the eye too.

[136] Described in an autosomal dominant tumour predisposition syndrome.

Many tools have been developed to help clinicians and patients identify lesions to evaluate further for melanoma. The term 'ugly duckling', the ABCDE rule of melanoma, and the Glasgow 7-point checklist can help identify them, so let's examine each in turn.

The ugly duckling sign refers to an ugly, pigmented lesion that looks different to surrounding naevi (moles), maybe brown or pink.

The ABCDE criteria is valuable for educating patients and clinicians:

'A' stands for asymmetry.

'B' stands for border irregularities.

'C' stands for colour variegation (different colours within the same region).

'D' stands for diameter of 6 mm or more.

'E' stands for enlargement or evolution of colour change, shape, or symptoms.

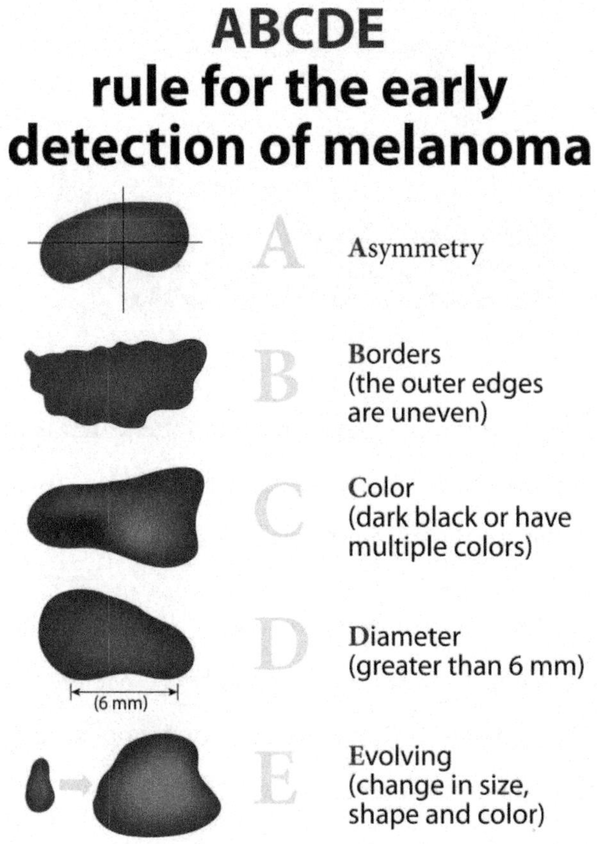

ABCDE
rule for the early
detection of melanoma

A — Asymmetry

B — Borders (the outer edges are uneven)

C — Color (dark black or have multiple colors)

D — Diameter (greater than 6 mm) (6 mm)

E — Evolving (change in size, shape and color)

For a patient with a lesion that meets at least one of the criteria, referral to a dermatologist for evaluation is indicated, and may include a biopsy being taken. However, melanomas in pre-pubertal and pubertal children often lack the conventional ABCDE criteria and may be clinically amelanotic (non-pigmented).

The Glasgow 7-point checklist is used as a tool for early detection of melanoma by both patients and clinicians. If a patient observes at least one major feature or at least three minor features detailed below, the patient should seek professional advice. If a clinician notes these during examination, then further evaluation of the lesion is warranted.

Major Features (Evaluate Further if at Least One is Present):

1) Change in size or a new lesion

2) Change in colour

3) Change in shape

Minor Features (Evaluate Further if at Least three are Present):

1) Inflammation

2) Bleeding or crusting

3) Sensory change

4) Lesion diameter 7 mm or more

Detecting melanoma in children and adolescents is tricky because their melanomas are different from adults (called the *spitz melanoma* type) and most of these will lack the conventional ABCDE features. In addition, the evolving lesion criteria may not be helpful at an age in which the occurrence of new, common naevi (moles) is normal. Additional paediatric criteria (paediatric ABCD and CUP criteria) have therefore been proposed to be used in combination with the conventional ABCDE rule:

Paediatric ABCD and CUP criteria

A = amelanotic (non-pigmented)

B = bleeding, bump

C = colour uniformity

D = de novo, any diameter

CUP: C = colour of pink or red or changing; U = ulceration, upward thickening; P = pyogenic granuloma-like lesion, pop-up of new lesions.

The ABCD CUP criteria are more useful for children than the adult criteria. For example, if a new pink or red papule (small pimple or swelling on the skin) is found on a child, it is important to consider associated features such as bleeding, history of trauma, itching or pain, growth or change over time, or similar lesions elsewhere, in the decision of whether to clinically monitor or biopsy a particular lesion. Excisional biopsy usually involves cutting out the melanoma, including the subcutaneous fat with a small 2 mm rim of normal appearing skin. The alternative, superficial 'shave biopsies', are not generally recommended because the full length of the lesion is required to determine maturation of melanocytes, to evaluate the base of the lesion, and to obtain and accurate measure of the tumour thickness.

If a melanoma is caught in the early stage when it is confined to the superficial layer of the skin it could be treated surgically and potentially cured by this treatment. The 5-year survival rate averages over 90%. The chance of survival is greater if the tumour is thin and not very deep.

In addition to the above guidelines for identifying melanomas, others are also produced by the American Cancer Society, the US Preventive Services Task Force (USPSTF), the American Academy of Dermatology, the Cancer Council of Australia, the Canadian Cancer Society, the Melanoma Genetics Consortium, and the American Society of Clinical Oncologists, all of which are helpful in guidance for screening and early detection of melanoma.

The next question to address is, what can we do to avoid or minimise the harmful effects of UV light exposure? There are some obvious, well-known ways, and some less obvious ones too, but how well do they really work?

8.2.3   Preventive Measures

The primary prevention of melanoma involves **reduction in exposure** to ultraviolet radiation from both natural and artificial sources. Public awareness through health campaigns has proved worthwhile. Since this intervention has been in place, a definite decline has been observed in incidences of invasive melanoma in Australia and the United States.

Tightly woven fabrics and dark colours confer the highest ultraviolet protection when outdoors. Specially designed ultraviolet **protection clothing**, having an ultraviolet protection factor (UPF) ranging from 15 to 50 are commercially available and can be worn while swimming or exposure to the sun. **Hats** are clearly useful, provided again that they are made from material that blocks UV. **Sunglasses** help to protect the eyes, provided they contain lenses with UV filters. Simply wearing shaded glasses (no UV filter) may, in fact, be more damaging to your eyes, as the shading encourages the pupils to dilate to let in more light, and so the exposure to UV may be increased if not filtered out.

Window glass provides a variable degree of ultraviolet protection. This has resulted in the introduction of special filters for ultraviolet A and infrared radiation. **Window films** can also be applied to windows of cars and are commercially available.

The major method of protection is the use of **sunscreens** (creams, oils, lotions) with a sun protection factor (SPF) of 15 for everyday use, and at least SPF 30 (better to use a higher SPF like 50) for intense sun exposure. The risk is highest during midday hours from **10 am to 4 pm**. To achieve the stated level of protection, sunscreens often have to be re-applied at intervals, or after swimming etc. Nowadays, cosmetics and moisturisers are made with broad-spectrum sunscreens too, which offer protection.

The question arises, how effective are using sunscreens?

Evidence from studies of Caucasian school children who were randomly assigned to receive either SPF 30 broad-spectrum sunscreens, with instructions to apply it if sun exposure was expected to last 30 minutes or longer, or who were not offered any intervention, showed that children using sunscreen developed fewer naevi (moles) over a 3-year period (median count 24 versus 28 without sunscreen). The use was more beneficial for freckled children in the intervention group. These children developed 30 to 40% fewer naevi than those in the control group.

Similar studies using a physical barrier (clothing) showed that 12-year-old children who had been followed up for more than six years developed fewer new naevi if they covered their backs all the time, compared to children who covered their backs less than 70% of the time.

Another study looking at children and their clothing pattern during holidays in sunny climates also confirmed that they developed fewer naevi if they were covered up well.

All these studies indicate that the use of skin protection, either by a sunscreen or clothing, reduces the hazardous effects of ultraviolet radiation exposure.

Now, here's a bit of a curved ball for you … **beards!**

There is strong evidence that a thick beard is capable of blocking out 95% of the ultraviolet rays from the sun. Not only do beards prevent the skin from getting burnt, they also help to protect the skin from getting cancer, including melanoma. Additional advantages include prevention of acne, being a natural filter by keeping out microscopic allergens from entering the nose (with a moustache) and hence preventing conditions such as hay fever and other allergies. Beards also keep some allergens and airborne bacteria out of the mouth, which could lead to better overall health. Hence facial hair acts as a filter. It also avoids discolouration of the skin, which stays healthier for longer. Beards are also associated with fewer wrinkles and give an impression of a younger look. There is evidence that it also helps lessen the possibility of gum disease by keeping the airborne bacteria out of the mouth.

In contrast, shaving opens up pores in the skin and can also cause cuts on the face that dry out the skin over time. Beards, on the other hand, keep the skin moist and avoid flaking of skin. However, growing a thick beard is not a practical possibility for everyone, especially younger women! Whether a face mask would offer the same benefit has not yet been studied.

Many vitamins, minerals, anti-inflammatory, antioxidant, and phytochemicals, along with targeted agents, are being studied for chemo prevention of pre-malignant lesions. They are thought to help stop progression of these lesions to invasive cancers, and have been evaluated as a means of primary prevention. So far, none have proven to prevent melanoma in clinical trials, but the search continues and in future we might be able to have effective agents available.

Vitamin D is known to have an antiproliferative and pro-apoptotic effect. Sun exposure is necessary for the synthesis of 25-hydroxyvitamin D in the skin. This intermediate is transformed to its biologically active form under conditions of physiologic demand for calcium and phosphorus. The potential health benefits of supplemental dietary vitamin D continue to be explored. However, so far studies have not shown any association between serum levels of vitamin D and risk of melanoma. At best, studies on the impact of dietary vitamin D and risk of melanoma have come up with conflicting results. When studied in the laboratory test tube (in vitro) and among animal models, like mice (in vivo), it has been suggested that there is protective effect of vitamin D on melanoma. In addition, some studies have shown that the risk of melanoma reduces for individuals who have high vitamin D intake. It is possible that the combination of calcium plus vitamin D might be more beneficial in a subgroup of patients, especially women with a history of non-melanoma skin cancer (NMSC). They might benefit from a combination of vitamin D[137] and calcium and have up 57% fewer melanomas than women who are not taking these supplements.

In one study, the use of oral vitamin B3 (nicotinamide) 500 mg supplements twice daily for 12 months interestingly resulted in a 13% reduction of actinic keratosis and a 23% reduction of non-melanocytic skin cancers. This has given rise to hope that it could also influence the risk of melanoma, but further research needs to be done in this regard.

---

[137] Vitamin D deficiency is one of the most overlooked health problems. Vitamin D plays an important role in bone health and immunity against diseases. Its deficiency leads to a multitude of symptoms such as generalised aches and pains, which often baffle the patients and doctors alike. The human body needs exposure to sunshine to make vitamin D. Our modern lifestyle of staying indoors in centrally heated/ cooled environment perpetuates this deficiency. This is most evident by studies from Saudi Arabia (a very sunny country) which showed that 60% of their healthy population (aged 18–80 years) suffers from Vitamin D deficiency.

Other candidates for therapeutic prevention of melanoma include pigmentation enhancers, DNA repair enzymes, additional vitamins and minerals, and phytochemicals (plant-derived biological active compounds), for which research is ongoing.

As it's always good to end on a positive note, I do have some good news. Use of non-steroidal anti-inflammatory drugs (NSAIDs), like aspirin, do seem to offer benefit. Several case-controlled studies found a protective effect of aspirin and other non-steroidal anti-inflammatory drugs for melanoma. The risk reduction ranged from 13 to 50%, depending on the frequency and duration of use. The greatest benefit was achieved for long-term, continuous use of low-dose aspirin, which is commonly prescribed for people to prevent the recurrence of heart attacks and in other conditions.

Even better, multiple combined analyses of large observational studies (including 850,000 patients) have shown a protective effect for caffeinated coffee (but not for decaffeinated coffee). Generally, the risk was reduced by 4.5% for one cup of coffee per day increment compared with no consumption. The protective effects of caffeinated coffee seemed to be more significant in women compared to men.

A discussion of UV light and melanoma wouldn't be complete without a brief resume of other risk factors that have emerged from various studies.

8.2.4 Other Risk Factors

1. PUVA Therapy

Oral methoxsalen (**psoralen**, a drug that sensitizes the skin to UVA radiation) and ultraviolet A radiation (together they are called 'PUVA') is used in the treatment of psoriasis and other skin conditions but is associated with a long-term increase in the risk of melanoma. The risk usually increases between 16 to 20 years after treatment and may be more than 12 times higher beyond 20 years after treatment. People receiving higher doses of PUVA treatment are at a higher risk.

2. Immunosuppression

People with suppressed immune systems can develop melanoma. These include those who've had an organ transplant and who are therefore receiving immunosuppressive therapy to prevent the rejection of their new organ. A study conducted with 90,000 renal transplant recipients in the United States, followed over a 10-year period, identified 246 patients with melanoma and a 3.6 times greater likelihood for the development of melanoma in organ transplant recipients compared with the general population.

3. Occupational exposure

Exposure to certain chemicals during work is associated with an increased risk of melanoma. These include polychlorinated biphenyls (PCBs are used in the manufacture of plastics), petroleum products, ionising radiation, and selenium.

4. Alcohol

A high consumption of alcohol compared with no or occasional drinking can increase the risk of melanoma. The risk was found to be 55% higher for individuals drinking 50 grams of alcohol per day in a combined analysis of 16 studies including a total of over 6,000 patients.

5. Citrus Fruits

An analysis of data from over 100,000 individuals participating in the well-known Nurses' Health Study[138] found a modest increase in melanoma risk associated with high dietary intake of citrus fruit or juice, after looking for recognised risk factors such as family history, number of naevi, and number of lifetime blistering sunburns. One explanation for this bizarre phenomenon is that citrus fruits are a source of psoralens (please see above, under PUVA therapy). Hence citrus fruit on its own may not be harmful but exposure to harmful ultraviolet radiation along with high intake of fruit could increase the risk.

6. Parkinson's Disease

Parkinson's disease has been associated with increased risk of melanoma. One study involving more than 14,000 patients with Parkinson's disease found a statistically significant increase in incidence of melanoma in this population compared with the general population. A separate, Swedish study of Parkinson's disease also found a 60% higher risk of melanoma compared to those without Parkinson's. The results did not show a family history association, as the risk of melanoma was similar in siblings of the Parkinson's disease patients and those of the Parkinson's disease-free individuals. Importantly, so far, there is no evidence that the treatments for Parkinson's disease have any role to play in the development of melanoma. The increased risk for melanoma precedes the diagnosis and treatment of the neurological disorder. This is still an unsolved enigma but hopefully in the near future we will resolve it.

---

[138] Nurses' Health Study is a large observational study first launched in 1976 by Dr Frank Speizer in the USA.

7. Endometriosis

Studies have shown a statistically significant increase of melanoma in women with endometriosis. This is a condition caused by the appearance of endometrial tissue outside of the womb and which causes pelvic pain, and which can be severely debilitating.

8. With a History of Prostate Cancer

The United States Health Professional Follow-Up Study, including over 40,000 participants, found that a personal history of prostate cancer was associated with an increased risk of melanoma, when adjusted for age, body mass index, smoking, use of sildenafil (Viagra), skin prototype, naevus count, family history of melanoma, and history of sun exposure. The underlying mechanism is unknown.

Before concluding our discussion of UV light, there are two further potential risk factors that warrant discussion. These are very much 'man-made' in nature, reflecting some individuals' behaviour, and so we should view them as being the exercising of their 'free will', despite the risks. Here, I'm talking about skin bleaching and indoor tanning.

8.2.5   Skin Bleaching

There is mounting evidence that skin bleaching can be hazardous to human health and one of the suspected risks is that it can cause skin cancers, including melanoma, but more research needs to be done on this matter.

Skin bleaching is a cosmetic procedure for lightening the skin colour. It is a global phenomenon, practiced by people living in communities far and wide, including Africa, North and South America, Asia, Middle East, and Europe.

Agents used in skin bleaching include hydroquinone, topical steroids, mercurials, kojic acid[139], and sometimes even products such as a battery fluid and cement. These measures can lead to irritation of the skin, allergic contact dermatitis, infections, and systemic problems such as hypertension, diabetes mellitus, and renal disease.

More recently, there has been increasing use of glutathione for skin bleaching, especially in the United Kingdom. Glutathione is a tripeptide (combination of three [tri] protein chains) consisting of the amino

---

[139] Kojic acid is made by several species of fungi during the fermentation of rice to make *sake*, the Japanese rice wine. It inhibits pigment formation in plant and animal tissue.

acids cystine, glycine, and glutamate. The skin-lightening effects of glutathione are probably due to its antioxidant properties, and its ability to switch eumelanin production to pheomelanin, the type of melanin found in individuals with lighter skin tones[140].

Not a lot of research has been done scientifically for the use of glutathione parenterally (injected into the blood stream) to lighten skin. A small study of 30 subjects who received an oral lozenge formulation containing reduced l-glutathione as well as selenium, vitamin C, vitamin D3, vitamin E, and grape seed extract, demonstrated skin-lightening effects. There are no published guidelines for the appropriate dosing or treatment duration when using this agent for skin lightening. Adverse effects reported include neurotoxicity (nerve damage), renal (kidney), and hepatic (liver) toxicity, transient headaches, and skin eruptions such as Stevens-Johnson syndrome and toxic epidermal necrolysis (a severe form of skin reaction in which the skin rots away). Last but not least, given that glutathione plays an important role in mediating the switch from eumelanin to pheomelanin synthesis, there are theoretical concerns about long-term skin cancer risk.

8.2.6   Indoor Tanning

Commercial tanning for cosmetic and aesthetic purposes has been in vogue for a long time (since the 1920s). It is estimated that nearly one third of white women aged 18 to 25 have indoor tanning sessions in the United States, with approximately 15% engaging in frequent tanning sessions (10 or more per year). Indoor tanning is positively associated with sunburn, with 82% of indoor tanners reported to have at least one sunburn in 2015. Evidence from multiple studies has suggested that tanning beds increase the risk of melanoma. In 2009, the World Health Organisation's International Agency for Research and Cancer (IARC) classified ultraviolet light emitted from tanning beds as a human carcinogen.

A 2014 combined analysis of 31 observational studies, including nearly 250,000 participants, found an overall 16% increase of melanoma risk versus those who never use tanning beds. The risk was increased by 61% for people who reported more than one year of use, and 34% for a lifetime exposure to more than 10 sessions. The risk was also increased by 35% for first use before the age of 25 years. The IARC concluded that there is a 75% increase in melanoma in those who first used tanning beds in their 20s or teen years, and hence have recommended that minors and young adults avoid the use of tanning devices, and supported moves to restrict access to artificial tanning facilities for individuals under the age of 18.

---

[140] It also has inhibitory effects on tyrosinase, a key enzyme involved in the process of melanogenesis. It also interferes with the transfer of tyrosinase to pre-melanosomes.

Another study of patients (less than 50 years of age) with melanoma, compared to those who did not have the disease, found that women who had ever tanned indoors had a two to sixfold increased risk of melanoma compared with women who had never tanned indoors, with the highest risk observed among those who were younger than 30 years at diagnosis.

In this study, among all age groups, the risk was consistently higher for women who started tanning indoors before the age of 25 and for those reporting more than 10 tanning sessions (in total). Based on these findings, individuals under the age of 18 years are banned from using tanning beds in France, Spain, United Kingdom, Denmark, Finland, Norway, Sweden, Iceland, Germany, and Lithuania.

In Canada, there is a ban for under 18s in Ontario, Quebec, and British Columbia, and under the age of 19 in Nova Scotia. Since 2008, New Zealand and Australia have banned sun-tanning units for persons under the age of 18 and for all persons with vulnerable skin type[141], known as 'skin type I', defined as the palest skin with abundant freckles that never tans but burns on exposure to sunlight.

From January 2015, tanning beds have been banned in the Australian territories of New South Wales, Queensland, South Australia, Tasmania, and Victoria. A similar ban was introduced in Brazil in 2009.

In the US, indoor tanning is banned for those under 18 in a number of states, including California, Hawaii, Texas, and Washington. In many other states, parental permission is required for minors. The US Food and Drug Administration has, since May 2014, requested that sunlamp products used in tanning salons carry visible boxed warnings that state that sunlamp products should not be used on persons under the age of 18 years. Increased risk for melanoma has been detected in individuals who began tanning in mid-adulthood.

There is an interesting theory about people who like to tan frequently. Evidence suggests that skin tanning can be due to an addiction. It has been proposed that ultraviolet-induced production of pro-opiomelanocortin products, including beta-endorphins (yes, I know, another mouthful of words to digest), may be a contributing factor to tanning addiction, as they give the tanner a happy buzz. This theory was supported by the findings of a trial in which a drug, naltrexone (used to treat opiate abuse), was associated with a reduced desire for ultraviolet exposure among frequent tanners. Naltrexone also led to withdrawal symptoms in four out of eight frequent tanners, while no withdrawal-like symptoms were seen in those who did not use indoor tanning sessions frequently.

---

[141] Thomas B. Fitzpatrick developed a scale with six types of skin based on the response of different skin types to ultraviolet light.

In fact, addiction to tanning may be common. In one study of college students, 90 of 229 students who reported tanning bed use (29%) met the diagnostic and statistical manual of mental disorders (DSM)IV–TR criteria for addiction. Tanning-bed addiction may be more common in individuals with anxiety, depressive symptoms, or substance abuse.

In a study of 389 non-Hispanic white women aged 18 to 30 who had used indoor tanning at least one time in the previous year, 23% screened positive for indoor tanning dependence. Factors associated with indoor tanning dependence included high frequency of use (20 times or more in the previous year), stronger belief about the benefits of tanning, greater perceived susceptibility to indoor tanning risks, stronger beliefs about physical appearance, and depressive symptoms.

8.3   Asbestos

Ninety percent of the Earth's crust is made of silicon and its different mineral forms.

If you were given the power to create life on Earth, the obvious choice would be a silicon-based life form. It makes sense – silicon is everywhere. Silicates forms part of the sand beneath our feet, and heating sand with soda and lime creates glass. And when creating artificial intelligence, we have used silicon for the microchips in our computers and mobile phones because of its semi-conducting properties. They don't call the hubs of modern technology 'silicon valleys' for nothing.

But for some unknown reason, all lifeforms on our planet are carbon-based. And, although we have dozens of elements in addition to carbon in living organisms, the one which is very noticeable by its absence is silicon. This has led some (including me) to believe that life did not start on this planet but was probably brought in from another part of the universe via comets or asteroids. Add to it the fact that if, by chance, we get silicon into our bodies, we react to it as a foreign chemical, and the argument sounds even more plausible.

The most common form of silicon is silicon dioxide, known to us as 'sand'. Rarely, silicate minerals occur in a fascinating form of long, thin, and fibrous crystals, which can be woven into a fabric, just like cotton or wool threads. These rare forms of silica (six naturally occurring types) are known as 'asbestos'. The best known of these are white asbestos (chrysotile), brown asbestos (amosite), and blue asbestos (crocidolite).

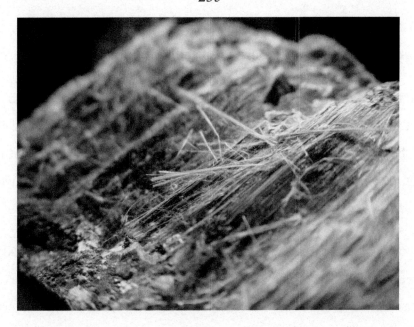

Asbestos fibres.

Asbestos has amazing, almost magical qualities, which have made it a cherished material for thousands of years. It is lightweight, flexible, fire-resistant, and an excellent insulator. Stone-Age man used it to make pottery which was durable and flame-resistant. Ancient Egyptians used it in the shrouds for their pharaohs. Persian kings made napkins out of it which did not need washing as, instead, they could be cleaned by throwing them onto a fire to burn off any dirt and grime. That must be an impressive trick at their dinner parties.

Pope Alexander III made a whole robe out of it. Emperor Charlemagne settled for a tablecloth.

The source of this magical material was kept secret and myths were promoted to mislead the people. One stated that asbestos came from the fur of an animal called a *samandar*, in Persian language, which lived in fire and died when exposed to water. Over the centuries, when such stories reached Europe via many travellers, including Marco Polo, the name *samandar* got corrupted to 'salamander', with the result that the poor, newt-like amphibian, the salamander, was considered fire-resistant and even believed to be created of fire. The fact that they lived in water and had no fur to provide asbestos fibres never crossed people's minds.

In the 1800s, asbestos mines were established all over the world and production started on an industrial scale to make fire-retardant coatings, cement, bricks, pipe insulations, plasters, brake pads, filters, shoes, clutch discs, fireproof materials, furniture, and many other products.

By the early 1900s, it was becoming obvious that asbestos caused lung disease among many, if not all, people exposed to it, decades after their initial exposure. This included plaques around the lung (in the pleural membranes) and sometimes a very aggressive tumour of the pleural membranes known as a *mesothelioma*. But the use of asbestos continued unabated, exposing millions of lungs to its deadly fibres.

Nowadays, it's astonishing to think that artificial snow was created out of asbestos for Christmas decorations, and used in homes and movie sets, including the famous movie *The Wizard of Oz*. Talc, contaminated with asbestos, was found in children's crayons as late as the year 2000. In 2018, the company Johnson and Johnson paid a record $4.69 billion US dollars compensation for their talc-based products, including baby powder.

In the 1940s, while conducting research on the safety of asbestos, Dr Leroy Gardner discovered that more than 80% of his experimental mice developed cancer after inhaling asbestos. He excitedly reported the findings to his sponsors, Johns-Manville Corporation, who very kindly kept it a secret for 40 … yes, FORTY … years. Dr Gardner begged them to make the news public, but the sponsors had made him sign a contract that they had the right to censor any information from the experiments, and reminded him that they had asked him to establish the safety of asbestos, not its dangers. So, asbestos kept being produced, sold, and used, causing cancer and generating billions of dollars for big fat greedy corporations. In the 1950s one or two people in a million got asbestos-related cancer (mesothelioma); by the mid-1970s it had risen to 15,000 per million.

The worst case of asbestos use was in 1952, when cigarette manufacturers Lorillard used asbestos in its cigarette filters (the 'famous microns filter' for its Kent brand) and produced billions of these deadly combination cigarettes up until 1956.

Dr Gardner's findings were only made public when litigation cases went to court in USA in the 1980s and the World Health Organisation finally issued its first warning in 1986.

Today, use of asbestos is banned or regulated in most countries, but historic use has left us with buildings and structures laden with it, and which continues to be a potential threat of asbestosis (a lung disease marked by fibrosis/scaring) and mesothelioma.

In the UK, the removal and disposal of asbestos has to be undertaken by licensed specialist operators, and it can prove expensive for house movers who discover that the old garage next to their new house was made of the stuff. Often, asbestos used in construction came in forms that were sealed (e.g., boards for insulation). As long as the seal remains intact, and so asbestos fibres and dust aren't shed into the air, the risk is low, and that's why some buildings containing asbestos have been left until demolition or refurbishment necessitates its controlled removal and disposal.

8.4   Arsenic

Among chemicals that can cause lung cancer, arsenic is an important element. There is increased risk with an increased amount of arsenic found in drinking water. The risk is higher due to synergistic effects of other risk factors, especially smoking. Arsenic has been used by man throughout history, from poisoning Napoleon Bonaparte to mass killings during warfare. It is a component of the chemical weapon, lewisite[142], also known as 'Agent L', allegedly used during the Vietnam War.

Interestingly, arsenic has been approved for the treatment of resistant acute promyelocytic leukaemia (APRA). It is also used for treatment of psoriasis in Fowler's solution. Arsenic-74 (a positron emitter) is also used for PET (positron emission tomography) scans, as it gives a clearer signal than iodine-124, which goes mostly to the thyroid.

8.5   N-nitrosodimethylamine (NDMA)

Do you live near to a rocket site? Thankfully, few of us do. Do you live in an area where your water supply is chlorinated? You do! Then read on.

Rocket fuel in the form of the asymmetrical dimethylhydrazine is a highly effective precursor to a compound called 'N-nitrosodimethylamine', or 'NDMA'. It is also known as 'dimethyl nitrosamine', or 'DMN'. Groundwater near rocket launch sites often has high levels of NDMA. It is an organic compound, a volatile yellow oil, and is known to be both hepatotoxic (toxic to the liver) and carcinogenic in laboratory animals.

The worrying fact is that it can be produced in the process of water treatment by chlorination or chloramination. Different governments have set varying allowable levels for this chemical, but a general consensus is lacking. For example, the United States Environmental Protection Agency (EPA) sets the maximal admissible concentration of NDMA in drinking water at 7 nanograms per litre. The US state of California allows a level of 10 nanograms per litre, whereas the Canadian Province of Ontario sets the standard at 9 nanograms per litre. No one knows what level cancer has set for NDMA!

The potential problem is greater for recycled water that can contain dimethylamine. It does not readily biodegrade, adsorb, or volatilize. It is also difficult to remove it from water. Low levels of NDMA are also found in cured meat, fish, beer, and tobacco smoke.

---

[142] Lewisite is called 'lewisite' because it was synthesised in 1904 by Julius Arthur Nieuwland, a Belgian priest and professor of chemistry as part of his PhD doctoral thesis. In 1918 a US soldier and chemist named Winford Lee Lewis read his work and decided to remake the chemical and acknowledge Julius by naming the compound after himself, 'Lewisite'.

The fact that NDMA can kill a person has been well known among criminals for a long time. There have been some notorious criminal cases involving this chemical. In 1978, a teacher in Ulm, Germany, was sentenced to life in prison for trying to murder his wife by poisoning, adding NDMA to jam and feeding it to her. Both the wife and teacher later died from liver failure. I wonder if she had added it to his bottle of jam too?

Also in 1978, Stephen Roy Harper spiked lemonade with NDMA at the Johnson family home in Omaha, Nebraska. The incident resulted in the death of 30-year-old Duane Johnson and 11-month-old Chad Shelton. For his crime, Harper was sentenced to death but committed suicide in prison before his execution could be carried out. What was it about that year and NDMA?

More recently, in another famous case in 2013 known as the 'Fudan poisoning case', Huang Yang, a postgraduate medical student at Fudan University, was a victim of a poisoning in Shanghai, China. Wuang was poisoned by his roommate, Lin Senhao, who had placed NDMA into the water cooler in their dormitory. Lin claimed that he was only doing it as an April fool's joke. He received a death sentence and was executed in 2015 for his foolish act.

Sometimes, small amounts of NDMA are found as an impurity in certain medicinal drugs, such as valsartan and other angiotensin II receptor blockers (ARBs), and the common antacid known as 'ranitidine'. Unacceptable levels of NDMA form in ranitidine over time, especially when these antacids are stored where it is warmer than room temperature (25 degrees centigrade). In 2019, ranitidine was recalled across the world due to contamination with NDMA.

Unacceptable levels of NDMA have also been found in the antidiabetic drug metformin by the FDA (the US Food and Drug Administration). In December 2019, FDA began testing samples of metformin for carcinogens and NDMA, and this led to the recall of three versions of metformin in Singapore. The European Medicines Agency (EMA) has requested that manufacturers routinely test for NDMA. Ironically, metformin by itself is a very useful drug with some anti-cancer effects.

The European Union's Committee for Medicinal Products for Human Use (CHMP) within the EMA has strong recommendations in keeping the amount of NDMA as low as possible. People should generally not be exposed to a lifetime risk of cancer exceeding one in 100,000 from nitrosamines in their medicines. Many drug manufacturers have been asked to recall their medicines when unacceptable levels are found.

The only effective methods for removal seem to be use of ultraviolet radiation and reverse osmosis (where molecules pass through a semi-permeable membrane). Relatively high levels of ultraviolet radiation in the

200 to 260 nanometre range break the nitrogen-nitrogen bond and can thus be used to degrade NDMA. Reverse osmosis removes approximately 50% of NDMA.

8.6   Outdoor Air Pollution and Diesel Exposure

Air pollution, especially from vehicle fumes and smoke from burning fossil fuel, can increase the risk of cancer. Natural pollutants such as dust and radon gas (already discussed in detail) can also add to the risk of developing cancer.

A specific type of pollutant known as 'particulate matter', found in diesel and petrol exhaust fumes, and tobacco smoke, has been shown to increase the risk of cancers, especially lung cancer, due to long-term irritation and damage to the airways.

Burning diesel is an unclean process. Combustion is often incomplete, generating carbon-containing particles (soot). Some of these are extremely tiny, known as 'nanoparticles' and can be easily inhaled and lodged into the lungs. Diesel oil has more than 30 components that can cause cancer according to the International Agency for Research on Cancer. Fortunately, filters known as 'DPFs' (diesel particulate filters) are valuable, and can remove most but regretfully not all of these particles. The levels of particulate matter tend to be higher in cities and can vary depending on traffic density and weather conditions.

Breathing air infused with toxic fumes from disaster sites or leakage from radiation sources, such as nuclear power plants which have been damaged, can increase the risk of cancer.

A study was carried out in New York City for the firefighters, office workers, and students who returned to downtown Manhattan in the days and weeks after the 9/11 attacks. It was found that they consistently had higher rates of roughly 70 different types of cancers, including breast, cervical, colon, and lung cancer. People who lived near the nuclear disaster site of Chernobyl in Ukraine in 1986 developed higher than usual rates of lung and thyroid cancers, as well as leukaemia.

8.7   Some Types of Plastic

Certain types of plastics have been associated with increased risk of cancer. For example, PBA (bisphenol A) is a primary building block used to make polycarbonate plastic and is associated with increased risk of cancer.

Bisphenol A prevents oxidation and acts as a kind of steriliser for plastics. It has been used in plastics and resins since the 1960s. It has a synthetic, oestrogen-like structure, and can leak through scratches or cracks in a container. It is also used in metal food cans as sealants, while polycarbonate BPA plastics are present in water bottles and food storage containers. BPA is even present on the shiny side of the receipt paper you get after shopping, where it is used to stabilise the ink. Due to its oestrogen-like nature, it can cause fertility problems, male impotence, heart disease, and also increase the risk of breast cancer.

8.8   Glyphosate

This is a common weedkiller[143] used by many farmers. Studies have shown that it is linked with a very high rate of non-Hodgkin lymphoma in farmers. However, it is not clear whether the potential trace amounts of this pesticide found in food that we eat are harmful enough to cause DNA damage and mutations leading to cancer.

8.9   Miscellaneous factors

Size Does Matter: Tall Stature and Risk of Cancer

You might be surprised to learn that being tall (having what we call *greater linear growth*) increases the risk of cancer. This might strike you as odd, if not a little unfair. We don't know exactly why this is so, but there are several aspects that hint towards an explanation. Firstly, taller people are usually so because at one time or another they've had a greater growth spurt than average. And, as they grow larger, they end up comprising more cells than the average person. For example, their bowel will be longer and bigger the taller they are.

When more cells are dividing at a faster rate or for a longer period of time, we know the chances of DNA damage are higher in them. So, although the DNA repair system in taller people is just the same as that in shorter individuals, the chances of unrepaired mutations will be higher compared to those who are less tall.

This is evident with a rare hormonal imbalance condition known as gigantism. In this condition there is an overproduction of a growth hormone. Growth hormone does exactly what it says, it makes us grow tall, and people with gigantism can grow very tall. Increased growth hormone production is also accompanied by an increased production of another growth factor known as *IGF1*, or *insulin-like growth factor 1*. You might recall from previous chapters that cancer cells have a lot of receptors dedicated to IGF1, using it to stimulate their growth.

---

[143] A broad-spectrum organophosphorus compound that kills many types of weeds.

Unsurprisingly, people with gigantism are known to have a twofold increased risk of colorectal cancer.

Solid Organ Transplants

Though successful and routine organ transplantation has only become feasible within the past 100 years or so, it has been a human dream since time immemorial.

Whether it was the Hindu legend of Shiva transplanting a baby elephant's head to his little boy, Ganesha, whom he had beheaded in a fit of anger (the first reported successful case of a xenograft between two species), or the Chinese clairvoyant physician Pien Chi'ao/Bian Que doing heart switching transplants between a man of strong spirit but weak will and a man with weak spirit and strong will, the desire has always been strong.

Third-century Saints St. Damian and St. Cosmos are also reported to have replaced the cancerous leg of a Roman deacon with the leg of a deceased Moor (a term initially used for people of North African origin and later to describe Muslims in general). Nowadays, such legs are treated with chemotherapy and radiotherapy, allowing the Moors to be buried with both legs.

Apart from deities, clairvoyants, and saints, mainstream physicians and surgeons also pursued the cause for thousands of years.

The first successful skin grafting procedure in recorded history was by the Indian physician and surgeon Sushruta, who did the procedure as part of a nose reconstruction for a patient in the 2nd century BC. This was the first rhinoplasty (nose job) and hence Sushruta is rightfully considered the father of plastic surgery. Sushruta used the skin from the forehead of the patient to reconstruct a severed nose and left a detailed account of how the procedure was done, including methods of making a skin flap, which are still used.

The practice of transplanting skin from one part of the body to another has been successfully carried out since. But challenges arose when surgeons tried to transplant skin or organs from one person to another. The grafts failed spectacularly, being rejected by the recipient.

Worse cases of rejection were seen in organ transplants, whether attempted in animals or humans. Soon, it was realised that the body identifies foreign material and launches an immune reaction against the transplanted tissue. This meant that if one could find a donor who was identical to the patient, a successful implant should be possible. And that's exactly what Dr Joseph Murray did, in 1954, at the Brigham and Women's Hospital in Boston, USA.

Dr Murray was treating a young man named Richard Herrick whose kidneys had failed. Fortunately for Richard, he had an identical twin brother, Ronald, who was willing to donate one of his kidneys to save his brother's life.

The operation was a historical feat because never before had a human voluntarily parted with a kidney or another human received it. These were unchartered waters and Dr Murray later admitted that he was afraid both the donor and the recipient might not survive.

Thankfully for the twins, the procedure was successful. More so for Richard, who got more than just a new kidney out of this operation. He also married his nurse and had two children with her. Dr Joseph Murray eventually received the Nobel Prize in 1990, which hopefully provided a belated compensation for losing his nurse.

The operation proved a landmark because it established the fact that organ transplantation was a possibility if the donor and the recipient were identical. But when tried for donors and recipients who were not identical twins, the transplant failed within weeks due to immune reactions. The hunt was on to find drugs which could suppress the immune system and allow the transplants to survive in their new environment.

The first breakthrough came in the form of soil samples collected by employees of a pharmaceutical company. Samples collected from Norway and Wisconsin USA grew fungi that produced a toxic chemical which suppressed the immune system. The drug was called 'cyclosporin' because it had a round or cyclical structure and came from fungal spores. This started a trend for digging up soil samples from all over the world in quest of new immunosuppressive drugs.

In 1964, a research expedition was sent to a remote volcanic island known as 'Rapa Nui' in the Polynesian language (you might have heard of its European name, Easter Island – we talked about it in an earlier section). The island is famous for its 900 monumental statues with oversized heads, known as *moai*, which are an archaeological enigma. Soil samples collected from the island contained a bacterium, *Streptomyces hygroscopicus*, which made a chemical that killed fungi. In honour of the island, it was named 'rapamycin'.

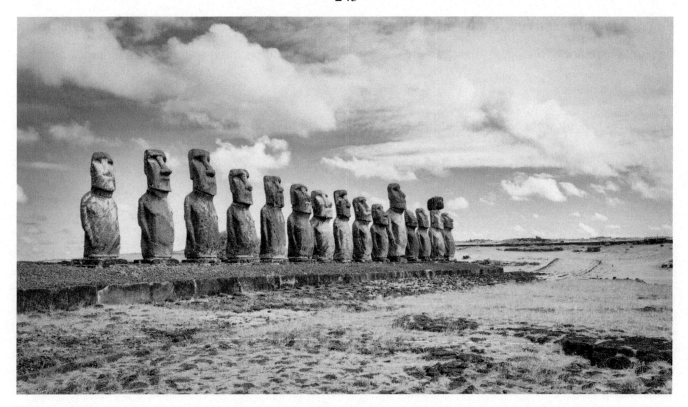

Stone statues on Easter Island.

Rapamycin had an unexpected action. It attached to and inhibited a protein in the cells which regulates cell growth, proliferation, survival, and motility. Scientists named it *mTOR*, this 'mammalian target of rapamycin' once again demonstrating their lack of ingenuity in naming cellular proteins.

By inhibiting mTOR, rapamycin not only suppressed immune cells but also cancer cells and soon a stream of related drugs came into production, which revolutionised transplant medicine and cancer treatment.

Nowadays, transplant recipients may receive a cocktail of immunosuppressive drugs which stop their immune system from attacking and rejecting the transplanted organs. Initially, the only challenge of using immunosuppressive drugs in transplant patients was the increased risk of infection due to a compromised immune system. This was successively managed by reducing the risk of infections and administering antibiotics. But over the decades doctors have realised that solid organ transplant patients or recipients (SOTRs) face an increased risk of dying from cancer, regardless of age, sex, the organ transplanted, or transplant period.

The increase in cancer mortality is multifactorial. As we've seen before, the human body has a remarkable immune surveillance system which detects cancer cells. When the immune system is dampened with effective immune suppression to facilitate graft acceptance, this surveillance process decreases. With immune suppression, patients are also unable to fight infections (such as certain viral infections) and this may be associated with some cancers, too.

Organ transplant patients are not only at risk of more cancers but also have a higher risk of dying from cancer. There are two leading theories why solid organ transplant recipients are at a higher risk of cancer death:

1) Cancer arising from an immunosuppressed environment may be more biologically aggressive.

2) Patients may receive less aggressive cancer treatment due to co-morbidities and the fear that transplant rejection may occur.

For example, oncologists may not, justifiably, be willing to give a full dose regimen of life-saving chemotherapy to a transplant recipient.

The incidence of cancer deaths in SOTRs is 2.84 times higher than that of the general population, according to a study published online in *JAMA* (*Journal of American Medical Association Oncology*). The study showed that cancer mortalities are the second most common cause of death in solid organ transplant patients.

Can the risk be reduced? The key probably lies in prevention or early detection through screening. For example, patients with risk of lung cancer, especially those who smoke, should undergo regular lung cancer screening. This can strike a healthy balance between the increased risk of cancer and organ transplant, which is a life-saving treatment.

Night Shift Work

There have been a lot of interesting studies regarding night shift workers. Some studies have suggested that working night shifts and being exposed to artificial light at night could increase the risk of cancer, especially breast cancer. However, many of these studies were looking at the risk of breast cancer in animals and not humans.

In 2007, the International Agency for Research and Cancer (IARC) concluded that working night shifts probably does increase the risk of cancer, based on the evidence available to them at that time. However, recently, a review of 10 different studies in humans has shown that night shift work is unlikely to increase the risk of cancer, especially breast cancer.

They looked at the confounding factors and found that women working night shift were more likely to be overweight or obese. These factors are associated with a higher risk of many cancers, including breast cancer, and this could explain the difference between higher incidences of breast cancer among women who are working night shifts. Another reason could be that the pattern of night shift work makes it more difficult for people to shop and cook healthy food, or take part in regular physical activity.

So, the conclusion for night shift work is that if you maintain a healthy weight, keep active, eat a healthy diet, do not smoke, and exercise regularly, the risk of cancer should not be any higher than those who work in the day shift.

8.10   Known Carcinogens: All Suspects, Big and Small

A list of all suspected carcinogens published by the International Agency for Research on Cancer (IARC) can be found on their website.

PART 9

SCREENING
A HISTORICAL PERSPECTIVE

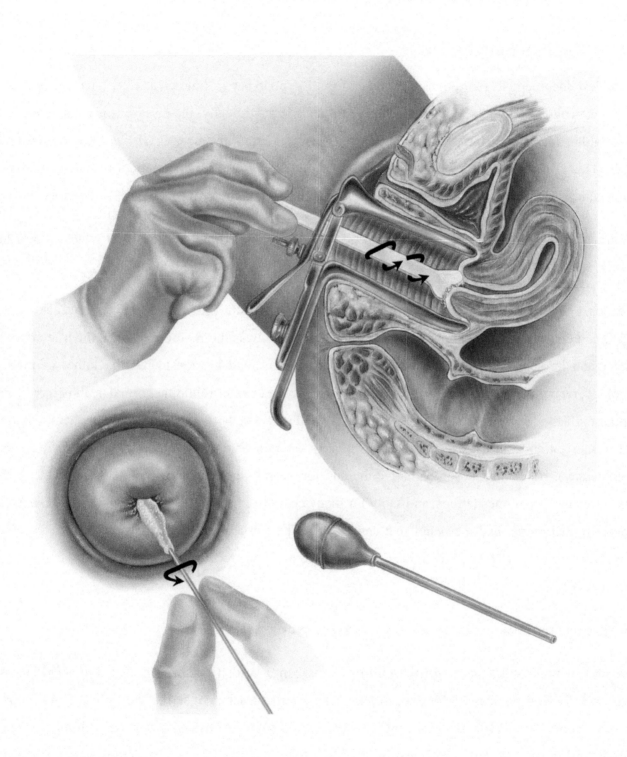

PART 9: SCREENING: A HISTORICAL PERSPECTIVE

9 Screening: A Historical Perspective

9.1 Establishing Links

The oldest documented record of cancer comes from Egyptian papyri (known as Eber's papyrus), written 2,600 years ago. Despite the Egyptians attempt to manage it surgically, the disease was considered as an untreatable curse. Hippocrates (circa 460 BC to 370 BC) referred to cancer as *carcinos* (Greek for 'crab' or 'cray fish'). Celsus (circa 25 BC to 50 AD) translated *carcinos* to *cancer* (Latin for 'crab'), and Galen (2nd century AD) first used the term oncos, from which the modern term 'oncology' is derived.

Treatment at the time consisted of dietary modifications, bloodletting, and laxatives which at best had little, if any, effect on managing or treating the disease, and probably made it worse.

The most practical approach to managing cancer came from Ibn Sina (circa 980–1037 AD; see also section 7.2). The Persian physician, known to the West as Avicenna, was the first to recognise the true nature of cancer and its spread through the venous circulation. He could be considered the father of modern oncology, recommending radical surgery (removing cancer and its surrounding normal healthy tissue, very similar to the wide excision margins given nowadays in surgery), herbal extracts (akin to chemotherapy), and cauterization (similar to modern techniques of radiofrequency ablation, laser therapy, and radiotherapy). He also proposed palliative therapy for treating the advanced stages of cancer. Until Ibn Sina's detailed recommendations, and sadly for many centuries afterwards, a large number of physicians, especially in Europe, had the belief that cancer could be flushed out of the body by use of laxatives. Ironically, even today some practitioners of alternative medicine recommend exotic enemas based on the same concept.

It took a long time before cancer was recognised as a preventable disease.

The idea of preventing cancer goes back to 1775, when a British doctor, Percival Pott, working as a surgeon at St. Bartholomew's Hospital, London, came across a series of scrotal cancer cases in his clinic. He noted something odd about his patients. Almost all of them were boys who worked as chimney sweeps. This involved them working nearly naked, exposing their bodies to the soot and gunk in chimneys. The cancer almost always occurred in the lower part of the scrotum and as the patients were all beyond puberty it was suspected of being a venereal disease. The cancer was preceded by a superficial skin wound known as a 'soot wart'. Unknown to Percival Pott, the soot these young children were cleaning from the chimneys contained a mixture of carcinogens. He did note, however, that the skin of the chimney sweeps carried traces of chimney soot. Percival published his findings, laying a foundation for prevention of cancer by avoiding a carcinogenic factor. However, this did not immediately resolve the problem for the poor chimney sweeps. Change came very slowly. In 1788, the Chimney Sweepers Act was passed, preventing children under the age of eight from being employed as chimney sweeps. In 1834, this age was raised to 14, and in 1840 to 16 years. It was not until 1875 that the use of boys was fully forbidden, and the incidences of scrotal cancers started to decline.

Fast-forwarding to the last century, 1948 was a landmark year, with far-reaching effects for mankind. Wars, turmoil – the expected and the unexpected, the exciting and the mundane – all were happening.

In the east, Burma (later renamed 'Myanmar') gained independence from the United Kingdom, as did Ceylon (later renamed 'Sri Lanka'). The republic of South Korea was established; laying the foundations for the soon-to-come Korean War.

In the Middle East, civil war broke out in Palestine, resulting in the exodus of hundreds of thousands of Palestinian Arab Muslims, and Christians. Almost half of their population fled or was expelled, an event still remembered as the Nakaba. By the end of the year, a fully fledged war between the Arabs and Israelis had begun and things have never been the same since.

Russia decided to launch Operation Vesna, with mass deportation of Lithuanians to Siberia. By this time, they had already successfully managed to deport many other nations from their homelands, including almost one third of the population of Chechens, Ingush, and Balkars, resulting in a death rate of around 25% (400,000 Chechens died, including a large number of small children, comprising 30-40% of the exiled population).

In India, Mahatma Gandhi was shot by a Hindu nationalist, Nathuram Godse, bringing to a violent end an era of peaceful political resistance.

In the Western hemisphere things were also getting exciting. Bill France Sr founded NASCAR. The Hells Angels motorcycle gang was established in California. Albert 1, the first monkey astronaut, was launched into space on 11th June.

On the health front, major developments were taking place too, which were to impact human history for decades to come. The World Health Organisation (WHO) was established on 7th April by the United Nations. Alcoholics Anonymous's first London group was started on 15th July.

But there were two other important events that year. And they were to have a long-lasting effect on cancer and its management.

In the UK, the National Health Service (NHS) was launched by Aneurin Bevan, the British health minister, on 5th July, 1948, undoubtedly the best thing gifted to the British nation since sliced bread, and rather more useful too. However, more importantly, earlier in the year, somewhere around May 1948, Richard Doll, a 36-year-old British medical researcher, quit smoking. The event would involve one of the most important landmarks in medical history, for the story of mankind and cancer was about to take a major turn. And here's how the story of Richard Doll quitting cigarettes started.

By 1948, Britain was facing an epidemic of lung cancer morbidity and mortality which had risen nearly 15-fold over the previous 20 years. The cases were higher in towns and cities compared to villages and hence it was thought that the smoke and pollution found in the cities, along with tar in the roads, automobile exhausts, and lack of sunshine (not uncommon in the British Isles) were to blame. Ironically, no one wanted to blame cigarette smoking for the increase in cancer rates. This is despite the fact that doctors performing autopsies on bodies of lung cancer patients had already evidenced the signs and stigmata of chronic smoking, in the form of blackened lungs and tar-stained airways. They had also seen cancer sprouting out of these contaminated lungs, which almost always belonged to smokers.

However, all of these signs were ignored. The reason was that scientists were using an old model designed by a microbiologist named Robert Koch to find a cause for cancer. This model had actually been designed to find a positive agent for infectious diseases. The model decreed that in a diseased human the causal agent had to be present. Secondly, that the agent responsible could be isolated from the diseased person and, when introduced to a healthy secondary host, be capable of transmitting the disease. This model utterly failed to work for identifying the causative agent behind any kind of cancer. The lag time between exposure to a carcinogen and development of fully fledged cancer could be years or decades, and by the time cancer develops as an aftermath of damage done by the carcinogen, the initiating factor is often long gone, leaving behind no trace, apart from death and destruction.

Outside of infectious diseases, the Koch's model fails in most circumstances. For example, you cannot apply the Koch's hypothesis to a fire that has burned a house down to ashes. Cancer is very much like the ashes of a burnt structure with no sign of the original fire. All you see is the result of an earlier event.

In 1948, the UK's Medical Research Council selected a renowned biostatistician, Austin Bradford-Hill, to look into the matter, and Hill hired the services of a medical researcher, Richard Doll, to help him out. Doll himself, a chronic smoker, continued to light up his cigarettes during breaks while working on the project. The project was simple. They studied patients admitted to 20 different London hospitals with and without lung cancer and asked them questions about different factors thought to influence the risk. These included, how far their homes were from factories and gas works, whether they ate fried fish or preferred fried bacon, whether they consumed sausages or ham for dinner, together with a cursory enquiry about their smoking habits. By May 1948, based on the 156 interviews, the only indisputable statistical association with lung cancer was cigarette smoking. This came as a great disappointment and personal shock to Richard Doll, who had always suspected road tar exposure as the cause of lung cancer. Even before the survey was complete, the data convinced him sufficiently to quit smoking for good.

Their findings were published under the title, 'Smoking and Carcinoma of the Lung', in the *British Medical Journal* and the results were further strengthened by a similar finding across the Atlantic, published in the *Journal of the American Medical Association* (*JAMA*) by Ernest Winder, an epidemiologist, and Evarts Graham, a physician and surgeon.

The establishment of the National Health Service in 1948 gave rise to another opportunity for Doll and Bradford-Hill. The NHS had a centralised registry of all doctors, comprising more than 60,000 names. Every time a doctor passed away, the registrar was notified with a description of the cause of death. This gave Doll and Bradford-Hill the idea of launching a simple but brilliant research study.

In October 1951, they sent out letters to more than 59,000 doctors requesting a quick five-minute survey about their smoking habits and the number of cigarettes they consumed per day. Fortunately for them, more than 41,000 wrote back. They categorised the doctors into two groups: smokers and non-smokers. Now the waiting game began. Every time a doctor passed away, they retrieved information about the precise cause of death. In the following 29 months, between October 1951 and March 1954, 789 deaths were reported and 36 of them were attributed to lung cancer. As expected, all 36 of the deaths had occurred in smokers. This left no doubt about the link between cigarette smoking and lung cancer. It was hard to blame any other factor like road tar, city smog, or lack of sunshine. The group of doctors was well balanced for all other characteristics. Here we had a group of people who belonged to the same profession and were exposed to similar environmental factors. The only difference was between smoking and non-smoking, and their addiction was costing them their lives.

This didn't go down well with cigarette manufacturers. In 1954, the tobacco industry published a full-page advertisement in more than 400 newspapers in America titled, 'A Frank Statement to Cigarette Smokers'. They conveniently ignored the findings by Bradford-Hill and Richard Doll and their own fellow Americans, Ernest Wynder and Evarts Graham, despite the latter being a renowned lung surgeon, and instead focused on different research done on mice, trying to divert the public's attention. The opening lines of this frank statement said, "Recent reports and experiments with mice have given wide publicity to a theory that cigarette smoking is in some way linked to lung cancer in human beings." They also formed the Tobacco Industry Research Committee (TIRC) to counter any evidence that emerged linking lung cancer and smoking. Despite the fact that the tar from cigarette smoke was shown to grow cancers on the backs of mice when their skin was exposed to it, defendants of the tobacco lobby nevertheless kept hiding behind Koch's hypothesis, that of the classical trio of association, isolation, and retransmission, and that it could not be demonstrated in human beings.

The solution to this issue came from Austin Bradford-Hill, the genius British epidemiologist we have already talked about, who presented a criteria of nine features (known as 'Hill's criteria for causation') establishing a link between cancer and its risk factors, as an alternative to the Koch's hypothesis:

1) Strength (effect size): Smokers had a five to tenfold increased risk of developing cancer, so the association was quite strong.

2) Consistency (reproducibility): The findings were consistent when studied in England and across the Pacific in America. These included vastly different populations.

3) Specificity: The association was specific between the factor (smoking) and its effect (cancer).

4) Temporality: The longer people smoked, greater was the risk of developing cancer and hence the findings were temporal.

5) Biological Gradient (dose-response relationship): The amount of cigarette smoke also mattered and the more one smoked in quantity, the greater was the risk for lung cancer, and hence possessing a biological gradient or dose-response relationship.

6) Plausibility: Cigarette smoke was inhaled, and cancer developed in the lungs, thus giving a plausible mechanistic link between the inhaled smoke and the malignant change.

7) Coherence: It was backed by experimental evidence of cancer developing in mice when exposed to cigarette tar and hence the findings were coherent.

8) Experiment: There was experimental evidence from mice of growing tumours when exposed to tar from cigarettes.

9) Analogy: Smoking had also been associated with lip, throat, tongue, and oesophageal cancer, which made the findings similar and analogous, showing that smoking behaved in a similar manner in analogous situations.

Finally, there were criteria[144] which could replace the Koch's hypothesis and be applied to cancer risk assessment.

But despite the mounting evidence, people still continued to smoke. In 1954, British minister of health, Iain Macleod, called a press conference on the subject and gave his famous statement, "It must be regarded as established that there is a relationship between smoking and cancer of the lung."

The journalists listened to him in shock, not because of his statement but the fact that he was smoking a cigarette at the same time.

In the 1960s, Oscar Auerbach, a well-known lung pathologist, completed a study comparing lung samples from 1,522 autopsies of smokers and non-smokers. His published findings showed that long before lung cancer grew there were a series of changes taking place in the smokers' lungs, starting with a thickening of the outermost layers of the airway passages exposed to smoke. Over time, this thickened layer developed atypical or abnormal-looking cells and started to show changes consistent with cancer. Eventually, these cells broke through the basement membrane, the barrier keeping them in place, and transformed into invasive carcinomas.

This was in stark contrast to the picture that the tobacco industry had been painting. The hallmark of their advertisement campaigns was exemplified by Philip Morris, when the company launched the Marlborough Man in 1955. The epitome of male health and style associated with smoking, the image increased sales of their brand by 5,000% over the next eight months. In addition, they added filters to the cigarettes to convince the people that anything harmful was being taken out of the smoke before it entered the lungs.

Political lobbying continued too. Despite nicotine being a drug, it has never been regulated by the Federal Food and Drug Administration (FDA); as such, cigarettes weren't classified as a drug. Instead, cigarettes are regulated by the Federal Trade Commission (FTC).

In 1964, the FTC proposed that cigarette packages should be labelled with, 'Caution: Cigarette smoking is dangerous to health. It may cause death from cancer and other diseases.' The tobacco lobby successfully

---

[144] The list of the criteria is now grown to 10. 1) Strength or effect size; 2) Consistency or reproducibility; 3) specificity; 4) temporality; 5) Biological gradient or dose-response relationship; 6) Plausibility; 7) Coherence; 8) Experiment; 9) Analogy; and 10) Reversibility – that is, if the cause is removed, the effect should disappear as well. Number 10 is key to the principle of preventing cancer.

convinced congress to change this warning to a much more benign phrase, "Caution: Cigarette smoking <u>may</u> be hazardous to your health", in 1965. This small, three-lettered word created a big doubt.

Over the decades, evidence emerged that the lag time between tobacco exposure and lung cancer could be as long as nearly three decades. By 1988, the tobacco industry had reversed their initial narrative. In an open letter from the tobacco industry, they shamelessly threw all the blame on their customers, stating, "Certainly, living in America in the last half of the 20th century, one would have to be deaf, dumb and blind not to be aware of the asserted dangers, real or imagined, of cigarette smoking. Yet the personal choice to smoke is … the same kind of choice as the driver who downed the beers and then the telephone pole."

In November 1998, an agreement known as a 'Master Settlement Agreement' (MSA) was signed between the major cigarette manufacturers, Philip Morris, R. J. Reynolds, Brown and Williamson, and Lorillard Tobacco Company, and the attorney generals of 46 US states, agreeing to restore restrictions to cigarette advertising, but also ensuring protection from future legal action, providing a virtual monopoly in return for regular payments to help meet the cost of the health crisis they create. The cost, of course, is easily and regularly passed on to their clients, the smokers, who end up paying a higher price for their cigarettes every year.

With time, the list of preventable carcinogens continued to grow. Asbestos was found to cause mesothelioma after decades of exposure. Some carcinogens behaved in a bizarre fashion, such as a synthetic hormonal medicine called 'diethylstilbestrol' (DES), prescribed to pregnant women in the 1950s to prevent premature deliveries. These women did not suffer from any adverse events but, a generation later, daughters born to those mothers who'd received diethylstilbestrol were found to have a very high incidence of vaginal and uterine cancers. Nowadays, the drug is banned for use in women, especially pregnant women, but is safely used in men for treatment of prostate cancer.

An interesting method of finding carcinogens was developed by Bruce Ames, a bacteriologist at Berkeley, California, in the 1960s. While working with bacteria, Ames found chemicals or agents that caused a mutation in the bacteria could also cause DNA damage, leading to cancer development, in humans. These included X-rays, benzene compounds, nitroso-guanidine, and chemicals found in cigarette smoke. He tried them on laboratory animals such as rats and mice and successfully induced cancers in them.

At around the same time, Baruch Bulberg discovered the link between the hepatitis B virus and liver cancer. In the 1970s, Harold Zurhausen discovered that the human papilloma virus (HPV) causes cervical cancer.

In 1984, Australian gastroenterologist Robin Warren and his colleague, Barry Marshall, working at Royal Perth Hospital, discovered the link between a bacterium, *Helicobacter pylori*, and stomach cancer, which usually develops in ulcerated stomachs. Earlier, they had discovered this bacterium growing in gastric ulcers and inflamed stomach lining. Using Koch's hypothesis, they isolated the bacteria, grew it in cultures and inoculated healthy pigs with it. However, weekly endoscopies on the pigs did not show any development of gastric ulcers or inflammation of the gastric lining (gastritis). This should not have come as a surprise, as pigs are notoriously good at ingesting and tolerating bacteria-laden, rotting food. By July, a much-frustrated Marshall took fate into his own hands and, after a period of fasting, drank 200 ml of a brown liquid containing the live bacteria.

Within days he started to develop symptoms of nausea, vomiting, sweats, and fever. Serial endoscopies and biopsies showed a highly active gastritis with live bacteria growing in his stomach among ulcerated lesions. Finally, the Koch hypothesis had shown a link between the cancer-causing agent and a pre-cancerous condition. Marshall treated himself with antibiotics and successfully cured the infection. Nowadays, the antibiotic regime is used all over the world for patients suffering from gastritis and gastric ulcers. Over the years, this led to a significant reduction in the incidence of gastric cancer, especially in geographical areas where the disease was rampant, such as the western coast of Japan.

9.2   Prevention by Screening

Perhaps the most amazing story of cancer prevention strategies comes from George Papanicolaou, a Greek cytologist at Cornell University in New York, who arrived in the USA in 1913. His job at Cornell involved an unusual study of the menstrual cycle in guinea pigs, a species of mammals that neither bleeds visibly nor sheds any tissue during menstruation. Papanicolaou had to scrape off the cervical cells from the guinea pigs' cervix using Q-tips and nasal specula, and spread them on glass slides to study. By studying these cells, he could foretell the stages of the menstrual cycle in guinea pigs. After a while, he extended this technique to a human volunteer (his wife, Maria) and was able to successfully identify the stages of her menstrual cycle from the cells scraped from the cervix. This amazing feat had no practical value as almost every woman is able to foretell the stage of her menstrual period without the need for her cervix to be scraped for cells. Therefore, Papanicolaou decided to extend his technique as a new test for detecting cancer cells. However, this too was not very useful, as getting a biopsy from the cervix is a much more reliable method of diagnosing cancer.

At a Christmas party in 1950, while being mocked by a colleague, Papanicolaou suddenly had the idea to use the technique for identifying pre-cancerous lesions on the cervix in women who had not yet developed cervical cancer. In 1952, he convinced the National Cancer Institute to launch a clinical trial involving 150,000 women. Studying their smears, he found evidence of invasive cervical cancer in 555 women but, more importantly, 552 women were found to have pre-cancerous lesions. These women were, on average, 20 years younger than the women diagnosed with full-blown cancer, indicating that the growth and development of a cancer in the cervix from pre-cancerous lesions took around two decades. Hence, the well-known PAP smear test was born, able to detect pre-cancerous lesions decades before a cervical cancer develops, enabling doctors to treat and cure the subject.

Breast cancer screening, now the norm, also started with an interesting story. In 1913, a Berlin surgeon, Albert Salomon, had been performing mastectomies (removal of the breast tissue) but, unlike other surgeons, after doing his procedures he took the resected breast and photographed them using X-rays (a technique known as 'mammography'). After carrying out mammographies for almost 3,000 amputated breasts, he found signs of microscopic sprinkles of calcium in the cancer tissue (described by radiologists as 'grains of salt'). However, his efforts were rudely interrupted by the Second World War.

By the 1960s, mammography was brought back by pioneering radiographers such as Robert Egan, who was able to identify pre-cancerous lesions appearing as trabeculae, "as thin as spiders webs", in the breast tissue. Egan's mammograms could detect tumours as small as a few millimetres and hence catch cancer at a very early stage. This led to many trials of mammography in the quest to identify and treat breast cancer as early as possible. One of these trials is known as the 'Health Insurance Plan trial '(or also known as the 'HIP trial') conducted by Sam Shapiro, a statistician, Philip Strax, a New York doctor whose own wife had suffered from breast cancer, and Louise Venet, a surgeon who specialised in breast cancer surgery.

After eight years of study, in 1971 the HIP trial showed that mammography could reduce breast cancer deaths by identifying the disease earlier and treating it promptly. There had been 31 deaths in the mammography screen group and 52 in the control group. This accounted for an almost 40% reduction in mortality for those who suffered from breast cancer. Similar trials were carried out at Edinburgh in the UK and in Canada. However, the trials were plagued with problems.

When it came to assigning women to the mammography group (rather than the control group who didn't have a mammogram), the researchers had a tendency to offer mammography to women with abnormal breasts or abnormal lymph node examinations. In other words, anyone with a suspicion of breast cancer was pushed into the mammography group. The same privilege was offered to friends and family members. This resulted in a high number of high-risk women in the mammography group. Overall, one would expect that this would lead to increased numbers of breast cancer detection in the mammography group, showing a superiority of this technique in breast cancer, but this selective bias also led to more women dying of breast cancer in the mammography group, and hence undermined any benefits from the technique of early detection.

Fortunately, a sensible and balanced trial was carried out by the Swedes. In 1976, they enrolled 42,000 women in a study known as the 'MALMO Mammography Study', named after the third-largest city in Sweden where the study was carried out. They used stringent and consistent methods for the study. Half of the women were screened with mammography and the other half were not.

The results at the end of 12 years of work showed that 588 women in the screening group were diagnosed with breast cancer, whereas 447 in the control group got a diagnosis of breast cancer. Early detection did not seem to make much of a difference on survival – 63 women in the screening group and 66 in the non-screened group died of breast cancer. When the study was analysed by sub-groups, the patients above the age of 55 years had benefitted from screening, with a reduction in breast cancer deaths by 20%, whereas women in the younger age group did not show any benefit. In 2002, a collective analysis combining all Swedish studies was published in the Lancet journal. Looking at the records of 247,000 women, it was obvious that mammography resulted in a 20–30% reduction in breast cancer mortality for women aged 55 to 70, but for women below the age of 55 the benefits were not significant. Hence, it was clear that screening is more effective in high-risk groups compared to low-risk age groups.

A similar pattern has been found for other cancers. Death rates from colon cancer can fall by nearly 30% and for cervical and uterine cancer by 20% due to screening, early detection, and treatment of disease. Introduction of more effective treatment techniques, such as a combination of surgery followed by chemotherapy (known as 'adjuvant chemotherapy') and radiation treatment (called 'adjuvant radiotherapy') for breast cancer has significantly reduced the mortality of this disease (almost 24%). Screening and detection of cancer early by itself is only beneficial when followed by effective treatment. Naturally, just finding a cancer early does not help the patient unless a curative treatment option is available. The more effective the intervention, the more the benefit. Cancer-specific treatment has reduced the stigmata of side effects associated with cancer treatment.

9.3   Detecting Cancer: Screening Tests, Bias, and Controversies

Cancer can be detected by different methods. Most usually it is found when a patient develops symptoms and signs of disease. This is known as 'clinically detected cancer'.

Sometimes it is a chance finding, incidentally detected when being investigated for other conditions.

Systematic searches for cancer by screening can detect cancer at an earlier stage. A good screening test has two prerequisites. Firstly, screening must advance the time of diagnosis of cancer that is destined to cause death. Secondly, early treatment of these cancers must confer some advantage over treatment at clinical presentation.

9.3.1   The Potential Bias of Cancer Screening

If treatment is not effective, or effective treatment is not available for the particular type of cancer, detecting it early can only make it look as if the patient has lived longer (a phenomenon known as 'lead-time bias'). This means that time from diagnosis to death is apparently increased, although treatment does not prolong life and patients do not live any longer. They are merely diagnosed at an earlier date, and it all looks good on paper.

Slow-growing or less-aggressive cancers, if detected early during screening, could create another bias known as a 'length bias'. More aggressive cancers present with symptoms are clinically detected and cause early death compared to a slow-growing, less-aggressive cancer detected on screening, and not posing a risk to the patient's life for a long time.

The benefit of screening is if it improves mortality, and not just the survival time, as survival could be falsely improved by a lead time or length bias.

One of the ways to achieve this is to identify high-risk groups for a type of cancer that can be effectively treated, ideally with a curative treatment, at an early stage of disease, and offer these subjects a highly sensitive and specific screening test. We call this an 'example of secondary prevention' (see below).

One study set up to examine this approach was the NELSON trial conducted by the Dutch-Belgian lung cancer screening team (Nederlands-Leuvens Longkankaer Screenings Onderzoek, a bit of a mouthful, so abbreviated to 'NELSON'). It was a population-based, randomised controlled trial initiated in the year 2000 with a clear aim: to show a reduction in lung cancer mortality of 25% or more with volume-based low-dose CT lung cancer screening in a high-risk male population at 10 years of follow-up. The screening arm was offered low-dose CT scans, whereas the control arm was only observed. The primary outcome measure was lung cancer-specific mortality. The screened group had 5.58 cases per 1,000 person years[145], compared to 4.91 lung cancer cases per 1,000 person years for the non-screened control group. This

---

[145] A person year is calculated by multiplying the number of people in a study by the amount of time each person spends in the study. For example, if a study follows 1,000 people for one year, the data collected would be called '1,000 person years' data.

translated into 341 lung cancers in the screened group and 304 in the non-screened group. With treatment, 206 men died in the controlled group, whereas 156 men died in the screened group. This translated into a 24% reduction in mortality. The trial concluded that a two-year interval between screenings is safe. Over-diagnosis was 10% at worst, and screening leads to an increased number of lung cancer patients' lives saved.

9.3.2 False and True Screening Tests

Screening tests also have issues of false positives and false negatives. An easy way of understanding this phenomenon is to take the example of trying to find a tiger cub which has escaped from the zoo and is hiding somewhere in the neighbourhood. We can use the neighbourhood CCTV cameras for checking out the area just like mammograms are used to detect breast cancers. However, when you see a small striped feline roaming around on the security camera, it could be the much sought-after, escaped tiger cub (a 'true positive' identification) or it could be a neighbourhood tabby cat, especially if it belongs to a breed with an almost identical pattern of stripes as the tiger[146], and this would be a 'false positive' finding. However, if you identified the feline on the surveillance camera as a tabby cat, but it actually *was* the tiger cub, this would be a 'false negative' finding. If the feline was identified as a tabby cat and on catching it indeed proved to be a tabby cat, this would be a 'true negative' finding.

Whatever the case might be, the fact of the matter is that there is risk of identifying non-cancerous lesions as cancers and ignoring cancerous lesions as benign. The ability of a screening test to detect cancer is known as the 'sensitivity' of the test. However, a very sensitive test might pick up a lot of cancerous lesions and anything else that looks like a cancer, but isn't.

The ability of the screening test to correctly identify the true positive cancer lesions is known as 'specificity', but a highly specific test risks missing those cancers which may not fit the stereotypical bill of a cancerous lesion.

9.3.3 Cancer Screening Controversies

Screening for cancer is an important method of early detection and prompt treatment can save lives. However, there are two schools of thought here – one believing that cancer screening has not shown to save lives, and others which swear by it.

---

[146] Such a breed does exist, known as a 'toyger', created in the 1980s by breeder Judy Sugden.

As noted above, there is little value in screening for an aggressive cancer for which interventions are unlikely to make a different in outcome, no matter how early the disease can be detected. So, if there is no effective cure, early screening can only add to the agony of the patient for a longer period of time. Equally, if the cancer is never going to kill you, no matter what the doctors do, screening will not help either. Once again, in such cases the person has to live for longer with the diagnosis of cancer compared to had he/she not been screened.

Hence, it is important to note that screening is only valuable if effective treatment strategies are available. In addition, screening also comes at a cost; not only financial but also of side effects of treatment.

Despite the controversies of whether screening improves overall survival or not, the good news is that screening can encourage people to have a healthier lifestyle. Findings published in the journal *Thorax* in 2016 showed that smokers who underwent a lung cancer screening programme were 50% more likely to have quit two years later. Screening programmes increase awareness about cancer risk and preventative measures because it seems to act as 'a close call' or close encounter with cancer.

Screening for prostate cancer has always been controversial. A massive British trial carried out prostate-specific antigen tests on 82,429 men aged 50 to 69 years and then randomised 1,643 to either active monitoring (545), surgery (553), or radiotherapy (545). There were 17 prostate cancer-specific deaths overall: eight in the active monitoring group, five in the surgery group, and four in the radiotherapy group. The difference among the groups was not significant.

Now, it is well-known that PSA screening detects very few cancers that are ever going to kill men, and that they will be equally alive 10 years later, whether you simply observe them, or operate, or give them radiotherapy. The PSA test looks for a prostate-specific antigen (marker) hence the abbreviation, *PSA*.

However, this does not apply to all types of prostate cancer, and all men with risk factors for prostate cancer. For example, the case is very different for people who have risk of prostate cancer associated with familial and hereditary cancer syndromes. A family history of hereditary prostate cancer conveys the greatest relative risk for all prostate cancer sub-types combined.

An important factor of screening is celebrity endorsement. An article published in the *British Medical Journal* (December 2016) looked at celebrity endorsement impact on screening. They carried out an observational study of BRCA gene testing and mastectomy rates after Angelina Jolie's *New York Times* editorial reporting her undergoing prophylactic treatment for breast cancer. Data was accessed from commercially insured United States populations of women aged 18 to 64. Results showed a 64% increase in BRCA testing rates occurred in the 15 business days after the editorial was published, and the rates were sustained throughout the year.

They concluded that celebratory endorsement can have a large and immediate effect on the use of health services, especially screening services. This is not only relative to preventative screening but also fad diets and supplements.

9.3.4   Cancer Screening for High-Risk Groups

To reduce the rates of cancer it is vital not only to identify the risk factors of cancer but also to find individuals who are at higher risk (for example smokers, hepatitis B and C patients) compared to the general population, and offer them effective preventive measures.

Recent research is also suggesting that screening intervals should be extended beyond five years in cervical screening programmes testing for high-risk human papilloma virus (HPV) infections. A study published in the *British Medical Journal* in 2016 showed that primary HPV screening provides better protection against cervical cancer than cytology testing (looking for changed cells). In HPV-negative women, extension of the screening interval beyond five years seems justifiable.

In 2018, the United Kingdom government dropped the age for bowel cancer screening from 60 to 50 years and would continue to screen people for them until the age of 74 years. Cancer prevention and screening is also important because, in the United States, cancer treatment now represents the major cause of personal bankruptcy. Add to this toxicity associated with cancer, treatment, and some of the toxicities can be potentially fatal.

9.3.5   New Screening Strategies

A sponge test has been developed for Barrett's oesophagus.

This condition can occur in patients with chronic reflux of stomach acid, which can damage the cells lining the oesophagus, increasing the risk of adenocarcinoma. Researchers used cytosponge, a pill on a string that expands when swallowed to collect throat cells, in nearly 500 patients with Barrett's oesophagus. They found that 35% were at low risk of developing oesophageal cancer by looking for genetic markers and cell changes, and combining these with information such as age and obesity. Compared with endoscopies performed in hospital, it is reported that the cytosponge causes minimal discomfort and is a quick and simple test that can be done by the GP.

PREVENTION STRATEGIES

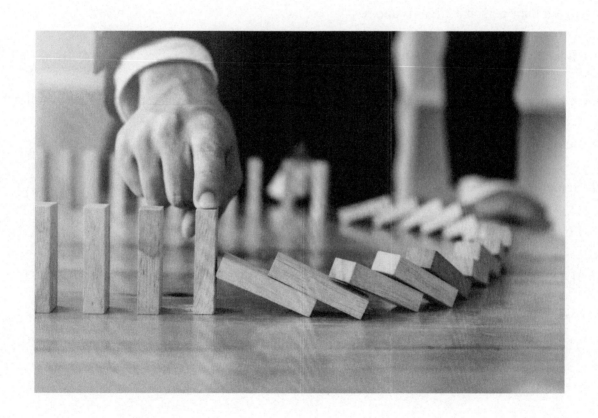

PART 10: PREVENTION STRATEGIES

10   Prevention Strategies

Have you ever wondered what the most important thing in life is? I have, and have asked around. People have given me all kinds of answers: love, money, kids, career, hobbies, and happiness. But the best answers have come from those who are looking death in the eye and have got their priorities right.

But before we start, please note that these are not rules written in stone. To every rule there are exceptions, and so that which applies to most in the general population may not apply to some or many individuals depending on their personal circumstances.

So here it is, my distilled down, '**Khan's philosophy of life**'.

The most important things in life in order of their importance (as a general consensus) are as follows:

1. Being alive.

2. Being in good health.

3. Love and being with loved ones.

4. Happiness (you need loved ones first; think about it, sharing happiness makes us happier).

5. Everything else: money, fame, status, career, living by a philosophy or faith, and the list goes on. These are the icings on the cake of life (1,2,3, and 4) and mean less on their own.

Let's analyse them one by one.

1. Being alive

For someone sentenced to death, no amount of good health, love, happiness, or wealth makes a jot of difference.

2. Being in good health

Suffering from disease or pain can seriously reduce the enjoyment of love, happiness, and all other worldly gains.

3. Love

Having love and loved ones (friends, family, pets … the list can go on, varying from one person to another) to share your happiness and success makes the experience more satisfying.

4. Happiness

If you are unhappy, no amount of money and status would compensate for it in life. It's no surprise that depression makes the very rich as prone to suicide as the poor.

5. Everything else

If you have 1–4, very little is needed from number 5 on the list to make life better.

Preventing cancer is important in life because it affects all of these factors. It's a major cause of death, disability, losing loved ones, and unhappiness. Number 5 on the list is not spared either. Almost every aspect of human life is affected by cancer. For example, it is the most common cause of bankruptcy in countries with a private healthcare system, like the USA.

10.1   The Components of Cancer Prevention

Everything in this world has risks associated with it. Life is all about taking calculated risks. What gives us life can also bring death. A glass of water comes with the risk of choking and death. Too much water can drown. Knowing the risks and risk reduction is essential for survival.

Differentiating between low and high risk helps to formulate effective screening programmes, and reduce the risk of cancer without compromising the quality of life. One should remember that 'low risk' does not mean 'no risk', but it is sensible to concentrate our efforts of screening and preventing cancer (for example, lung cancer) for high-risk factors (like smoking) among high-risk groups (e.g., smokers).

10.2   Approaches to Prevention

Contrary to the common misconception, preventing any disease, including cancer, is not only important before the onset of disease but also after it has occurred, to reverse the process, if possible, by using curative interventions or reduce the pace of its destruction.

When it comes to cancer, this strategy is even more important, because often the risk factors causing cancer in the first place, if not avoided, can make it worse and reduce the efficacy of treatment. Continuing to smoke, for example, creates an environment in which cancer cells prosper and treatment strategies such as radiotherapy become less effective.

The modern concept of preventing any disease is to work at different levels, as follows:

1) **Primary Prevention** – This is the classical concept of disease prevention by measures to avoid development of disease. Examples include health promotion measures, like anti-smoking campaigns and legislating for an asbestos-free environment.

2) **Secondary Prevention** – Secondary prevention strategies involve early diagnosis and treatment of cancer to avoid significant suffering and morbidity. For example, screening programmes for breast, lung, and colon cancer, followed by radical (curative) treatment such as surgery in combination with chemotherapy, radiotherapy, and hormone therapy including neoadjuvant (additional treatment given before the main curative treatment to shrink the cancer and make the main treatment more effective) and adjuvant (add-on treatment given after the main curative treatment to mop upon any left-over cancer cells) forms.

3) **Tertiary Prevention** – This involves treatments that aim to reduce the negative impact of established disease by restoring function and reducing disease-related complications. Examples are use of palliative chemotherapy and radiotherapy for metastatic cancers.

4) **Quaternary Prevention** – This is a new concept of health activities that mitigate or avoid the consequences of unnecessary or excessive interventions, like over-treating and over-investigating that do not confer a benefit to the patient.

Applying this multi-level prevention (primary, secondary, and tertiary) to the 20 most common cancers in the United Kingdom can be summarised as follows.

Cancers	Primary Prevention	Secondary Prevention	Tertiary Prevention
1. Breast	Health promotion, especially exercise	Screening (mammography)	Chemotherapy, hormone therapy, & radiotherapy
2. Lung	Health promotion, especially smoking cessation	Screening (low dose CT scans)	Chemotherapy & radiotherapy
3. Colorectal	Health promotion, NSAIDs	Screening	Chemotherapy & radiotherapy
4. Prostate	Health promotion, especially diet	Screening (controversial)	Chemotherapy, hormone therapy, & radiotherapy
5. Non-Hodgkin's Lymphoma	Health promotion	None at present	Chemotherapy & radiotherapy
6. Malignant Melanoma	Health promotion, especially UV protection	Screening (self-examination of moles in high-risk population)	Chemotherapy & radiotherapy
7. Bladder	Health promotion, especially smoking cessation and avoiding occupational exposure to carcinogens	Screening tests under development	Chemotherapy & radiotherapy

Cancers	Primary Prevention	Secondary Prevention	Tertiary Prevention
8. Kidney	Health promotion, especially smoking cessation and avoiding occupational exposure to carcinogens	Screening for genetically predisposed population	Chemotherapy & radiotherapy
9. Oesophagus	Health promotion, especially smoking cessation and alcohol avoidance	Screening for high-risk patients (especially Barrett's oesophagus)	Chemotherapy, stenting, endoscopic laser therapy & radiotherapy
10. Stomach	Health promotion, especially *H. pylori* eradication	Screening in high-risk populations (Japan)	Chemotherapy & radiotherapy
11. Pancreas	Health promotion, especially smoking cessation and balanced diet	Screening (potential for microRNA, miR-155 detection)	Chemotherapy & radiotherapy
12. Uterus	Health promotion, avoiding oestrogen-only treatment	Screening for high-risk population groups	Chemotherapy & radiotherapy
13. Leukaemia	Health promotion, smoking cessation, and avoiding known carcinogens	No effective screening at present	Chemotherapy & radiotherapy
14. Ovary	Health promotion, oophorectomy in high-risk groups	No effective screening at present but women with BRCA gene mutations can be offered preventive surgery	Chemotherapy & radiotherapy

Cancers	Primary Prevention	Secondary Prevention	Tertiary Prevention
15. Oral	Health promotion, especially smoking and alcohol cessation	Screening for high-risk groups (regular clinical examination)	Chemotherapy & radiotherapy
16. Brain with CNS	Health promotion, smoking cessation, and HIV prevention	No effective screening at present	Chemotherapy & radiotherapy
17. Multiple Myeloma	Health promotion, especially avoiding known carcinogens	No effective screening at present	Chemotherapy & radiotherapy
18. Liver	Health promotion, especially HBV and HCV prevention	Screening in high-risk groups especially those with chronic hepatitis	Chemotherapy & radiotherapy
19. Cervix	Health promotion, especially HPV vaccination, safe sex, and smoking cessation	Screening in females above the age of 25 by pap smears	Chemotherapy & radiotherapy
20. Mesothelioma	Avoiding asbestos exposure	Screening in high-risk groups with asbestos exposure	Chemotherapy & radiotherapy

10.3   The Dos, Don'ts, And Cant's of Cancer Prevention

In terms of what you can do to help reduce your risks for any given cancer, our current state of knowledge on risk factors allows us to recommend both positive actions (dos) and things to avoid (don'ts). There are also some things that are largely beyond our control (can'ts). Awareness of 'can'ts' may at first glance seem pointless, but often they are actually very important indeed. For example, knowing of a family history of a disease, or condition, that places you at an unavoidably higher risk may therefore encourage you to seek screening or monitoring where available, and this might be crucial to catching the disease in its early stages, allowing more effective treatment and a better outcome.

Here's a summary for the top 15 most common cancers. You will see there are some recurring 'dos' and 'don'ts' and so these are probably the most significant actions you can take to 'generally' reduce your risk.

(i) Prostate Cancer

Do exercise; have regular and frequent (consensual) sex; have a diet of rich in tomatoes and vitamins, especially vitamin E and mineral Selenium; consult a doctor to see if you can have low-dose aspirin and get sexually transmitted diseases treated promptly.

Don't be a couch potato; put on weight; have sex with someone who has *Trichomonas vaginalis* (if you find out too late, get treatment for both of you); or have a diet rich in calcium or dairy.

Can't help it if you are a male; very tall; and/or have a family history of prostate cancer (e.g., BRCA mutations); but you can compensate for it by minimising other risk factors.

(ii) Breast Cancer

Life Events – Events that increase the exposure to female hormones, oestrogen, and progesterone increase the risk of breast cancer. These events include:

1) Early menarche before the age of 12 (menarche is the first occurrence of menstruation)

2) Late menopause (after the age of 55)

3) Not bearing children

4) Having first pregnancy over age of 30

Conversely, the opposite of these life events, including late menarche, early menopause, bearing children and having pregnancy before the age of 30, reduces the risk of breast cancer.

Family History – The risk of breast cancer is higher for people who have a family member, especially a first-degree relative with breast cancer. The risk increases with the number of relatives with the disease. For example, with only one first-degree relative, the risk is twice as high compared to general population, but with more than one relative the risk increases three to fourfold. The younger the age of the relative with breast cancer, the greater is the risk of developing the disease for other relatives.

Do exercise; have a diet of rich in fruits, vegetables, carotenoids, and calcium after menopause; lose weight if indicated; have babies, and breastfeed if you can.

Don't drink alcohol; be a couch potato; put on weight; be exposed to chest X-rays unnecessarily; have a dairy-rich diet; or take medications containing oestrogens and progesterones.

Can't help it if you are a female; were born a big baby; grew to be very tall; had early menarche and/or late menopause; have no babies or had baby/babies after 30 years of age; or have a family history of breast cancer such as BRCA1 or BRCA2 mutations but you can compensate for it by minimising the risk factors. Especially if there is a family history of breast cancer, including BRCA mutations, you can enrol in a screening programme and possibly undergo prophylactic (preventive) surgery (removal of breasts and ovaries) if advised by your doctor.

(iii) Melanoma

Do drink coffee; grow a beard (if you can); use sun blocks (clothing and suntan lotion); have screening for melanoma if in a high-risk group; and consult a doctor to see if you can have low-dose aspirin.

Don't drink alcohol; expose yourself to ultraviolet rays, natural or manmade, petroleum chemicals, selenium, or skin-bleaching agents.

Can't help it if you are unable to grow a beard (for example, being a woman); have naevi (moles); congenital melanocytic naevi; atypical naevi; FAMM syndrome, atypical mole syndrome; a history of skin cancer, including melanoma; genetic history of melanoma; are immunocompromised; have/had endometriosis or prostate cancer, but get them checked out.

(iv) Bladder Cancer

Do exercise; have a diet of rich vitamins, especially vitamin D and C; eat fruit and vegetables, especially cruciferous vegetables; drink tea; and get any infections treated.

Don't smoke; drink alcohol; have arsenic in food or water; get urinary tract infections, and if you have them, get them treated early and don't let them fester.

Can't help it if you have mutations of the P53 gene; work with metal works, electronics and textile manufacturing, or industrial chemicals; are very tall; but you can compensate for it by minimising the risk factors.

Although there are no effective screening programmes for early detection of bladder cancer at present, for high-risk groups checking the urine for blood can be a good starting point. If blood is detected in the urine, an examination of the bladder (cystoscopy) by a urologist is helpful in detecting the cancer in its early stages. If found early, before it has spread outside the bladder, curative treatment can be offered.

(v) Brain Tumours

Do exercise; have a diet of rich in vitamins, especially vitamin C and E, fruits, vegetables, dietary fibre, whole grain; lose weight if indicated; and consult a doctor to see if you can benefit from low-dose aspirin (it doesn't help everyone, and the benefits have to be weighed against the risks).

Don't smoke; drink alcohol; get exposure to radioactivity, herbicides, insecticides; get a head injury[147]; get infected with *Toxoplasma gondii*[148]; have food or products with nitrosamines.

Can't help it if your mother didn't have a diet rich in vitamin A, C, folate and vegetables when expecting you; if you don't have frequent colds and flus; don't suffer from asthma and allergies; never had chicken pox (frequent colds and flu, asthma, allergies, and chicken pox reduce the risk of brain tumours); if you have a family history of certain conditions like Gorlin syndrome, familial glioma, Lynch syndrome (HNPCC); familial adenomatosis polypi (FAP); neurofibromatosis type 1 or 2; Li-Fraumeni syndrome or Von Hippel-Lindau (VHL) disease; or have been exposed to radiation after a head injury or in your childhood; BUT you can minimise the risk by avoiding other risk factors.

---

[147] Wear a helmet during high-risk activities.
[148] Use barrier contraceptive like a condom.

(vi) Colorectal Cancer

Colorectal cancer is the third-most common cancer in the world, and accounts for almost 10% of new cancer cases.

The survival from colorectal cancer depends on the stage of detection. If found at an early stage, the 5-year survival is around 90%, but at later stages, when the cancer has spread to other organs of the body, the survival at five years drops to around 13%. Hence, it is important to screen and detect it as early as possible, especially in high-risk groups.

Do exercise; have a diet of rich in calcium and vitamins, especially vitamin D and C; eat fish, dairy, fruits, vegetables, dietary fibre, whole grain; lose weight if indicated; consult a doctor to see if you can have low-dose aspirin and if suffering from inflammatory bowel disease, get it treated.

Don't smoke; drink alcohol; be a couch potato; put on weight; eat processed meat, red meat and food containing too much iron (especially haem iron).

Can't help it if you have FAP; HNPCC; or are very tall; but you can compensate for it by minimising other risk factors.

(vii) Endometrial (Womb) Cancer

Endometrial cancer, or cancer of the womb, is the sixth-most common cancer among women. The endometrium, the lining of the uterus, undergoes cyclical changes throughout the fertile years, almost on a monthly basis. This repeated activity of cell division puts it at risk of DNA damage and mutations that can lead to cancer.

The risk increases with age and is most common after menopause.

Life Events: The following life events have an impact on the risk of endometrial cancer:

1) Not bearing children – This increases the risk.

2) Late menopause – This increases the risk.

3) Early menopause – This reduces the risk.

4) Bearing children – This reduces the risk.

Medications - Medications which contain oestrogen or oestrogen hormone-like substances increase the risk of endometrial cancer. Oral contraceptive pills which contain oestrogen and progesterone reduce the risk, as does the use of progesterone-only medication.

Do exercise; lose weight; drink coffee; have kids (the more the better); if indicated, consult a doctor to see if you can avoid oestrogen-only hormone therapies.

Don't be a couch potato; put on weight; have a sugar or carbohydrate-rich diet.

Can't help it if you are very tall; or not having any kids; but you can compensate for it by minimising other risk factors.

(viii) Gall Bladder Cancer (Cholangiocarcinoma)

Gall bladder cancers are very rare, accounting for only 1% of all human cancers. However, they are difficult to treat and are associated with high mortality. They are more common in women than men, accounting for 57% of the total cases.

The gall bladder is a sack-like organ attached to the liver by ducts known as *bile ducts*. Its function is to collect, store, and release liver bile into the small intestine. Most of the gall bladder cancers are adenocarcinomas (90–95%), but some could be squamous cell carcinomas.

Do exercise; lose weight if indicated.

Don't be a couch potato; and put on weight.

Can't help it if you have gallstones despite having a healthy lifestyle.

(ix) Gastric (Stomach) Cancer

The most common risk factor of stomach cancer is infection with *Helicobacter pylori* (*H. pylori*), a bacterium[149] that likes to live in the stomach lining (gastric mucosa). This bacterium causes inflammation and an immune response in the stomach, resulting in the release of various bacteria and host-dependent cytotoxic substances. Usually, the infection is asymptomatic and spreads from one person to another through saliva and faeces.

---

[149] Belonging to the group of bacteria known as 'gram-negative'.

It is crucial that the pre-cancerous stage should be detected in high-risk individuals and treated with antibiotic therapy to eradicate the *H. pylori*.

The bacterium *H. pylori* is classified as a class 1 carcinogen.

Around 10% of the gastric cancers are associated with EBV (Epstein-Barr virus) infection. Infection with EBV is romantically referred to as the 'kissing disease', the only time a kiss is associated with disease. In reality, the infection spreads more by sharing utensils like cups and glasses which have not been washed (or not properly washed) and are awash/contaminated with human saliva.

Do exercise; have a diet rich in vitamins, especially vitamin C; fruits, especially citrus fruits; lose weight if indicated; and consult a doctor if suffering from gastritis, reflux, or *H. pylori* infection, and get it treated.

Don't smoke; drink alcohol; be a couch potato; put on weight; eat processed meat, grilled and barbecued food, salt-preserved food and fish; work with wood processing, rubber manufacturing, metal processing, and coal mining; avoid using unwashed utensils contaminated with saliva from other people, especially those with EBV or *H. pylori* infection, and don't kiss them, either.

Can't help it if you have high-risk mutations such as GTSM1[150], but you can compensate for it by minimising other risk factors.

(x) Kidney (Renal) Cancer

Kidneys are the filtration centre of the human body. They excrete unwanted stuff, be it excess water, salt, or toxins either consumed from our environment or produced within our cells. If the toxins are water soluble, they will simply get filtered out of the kidney. If they are not water soluble then the liver breaks them down into water-soluble components which are then excreted by the kidneys. For some chemicals, the kidneys also have special pumps which pump them out of the cells into the urine.

In light of their function of excreting toxins from the body, the kidneys are inevitably exposed to toxic chemicals more than other organs. Some of these toxins can cause DNA damage leading to mutations and formation of kidney cancer. Kidney cancer is the twelfth-most common cancer. The incidence is higher among men compared to women and more common in the Western world compared to Africa and Asia.

Do exercise; lose weight if indicated; and consult a doctor if suffering from hypertension, and get it treated.

---

[150] Glutathione S-transferase gene mutation, which can affect the risk of gastric cancer.

Don't smoke; drink more than 30 grams of alcohol a day; be a couch potato; put on weight; consume food or drinks with arsenic; use phenacetin, a painkiller and fever-relief medicine (Luckily, it's not available in the market anymore so don't worry about taking it by mistake. However, it is still, sometimes, used to adulterate cocaine).

Can't help it if you have polycystic kidney disease; tuberous sclerosis, Von Hippel-Lindau disease; and or are very tall; but you can compensate for it by minimising other risk factors.

(xi) Hepatocellular (Liver) Cancer

Liver cancer may not be the commonest cancer, but due to its deadly nature it is the second-most common cause of death from cancer worldwide.

Even with the best treatment, the survival rate for people with liver cancer at five years is quite low (12%). Unfortunately, the number of new cases is increasing every day and although in the Western world it is a disease associated with old age (above the age of 75), in developing countries, especially Asia and Africa, the patients tend to be much younger (typically around the age of 40 years).

Preventing liver cancer is probably one of the easier tasks compared to preventing other cancers. The basic rule is to be kind to your liver and not expose it to unnecessary toxins. It can cope with small amounts of insult and even regenerate its dead cells, but the capacity is limited and with advancing age it reduces further. In addition to the general preventative measures and a healthy lifestyle, there are some secrets which can help promote our health in general and reduce the risk of liver cancer. These are as follows:

Do exercise; have a diet of rich in vitamins; eat fish, nuts, fruits, vegetables; drink coffee; lose weight if indicated; consult a doctor to see if you can have low-dose aspirin and if suffering from hepatitis B, C, D, alcoholic liver disease or any other kind like non-alcoholic fatty liver disease, get it treated.

Don't smoke; drink alcohol; be a couch potato; put on weight; use oral contraceptive pills (use an alternative if possible); get exposure to hepatitis viruses or aflatoxin.

Can't help it if you already have had hepatitis and resulting scarring of the liver (cirrhosis) but you can compensate for it by minimising other risk factors.

(xii) Lung Cancer

Lung cancer is the third-most common cancer in the world accounting for about 13% of cases. If detected at an early stage, the 5-year overall survival is around 55%. However, if detected at a later stage, when it has spread to regions outside the lung, the survival rate is much lower, at between 10-17%. Unfortunately, 70% of the lung cancers are detected at a later stage.

Do exercise; have a diet of rich in vitamins, especially vitamin C, isoflavones, folate, fruits, vegetables; lose weight if indicated; consult a doctor to see if you are suffering from COPD (emphysema and bronchitis), tuberculosis, recurrent pneumonias, rheumatoid arthritis, scleroderma, sarcoidosis, lung fibrosis, or HIV and get it treated; and open those windows for a few hours every day to let the radon gas out.

Don't smoke, don't smoke, don't smoke … that's 95% of the lung cancers avoided.

In addition, don't drink alcohol; be a couch potato; put on weight; eat processed meat and red meat; get exposed to second-hand cigarette smoke, coal tar, asbestos, smoke from burning of wood and coal arsenic, crystalline silica, radon gas, mixtures of polycyclic aromatic hydrocarbons, uranium, nickel, and heavy metals[151].

Can't help it if you have Werner's syndrome, xeroderma pigmentosum, Bloom's syndrome, TP53, or RB gene mutations, but you can compensate for them by minimising other risk factors.

(xiii) Oesophageal Cancer

Oesophageal cancer is the eighth commonest cancer worldwide and accounts for 3% of all new cases. Men are twice as likely as women to develop this cancer. The 5-year survival for oesophageal cancer is quite poor, being about 20% in North America and 10% in Europe, and far less in the developing countries.

Do exercise; have a diet of rich in vitamins, especially vitamin C; eat fruits, vegetables; lose weight if indicated; consult a doctor to see if you are suffering from Barrett's oesophagus[152], oesophageal achalasia[153], tylosis[154], Plummer-Vinson syndrome[155], or GORD (gastro-oesophageal reflux disease), and get them treated.

---

[151] The musical rock 'n' roll type is safe from the lung cancer prospective. OK for brain tumours, too, unless you take the term 'headbanger' in a literal sense.

[152] An inflammatory condition of the oesophagus.

[153] A condition in which the lower end of the oesophagus goes into a spasm.

[154] A hereditary condition in which the skin of the palms and soles of feet is thickened and there is an increased incidence of oesophageal cancer. The reason is a defective tumour suppressor gene which causes extra growth of skin layers and development of cancer in the food canal.

[155] A rare disease, causing strictures/narrowing of the oesophagus. The exact cause is unknown. Fortunately, it is becoming rarer as time goes by and maybe, one day, we may never need to know what causes it.

Don't smoke; drink alcohol; very hot beverages; hot mate leaf drink; be a couch potato; put on weight; and eat processed meat.

Can't help it if you have HPV infection, but you can compensate for it by minimising other risk factors.

(xiv) Ovarian Cancer

Ovarian cancer is the seventh-most common cancer in women. It comes in two types: epithelia, from the epithelial cells in the ovary, and germ cell type, from the germinating cells.

The risk increases with age and after menopause for the epithelial ovarian cancers. However, the germ cell tumours peak between the age of 15 and 35. Ovarian cancers are usually quite advanced when they are diagnosed and hence the overall survival at five years with treatment is between 30–50%.

Do exercise; lose weight if indicated; have babies; breastfeed; use the oral contraceptive pill if needed; and if you have a family history of BRCA1 or BRCA2 gene mutations, consult a doctor to see if you can benefit from prophylactic surgery to remove the ovaries.

Don't be a couch potato; put on weight; have hormone replacement therapy (consider an alternative).

Can't help it if you are a female; don't have babies; had early menarche and/or a late menopause; are very tall; but you can compensate for it by minimising other risk factors.

(xv) Pancreatic Cancer

The pancreas is an important gland in the human body that lies behind the stomach. It has a dual function. Firstly, it produces digestive enzymes which are made in a part of the gland known as the *exocrine pancreas*. The second function is to produce hormones which regulate metabolism, especially glucose metabolism, such as insulin and glucagon, and these are produced by endocrine cells. Most pancreatic cancers occur in the exocrine tissue, accounting for approximately 95% of cases.

Pancreatic cancers are relatively rare and constitute only 2% of all cancers, but they account for 3% of all cancer deaths; indicating that survival rates are quite low. This is because the disease is often found late in the course of its development, and by the time the cancer gets diagnosed it has progressed to an advanced stage and spread to other parts of the body. The incidence of pancreatic cancer is higher among men.

Do exercise; lose weight if indicated; drink coffee; and consult a doctor to see if you are suffering from diabetes, and get it treated.

Don't smoke; drink alcohol; be a couch potato; put on weight; eat processed meat, red meat, and food containing too much fructose and fat.

Can't help it if you have a family history of pancreatic cancer or are very tall but you can compensate for it by minimising other risk factors.

10.4   Exercise (the New 'Chemotherapy')

'Tertiary prevention' with exercise is the new frontier of cancer treatment. Thierry Bouillet MD, an oncologist at Avicenne Hospital in Paris, believes that physical activity should be prescribed to women with early breast cancer, along with their regular therapeutic regimen of chemotherapy. This is based on the results of an analysis published in April 2015 from the Scientific Commission of the National Federation Support and Cancer (CAMI), in France.

His review of eight studies looked at how physical activity affected survival in patients with localised breast cancer. Led by Dr Bouillet, the author reported that physical activity higher than 8–9 metabolic equivalent task (MET is a measure of the rate at which a person expends energy relative to their build) hours per week was associated with a 50% reduction in mortality from both cancer and all other causes. This translated into the same benefit as from chemotherapy.

The CAMI federation began in 1998, with Dr Bouillet as one of the founding members. It now has 60 partner institutions across France that run courses with a variety of different physical activities. These programmes are increasingly being offered by hospitals, such as the Institute Gustave Roussy in Villejuif, France, which now hold dance and martial art classes. The French have introduced a new piece of health legislation called the *loi de la sante*. This amendment sets the framework for providing the service, including the responsibility for training physicians to prescribe adequate physical activity. However, more research is needed to study the benefit of physical activity and exercise in cancer patients receiving active treatment such as chemotherapy and radiation.

Let's admit it, most of us don't exercise (enough).

In fact, most people do have a strong desire to exercise but just won't do it. And there is a good reason why we won't exercise. But let's first analyse why we have a desire to exercise in the first place.

Humans are hunter gatherers, walkers, stalkers … stalkers of animal prey for food that is, not the psychotic kind! Exercise is very important. Our body is designed to stand and walk, not sit and watch. We are the only upright creature on the planet, not only in body but also mind. We stand up for justice, morality, and rights, human and animal. We walk upright in an unusual way. Other animals like bears, monkeys, gorillas, and meerkats – to name but a few – do so in short bursts, swaying clumsily before going back on all fours. We do it in a very dignified and sustained manner, apart from the occasional wobble.

Our body is destined not only to walk but also run. Everything about it – the skeleton, bones, muscles, bone alignment with the muscles and each other, joints, even the angles at which bones are attached to each other and the muscles, are designed for us to walk and run upright. Our strength is not in running faster but longer. Usain Bolt would definitely lose to Elsa the lioness, but I reckon Mohamed Farah would easily beat her long distance.

In the late 1940s, Jeremy Morris, a brilliant British doctor, carried out a clever study of 35,000 London double-decker bus drivers and conductors. Both professions were matched for all possible risk factors with only one difference. Conductors climbed 600 steps per shift compared to the drivers who just sat at their seats. The results showed that drivers were twice as likely to suffer heart attacks than conductors. This was the first time that advantages of exercise were proven on scientific grounds. This landmark study was expected to have a major impact on government policy for health but the outcome was totally unexpected. They introduced ticketing machines and got rid of the conductors.

A later, larger study of more than half a million people in 2012 showed that those who exercise just a mere 11 minutes per day after the age of 40 live 1.8 years longer than those who don't. An hour or more every day adds 4.2 years. Not a bad investment if you ask me. It also reduces suffering, by decreasing the risk of cancer, heart disease, diabetes, and strokes.

Despite all this, ask humans to work out in a gym and for many their hearts sink. Which raises the question, why?

And you would be glad to know that after much searching, I have found the answer to this question. So, brace yourself, for this is an exclusive.

Humans do physical activity for a material incentive, especially food and survival. It's against our nature to exercise without a material reward that can translate into either sustenance or survival. Our ancestors did not exercise to look good in the mirror, because there were no mirrors. They feasted their eyes on other people's beauty, not their own. Narcissism is a relatively new concept. And it cannot be a positive driving force for health. Maybe for some select individuals, but definitely not for the masses.

Humans will exercise, regularly and religiously, if they are paid for it because our instinctive nature is to work for material gains. Remember the research in the 1940s by Jeremy Morris? The bus conductors were blissfully unaware of the level of exercise and its beneficial effects, yet did it regularly and effortlessly because it was part of their job, which generated a salary.

Lack of exercise and our modern lifestyle are both toxic to anyone who indulges in them. Nowhere is the effect of lack of exercise and modern lifestyle more evident than among man's best friends, dogs, and their nemesis, cats. Both species have a higher rate of a myriad of diseases including cancers compared to their wilder counterparts. Cancer is the leading cause of death in dogs at 47%, the highest among any mammals on the planet, and 32% among cats.

We have to remember that health and longevity come at a price, and a big part of that price is exercise.

PART II

LIVE
LONGER

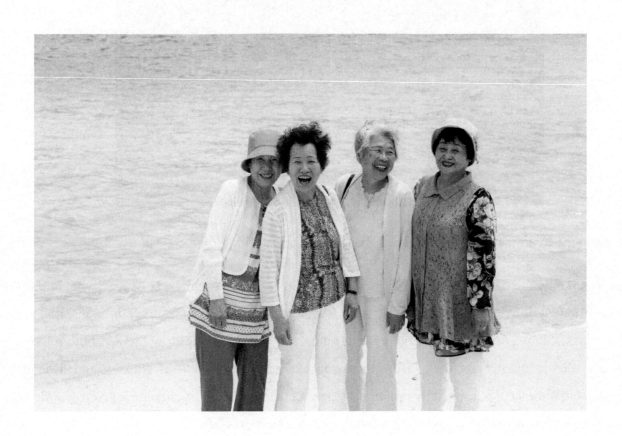

PART 11: LIVE LONGER

11   Living Longer: Lifestyle & Mind Over Matter

11.1   Living Longer and Healthier

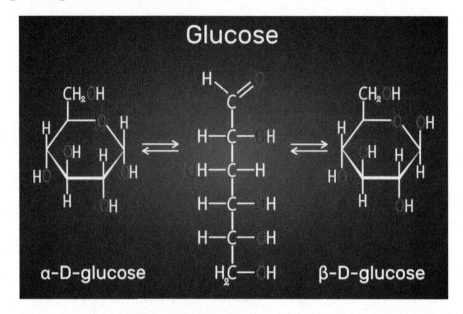

If you asked me to define ageing in three words, I would call it 'chronic glucose poisoning'.

Glucose is not only the fuel for cells but is also used to build cellular structures. However, what builds the body also brings it down. Glucose is a sticky stuff, literally; just as sugar sticks to your hands, it also has a tendency to stick unnecessarily. If the body needs glucose attached to proteins or fats as a building block, it uses enzymes to incorporate them. But glucose in excess has the habit of sticking and denaturing (damaging) other molecules, especially proteins, by a process known as *non-enzymatic glycosylation*. The end products are known as *advanced glycosylation end products* or *AGEs*.

It's these AGEs which are the major cause of ageing.

AGEs damage proteins, especially the structural proteins like collagen, which gives skin its elasticity and bounce. With AGEs, collagen becomes stiff and breaks easily. In a younger person, damage can be repaired but with advancing age and/or increased glucose in the body, the capacity of the repair mechanisms is reduced and easily overwhelmed. This is evident in younger people suffering from uncontrolled diabetes who, despite their youthful age, have problems with cataracts, and nerve and kidney damage, all usually associated with older age.

So, the key to staying younger is striking a balance between carbohydrate intake and our body's repair capacity. As we advance in years it becomes even more important to reduce our carbohydrate intake.

Living longer and healthier is an important way to prevent cancer. It may sound like stating the obvious, but there is a hidden truth to it. Most factors that help you live a long and healthy life also prevent cancer. Many years ago, scientists carried out a study funded by the US National Institute on Aging, looking at the different parts of the world where people had a tendency to live longer.

They chose three geographic localities: Sardinia in Italy, Okinawa in Japan, and Loma Linda in California, USA. All three are renowned for having a high rate of centenarians who suffer a fraction of the diseases that commonly kill people in other parts of the world, and who therefore enjoy more healthy years of life.

11.1.1 Sardinian Centenarians

In Sardinia, they focused on a community of 2,400 people living in a cluster of villages on the sloping fringes of the Gennargentu mountains in central Sardinia. Genetically, these people belong to a group of hunter-gatherers who, about 11,000 years ago, left the Iberian Peninsula and made their way eastwards to Sardinia. With advancement of other nations, such as the Phoenicians and Romans, over the centuries these Sardinians were driven deeper and deeper into the mountainous highlands, where they lived in relative isolation from other communities. Roughly 80% of them are directly related to the first Sardinians who moved there 11,000 years ago. So, their gene pool has been largely ring-fenced, with little influence from the outside world.

A peculiar finding among the Sardinians is that not only are they twice as likely as other Italians to reach their 100th birthday but also that the chances of doing so are similar for males and females. This contrasts sharply to the rest of the world where women tend to live longer than men. In the United States, for example, 80% of the centenarians are females.

Researchers found several important distinguishing characteristics among this population. Firstly, men and women had a very active lifestyle, working hard into the later years of their life. Reports of suffering from stress were very low. Their diet was usually based on home-grown fruits and vegetables, such as tomatoes, fava beans, eggplant (aubergine), and zucchini, all of which are associated with a reduced risk of heart disease and colon cancer. They consumed dairy products from grass-fed sheep and ate pecorino cheese, high in protein and omega-3 fatty acids. Sardinians do consume wine, but the grapes grown in this mountainous region have 2–3 times as much of the compounds found in other wines that may prevent cardiovascular disease. The researchers observed that obesity was virtually non-existent before 1940 among the Sardinians, and even at the time of the study it only affected about 10% of the population. It was observed that they eat a very thin, flat bread known as *carta da musica*, which means as thin as a 'sheet of music'. This obviously has fewer calories compared to other bread. Having a very close-knit family system, the concept of putting elders into a retirement home was almost unheard of. In fact, it is considered to be dishonourable for the family to do so. Their positive attitude towards life was noted. A typical Sardinian greeting is *a kent'annos*, which means 'health and life for 100 years'. Finally, it seemed that Sardinians do not get bored of life. They love living within their means and usually are very happy and satisfied with whatever they have.

11.1.2 Growing Old in Okinawa

The study of Okinawans in Japan was carried out because this island has one of the world's longest-lived people, with an average life expectancy of 78 years for men and 86 years for women. Research showed that they enjoy years free from disabilities and have a fifth of the heart disease, a fourth of breast and prostate cancer, and a third less dementia, than Americans. The important factors relating to their longevity are as follows:

1. *Ikigai*, which roughly translates to a quote meaning, 'what makes one's life worth living', is the main theme of Okinawan life. Hence, they have a purpose of life, making it worth living and they look forward to every coming day.

2. Seaweed is an important part of their diet, which is a very low calorie, plant-based source of nutrition.

3. Okinawans are physically very active, indulging in all kinds of exercises such as yoga, swimming, diving, and fishing.

4. Senior Okinawans have a very low incidence of obesity. Unfortunately, the newer generation indulges in fast food and the younger Okinawans now have one of Japan's highest rates of obesity.

5. Okinawans love to stay in contact with family and friends, and are very social people. This makes them less prone to depression and heart diseases.

6. Okinawans have a mutual support network called *moai*, providing emotional, social, and financial help throughout life.

7. The Okinawan diet is a low-calorie diet rich in vegetables, miso soup, and tofu with little fish or meat.

8. They live by the Confucian (Confucius was actually never called 'Confucius'; he was known as 'Kongfuze', meaning 'Master Kong') inspired saying *hara hachi bu*, which means 'eat until your stomach is 80% full'. This is similar to the ancient Arabic saying by Prophet Mohammad (may peace be upon him) which advises to stop eating while you are still hungry.

9. Okinawans have home gardens where they grow herbs and spices, fruits, and vegetables, such as garlic, Chinese radishes, cabbage, turmeric, and tomatoes. All contain antioxidants that can block cancer before it gets started.

10. Okinawans tend to stay outdoors quite a lot, exposing themselves to healthy sunshine which is a source of vitamin D and can help prevent osteoporosis, boost immunity, and reduce risk of diseases.

11. They tend to have a strong motive to keep living, which is especially based around friends and family.

11.1.3 Living Long in Loma Linda

The study of Seventh-day Adventists in Loma Linda, California, half way between Palm Springs and Los Angeles, showed that the average Adventist lives 4-10 years longer than the average Californian. This does not come as a surprise because the Adventist Church was formed in the 19th century on health-based reforms and has popularised organised vegetarianism. A renowned member was John Harvey Kellogg, whose name has been immortalised in breakfast cereals.

The Adventist Church forbids alcohol consumption, smoking, and eating pork. It also discourages consumption of other meat, caffeinated drinks, and stimulating condiments and spices. Their diet is mostly based on grains, fruits, nuts, and vegetables. In other words, they religiously consume a healthier diet. Important factors identified among the Seventh-day Adventist are as follows:

1) They put family as a priority.

2) Physically, they are very active on a daily basis.

3) They keep socially engaged.

4) Their diet is rich in fruits, vegetables, and whole grains.

5) They consume nuts and beans.

6) They observe the Sabbath (Saturday) reserved for religious activities, family, charity work, and nature walks, and have a strong faith.

7) Their food is often rich in soya milk, tomatoes, and other foods which lower the risk of developing certain cancers.

8) They eat whole-wheat bread.

9) Drinking five glasses of water a day is done with a religious regularity.

10) They consume at least four servings of nuts a week, reducing the risk of heart disease.

11) They do not eat red meat, which helps to avoid heart disease and cancer.

A study conducted from 1976 to 1988 by the National Institute of Health (NIH) looked at 34,000 Californian Adventists and observed their health-oriented lifestyles. They found that their life expectancy was higher, and risk of heart disease and cancer was significantly lower, than other Americans. It also helps that the Seventh-day Adventists associate with people who reinforce their healthy behaviour. Hence the key to their success is faith, food, and community.

Looking at these three populations and other communities which have a healthier and longer life, the following conclusions can be drawn (some of which would sound familiar from our discussion above).

1) Have a purpose of life, and love to live.

2) Put your family first, providing mutual support and love.

3) Be physically active every day.

4) Keep socially engaged, especially deriving support and company from like-minded people who have a healthy lifestyle. As an old Arabic saying goes, you end up with the same way of life as your friends[156].

---

[156] Book of General Behaviour, (*Sunan Abi Dawud)*, sayings of the Prophet Mohammad, may peace be upon him, number 4833: "A man follows the way of life of his/her companion/friend so each one of you should consider whom he/she makes his/her friend."

5) Eat food rich in fruits, vegetables, nuts, and whole grains.

6) Do not eat to fill your stomach and always stop eating while you are still hungry. This takes a bit of effort because our brains only get a signal from the stomach to stop eating 15 to 20 minutes after we have filled up our stomachs. This is probably an evolutionary mechanism to ensure that we have extra nutrition, as our ancestors never had access to ample food like we do. However, in the modern-day lifestyle it has negative connotations, and the end result is obesity.

7) 'The more you eat, the sooner you die,' goes an old Arabic saying. It seems like every human being is destined to have a certain number of calories in their life. Consuming those calories quickly over a short period of time is associated with a shorter lifespan. Observational studies show that if you spread out the calorie consumption, over the years you tend to live longer.

8) Have a low-calorie diet which should be rich in vitamins, minerals, and antioxidants.

9) Eat food which is rich with omega-3 fatty acids.

10) Eat small portions of food.

11) Find a purpose for life. This is a common recurrent theme among all three long-living communities studied in Italy, Japan, and America.

12) Have faith and belief (if you want to; remember, there is no compulsion in faith). Evidence from studies has shown that belief in God or a transcendental force helps people cope with depression and stress more easily compared to those who do not have such a belief.

13) Eat nuts and beans.

14) Keep life-long friends, as done by those who live long in Japan, Italy, and America.

15) Reduce stress and increase love in your life[157]. Stress is known to reduce immune response, and impaired immunity is associated with an increased risk of cancer.

16) Look after yourself. Life is worth more when healthy. Seeking treatment is a sign of intelligence. Take medications if you need them; seek medical help if indicated.

---

[157] Easier said than done.

17) Life can be defined as a sexually transmitted terminal condition. Like all sexually transmitted conditions, it's a gift that keeps giving. Pass it on if you can. It's one of the greatest joys of life.

18) Studies show that married people live longer. Experience says it makes life seem longer too.

19) Breath fresh air, not smoke – your lungs are not made for it.

20) Be happy without taking drugs. They can't 'make' you happy. All they do is bring out the happiness you already have inside. Find a way to unlock that happiness without drugs. Friends and family, exercise and love, altruism and sacrifice are some of the ways to do so without getting stoned.

11.2   Mind Over Matter

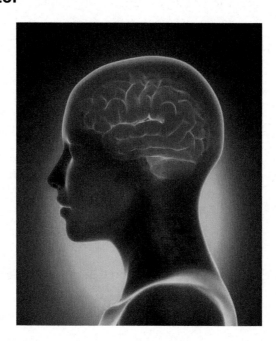

11.2.1 The Human Brain

Ingredients: 75-80% water, 20-25% protein and fat, no added sugar.

The human brain is the most important and least understood part of our body.

Its importance can be gauged by the fact that it is located in the most secure part of the body, a bony vault known as the *skull*, unlike some other organs[158] which are left hanging outside. Yet we know more about them than the brain.

---

[158] Nose, ears, lips, hair, hands, and the ones you are thinking about … feet.

Neuron and Glial cells

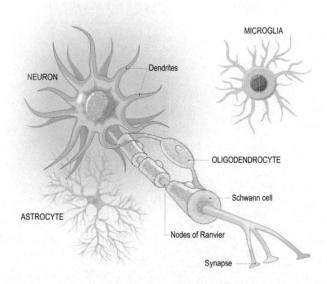

Brain cells. The heads of the neurons lie in the grey matter whereas the long tail and other cells extend to the white matter.

There are two main types of cells in the brain:

1. **Neurons**: These are the nerve cells of the brain. They have a small body with a nucleus and a relatively longer tail-like stem, known as an *axon*. The axon can be very long and has root-like extensions, called *dendrites*, at its ends for connecting to other neurons. These dendrites can number in the hundreds of thousands.

2. **Glial cells**: These outnumber neurons tenfold. They support, protect, and insulate the neurons, making sure the electric impulse in a nerve cell travels rapidly and safely from one neutron to another.

If you see a cross-section of a brain, you will find an outer thin veneer of greyish tissue, known as the *grey matter*, and an inner bulk called the *white matter*. They are known by their colour.

Grey matter is the part where the neuron body and nucleus are located. All the brain's function, thinking, memory, emotion, you name it, happens here. It's a humbling thought to realise that all of our wisdom and intelligence is only 4 mm deep[159] – that's smaller in size than an average human's smallest toenail.

---

[159] That's almost as thick as two British 10-pence coins stacked on top of each other. American readers can stack two nickels and that would be the approximate thickness of the grey matter in the brain.

Come to think of it, if beauty is skin deep, intelligence is hardly nail-depth even. Deep down, all of our thoughts are very superficial, in the literal sense. Yet, it's amazing what we humans have achieved by using such a thin layer of cells.

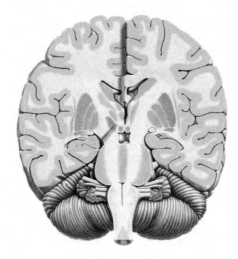

Cross-section of brain showing a thin layer of outer grey matter and inner white matter.

White matter is all axons and their connections, the wiring of the brain. And there are lots and lots of connections, and I mean *lots*, literally trillions and trillions (a trillion is a million million).

The most humbling fact about the human brain is that over the last 10–12 thousand years it has shrunk by 10%. Yes, really. Common sense says that this should have resulted in a dumbing down of our race but, while some may be nodding in agreement having spent the last hour watching YouTube videos of cats doing stupid things, to the contrary, we have not only maintained the intelligence and skills of our ancestors but have also improved on them tremendously. After all, if you showed Neolithic man a YouTube video of a dancing cat, I suspect he would be impressed and full of wonder. He might, of course, also be confused, wondering what happened to the cat after he'd smashed your iPad with his stone axe.

The secret lies in those trillions of connections in the white matter. Over time, our brains have become more efficient due to better wiring and connectivity. It's like mobile phones. In the 1980s, they used to weigh 5 kg[160], came with a carrying handle, and had no smart features. Today, they are much lighter and far more advanced. So, when it comes to the brain, bigger is not necessarily better, and humans have known it for centuries. It's even reflected in our literature. Think of fairy tale characters. Ogres are big on brain size but not brilliant, whereas goblins and leprechauns have smaller but smarter brains.

---

[160] Vodaphone VM1 model 1985 had a carrying handle and cost £4,400 in today's money.

An interesting quirk of the brain is that the right side controls the left side of the body, and the left side controls the right, and there is a method to this madness. The axons from the right have to cross over to the left to connect with the left side of the body and the ones on the left cross over to the right. In doing so they connect to each other in the middle and hence enable us to carry out coordinated movements of the two sides with precision and ease. How clever is that?

11.2.2 Mental Health

Devil Thy Name Is Despair

Legend has it that before he fell from grace, the devil as we know him now was heading all the angels and was known by the title of 'Azazel'[161] or 'the one dear to God'. Once he lost his place and title, he was named 'Iblis' (meaning 'the one who is in despair'). And this is said to be his main weapon against humans: he makes them depressed and pushes them to despair. It's clear from this concept that humans have long identified depression and despair to be the worst of evils which plague our lives.

But sadness, anxiety, and happiness are part of our normal life and mood. It's only when they reach an extreme – depression, mania, or despair – that they become problematic. Our mind has the capacity to deal with them and treat them, but sometimes these mechanisms are inadequate and require extra help in the form of professional advice and medications.

Depression and despair, a feeling of helplessness, are food for many diseases including cancer. They help them progress and this in turn feeds the despair, a vicious cycle where it becomes difficult to discern between the cause and the effect. Forget the seven deadly sins; the deadliest weapon in Mr de Evil's (aka, the devil's) arsenal is despair. Studies conducted at the University of Pennsylvania have shown that animals suffering from stress are less capable of fighting cancer than those who are unstressed. In humans, studies have shown a longer survival among cancer patients who were provided emotional support. Similar studies from Finland showed that the feeling of helplessness (despair) is associated with a higher mortality rate no matter what the cause was (e.g., heart disease, cancer, or another disease). To be alive, we not only need a healthy body but also a healthy mind full of hope and a will to live.

Let me tell you a little tale from a far-off land in the Himalayas where I come from.

Once upon a time in a far-off land, the *story* goes, there was a king.

---

[161] A combination of two words, 'Aziz' for 'dear' and 'EL' for 'God'.

Let's call him Mike (not his real name[162]).

King 'Mike' was bipolar[163].

Type 2 to be precise, part genetic, part PTSD (post-traumatic stress disorder) induced.

An exact estimate is not known, but it is rumoured that he suffered from 3–4 bouts of hypomania and a few major depressive episodes, which worried him no end. Being an intelligent person, as most people suffering from bipolar disorders are, he sought treatment. Due to a lack of lithium and electroconvulsive therapy (fortunate for the king), he was treated with potions, elixirs, and concoctions, mostly containing varying amounts of alcohol. Needless to say, they had little if any benefit.

Then, one day, he met a wise man who said he knew the secret to eternal happiness. Naturally, the king asked him for help. The wise one listened to the king patiently, told him that his hour was up, and gave him a follow-up appointment for the next clinic[164]. At their next meeting, the wise man presented the king with two (bipolar) boxes, one labelled 'Mania/ Hypomania' and the other 'Depression Major/Minor'. He advised the king to open them accordingly during his next mental episode and gave him a BOGOF deal (50% discount, or buy one get one free) on the advice.

Sure enough, in the next few days, the king had his next major depressive episode for no obvious reason. In the throes of misery and melancholy, he remembered the boxes and opened the one labelled 'Depression Major/Minor'. Inside he found an envelope. He opened the envelope to find a note that read, 'This won't last forever'.

The king felt calmer and started to distract himself with domestic and government affairs. A few days later he was back to normal.

Some weeks later, however, people around the king noticed an unprecedented mood of elation. Nothing seemed to bother him, especially the miserable condition of his subjects. After exhibiting a few inappropriate displays of euphoria, the king was diagnosed as suffering from a hypomanic episode. The

---

[162] His real name was Mahmud, King of Afghanistan, Pakistan, Iran, and Central Asia from 999 to 1030 AD ... but don't tell anyone (we must maintain patient confidentiality).
[163] A bipolar mental disorder is characterised by periods of depression and abnormally elevated moods. There are three forms: Type I, presenting with manic episode with or without depressive episodes; Type II, with one or more episodes of hypomania and one or more major depressive episode; and a third subtype, cyclothymia, which presents with hypomania and periods of minor depression with no major depressive symptoms. It effects 1% of the global and 3% of the US population.
[164] Some medical practices have not changed in more than a thousand years.

'Mania/Hypomania' box was brought with much fanfare (the king insisted on it and would have no less) and it was opened. Inside was an envelope with a note that said, 'This won't last forever'.

This non-pharmaceutical psychotherapy had a profoundly positive impact on the king's mood[165]. In due time, his bipolar disorder was downgraded to cyclothymia (mood swings), and he ruled, raided, looted, and plundered[166] happily ever after, albeit with minor symptoms.

The moral of the story, apart from the obvious shortcomings of non-pharmaceutical monotherapy (his disease wasn't cured, only downgraded) is that life is a rollercoaster, full of highs and lows – many of which may come expectedly or unexpectedly, but mostly never last. This open secret is lost to most. Mental health problems haunt us no end. Even the cleverest and the wisest among us are its victims.

In 2018, the American Psychiatric Association (APA) reported that, in the USA, one doctor commits suicide every day, the highest rate of any profession. In the general population, the suicide rate is around 12.3 per 100,000, but among doctors it ranges between 28 to 40 per 100,000. The top place within them went to psychiatrists. Some 87% of psychology graduates have anxiety, 68 % suffer from depression, 30% have felt suicidal, and 4% have attempted it. And these are the crème de la crème of human minds who have the greatest insight into mental health and its treatment.

Before we mull over mental health and the lack of research and treatment into the field (and I promise not to deny you the pleasure of mulling) let's take a look at the world around us.

The world we live in is a product of the human mind. Cars, trains, planes, automobiles, electricity, computers, food, running water, houses, shops, the internet, entertainment, and the list can go on and on. The human brain is behind all these phenomena of life, not the bowel or the bladder. Yes, they did have a supporting role, but if it was not for our superior brains (other animals have superior bowels and bladders) we would not have survived on this planet, let alone achieved great technological advancements that have made us the uncontested rulers of the world.

Sadly, and ironically, the one thing we lack knowledge of most is our brain. Very little research and technology have been dedicated to this field. More has been done for diagnosing and treating bowel and bladder (and other organ) ailments than the brain. When it comes to health, science, diagnostics, and therapeutics, the brain and mental health are the most neglected. We have yet to understand the purpose and function of most parts of our brain. On the other hand, we have discovered taste receptors in the

---

[165] He also understood why the wise man had only charged him 50%. It was the same advice given twice. "Fair play," said the king.

[166] Like most rulers used to do then, and some still do it now.

lungs[167], giving them a hitherto unknown functionality. Some of our neurosurgical procedures, like burr hole craniotomy[168] are more than 5,000 years old. Only the people doing them are new. There's a dearth of medication for almost all mental illnesses and the research for new drugs in this field is next to zero. It is as if we are putting voluntary effort into ignoring the brain and its functions, because we tend to ignore what cannot be seen. Be it God, soul, mind, or thought.

But the fact is that mind rules over matter.

Almost all the risk factors associated with cancer are associated with the mind. Smoking, alcohol, overeating, sedentary lifestyle, junk food, high-calorie diet, preservatives in food to extend shelf life, corporate greed at the expense of human life and health etc. Take the first two, for example. No one has ever smoked cigarettes or drank alcohol to please their lungs and liver. In fact, we make them suffer to pleasure the brain. And the consequences of cancer are as much mental as physical, if not more. Here, once again, we overlook and ignore the mind and mental health.

Our focus is on pharmaceutical products, often with a total disregard to the patient's feelings. For some odd reason we are ashamed of our feelings, especially those associated with perceived weakness – for example, depression or anxiety. And here's another irony. When a human is tired or sprains an ankle after running a mile or working out in the gym, it's not considered to be a weakness; it's a testament to physical fitness. But if the same person has a mental breakdown due to overwhelming stress, it's perceived as a weakness to be ashamed of.

Our mind is a functional product of our brain, just like digesting food is for the stomach or making urine for the kidneys. And the brain's function is as prone to malfunction as any other organ. When it comes to cancer and the mind, there are many unknown and unexplored links that can play a key role in preventing, treating, and curing this disease. For example, we know that our immune system has an inbuilt mechanism which can detect and destroy cancer cells. Our mental health has a direct influence on the immune system. Stress and depression can make the body release endogenous steroids which can suppress immunity and make the immune surveillance less effective. This is just one aspect of the mind-body interaction that is known to us. There are many more unexplored and unknown phenomena waiting to be discovered.

---

[167] Which explains why you can 'taste' the food just by its smell.

[168] Drilling a hole in the skull to drain out any blood that has collected around the brain after injury, to relieve the pressure.

The war on cancer will only be won when we open this new frontier against our worst enemy. I sincerely hope that by the time this book[169] undergoes its second edition we will have more information to share in this section.

For now, let's talk about the one mental health challenge that is well known to us all and can increase the risk of cancer by weakening our immune system (which carries out a surveillance for abnormal cells including cancer).

Let's talk about dealing with depression.

Sadness In the Sinai

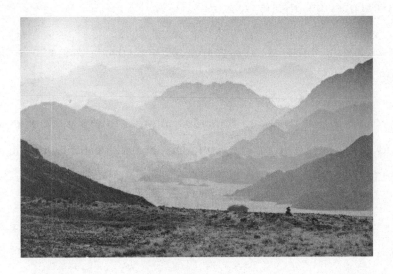

Sun rising in the Sinai.

It was no surprise that soon after arriving in the wilderness of the Sinai desert, the Israelites became depressed. It was a stark contrast to the lush green fertile Nile delta they had left behind. Naturally, they turned to Moses for advice (psychotherapy session) and Moses in turn sought solace consulting God.

And God said[170], "If you are grateful, I shall most certainly give you even more than you deserve."

Now, this sounds like difficult advice to follow, being grateful when you are feeling miserable, but when the advice is delivered through Moses, one of the prophets of God, well known for his temper – carrying a staff that could produce water from a stone, transform into a serpent and part the Red Sea – it wouldn't come as a surprise that nobody argued the case.

---

[169] God willing.
[170] Quran, 14: 7.

However, prophet Moses, may peace be upon him, is not among us anymore. Psychologists/psychiatrists are not allowed to carry a staff, let alone have a temper during a consultation, and hence they find it very hard to sell the concept of gratitude in the face of depression and despair. But, believe it or not, scientific studies have shown gratitude to be the most effective cure for sadness. However, it's not the only way to deal with depression.

There are the well-known and commonly applied tactics, like comfort eating, especially sugar-rich food (glucose acts as a short-acting anti-depressant), distraction strategies like watching TV and going for a walk, sleep, smoking, drinking alcohol, using mood-elevating drugs of the prescription or non-prescription type, and even retail therapy. But these are all short-term fixes and often people end up with a rebound attack of worse depression once the effects wear off.

Three things, say experts, are the most effective in treating and curing[171] an attack of depression, and they are backed by scientific evidence.

1. Being grateful for what you have and remembering that things were or could have been worse. Moses had used the same tactic[172] and reminded the twelve tribes of the torture, torment, and cruelty they had faced under the Pharaoh in the lush green pastures of Nile valley.

2. Helping others, especially those who are less fortunate than us. Remember, just like beauty, fortune or misfortune is a relative concept. There's always someone worse off than you and me in one way or another.

3. Believing in a benevolent, transcendental heavenly power (e.g., Almighty God) who is always looking after and protecting you. Now, this does not mean that we all *must* believe in God; nor am I trying to preach you to do so through this book[173]. It's just an evidence-backed fact that people with a strong belief in God, no matter what name they call Him by, can deal with depression better than those who don't believe. And there must be a lot of benefit in this belief, for almost every human society and race to come up with one, in one form or another, no matter how isolated they might be from the rest of the world.

---

[171] As with all rules, there are exceptions in this case, too. There are patients who will need additional therapy including regular medications for an effective treatment.

[172] Quran 14: 6.

[173] There's a separate YouTube channel for that purpose. Feel free to watch it, or not.

The future of cancer management is intertwined with the future of mental health. Not only for therapeutic but also preventive measures. We need a change of hearts and minds to transform and win the war against cancer.

And speaking of the future, let's see (in the next section) what it holds for us when it comes to treating and curing cancer.

CURING CANCER

THE FUTURE KHAN PLAN

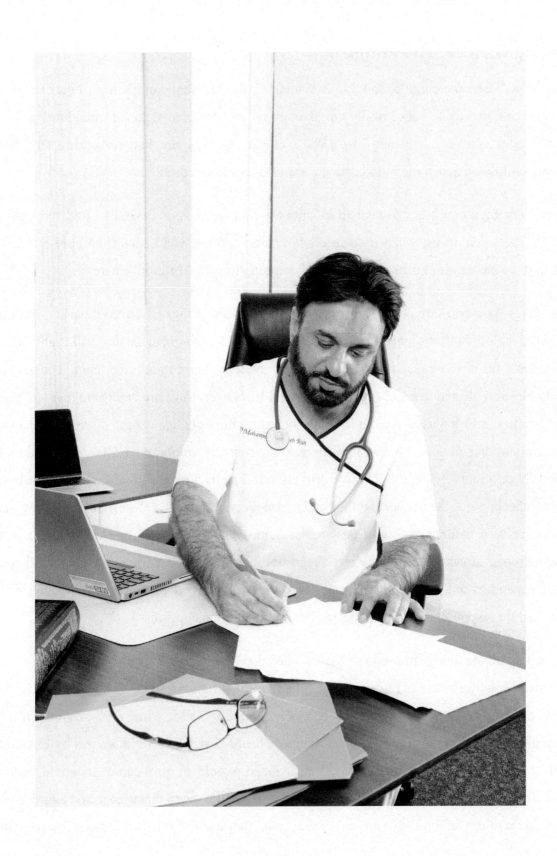

PART 12: CURING CANCER: THE FUTURE (THE KHAN PLAN)

12   Curing Cancer: The Future

I believe cancers will become curable, and this is evident by the fact that some kinds of cancers, such as testicular cancer, can already be successfully cured, even in the advanced stages. Depending on the type and stage, cure rates can vary between 70–90+%. Not bad. In fact, not bad for curing any disease. Similarly, many childhood and some blood cancers are also regularly cured.

The reason for very high cure rates in testicular cancer is that we have managed to find the right drug combination[174]. The same drugs, when used in other cancers, do not yield such high cure rates, which clearly show that we have to find different drugs and combinations for different cancers.

Conventional drugs, however, are not the only way to cure cancer. As we discovered earlier, our bodies have many remarkable inbuilt systems which are combating and curing cancer day and night. It's only when these systems fail that a cancer becomes clinically evident and requires treatment. These systems can and should be strengthened to make them more effective. Newer drugs are emerging that work not by directly killing cancer cells but assisting our immune system in the fight against the disease. One group of these cancer immunotherapies is the so-called *immune checkpoint inhibitors* (ICIs). Our bodies have controls called 'checkpoints' which affect how strongly our T-cells attack tumour cells. By disabling or inhibiting these checkpoints, the idea is that the 'brakes are taken off' the T-cell response, causing greater killing of cancer cells. A number of these drugs are now approved for use in Europe and the USA, and for an ever-growing range of cancers, and they are often used in combination with existing chemotherapies. They represent a step forward, but responses can be variable, and often only a minority of patients actually achieve a true lasting response, so it's best to treat them with cautious optimism.

As we have seen, there are many simple steps that can be taken to lessen the risk of developing cancer, be they lifestyle, diet, or being aware of our environment and mitigating for known risks and hazards. As the old, early 17th century saying goes, *prevention is better than cure*, and it's true. For example, if no one smoked cigarettes and made sure they minimised their exposure to radioactive radon gas by getting their houses checked out, the vast, vast majority of lung cancers would be prevented. It would become a relatively rare disease, not a major killer. And not smoking would lessen the incidence and aggressiveness of many other forms of cancer too. What an easy, quick 'win' that would be in our fight against the disease.

---

[174] A three-drug cocktail of bleomycin, etoposide, and cisplatin chemotherapy.

Current medicine is good at curing infectious diseases with antimicrobial agents, like antibiotics. Well, as long as the infections are bacterial, fungal, or parasitic. Our record against viruses is nothing to be proud of. We can't even cure the common cold. It takes seven days to recover from a cold if you have no treatment; with treatment you get better in a week! The only viral disease we have managed to cure so far, and that only in the last few years, is the hepatitis C virus. In other cases, we've striven to develop vaccines, to prevent infection, or lessen the severity should we get infected.

We learned in Part 5 of this book how the human papilloma virus (HPV) causes a number of cancers. We have no 'cure' for HPV infection but we can vaccinate against the virus, so avoiding many cancers arising in the future.

Globally, vaccines have made a major contribution to human health by preventing or eradicating polio and smallpox, and preventing many cases of, for example, tuberculosis and measles, both of which can lead to serious illness, disability, and death.

Caught in the early stages, cancer cure rates are impressively high and even in late stages some cancers can be cured with multiple modalities of treatment. We have already talked about the spectacular cure rates for testicular cancer but more common cancers such as breast and prostate cancer also have good cure rates too. Even the notorious lung cancer can be cured successfully with use of radiotherapy in its earlier stages.

And the future looks bright. With new research and drug developments, more and more cancers will become better manageable and curable. And new strategies are what we need, because conventional cancer treatments have some serious shortcomings. So, let's talk about these. Friends, Romans, countrymen (and non-Romans), lend me your ears ….

The Trouble With Treating Cancer Is That It's a Bit Like Killing Cornelius Cinna

Lucius Cornelius Cinna, member of the Roman Senate, was a brother-in-law of Julius Caesar (his sister Cornelia was married to Caesar). He became a critic of Caesar and gave an inflammatory speech just one day before Caesar was killed.

Gaius Helvius Cinna (known as 'Cinna the poet') belonged to a movement of unorthodox 'new poets' (Greek: *neoterikoi* or *neoterics*, 'new poets') who turned away from the classic Homeric-style epic poetry which focused on the feats of ancient heroes and gods.

Lucius and Gaius had two things in common, they were both Romans and called 'Cinna'.

After Julius Caesar was murdered, Mark Anthony gave an emotive and inflammatory speech at his funeral[175], which charged the crowd against his opponents. A murderous mob went looking for them, especially Cinna the senator, but instead found Cinna the poet. When they found out he was called 'Cinna', they decided to kill him.

"Tear him to pieces; he's a conspirator!" they cried.

"I am Cinna the poet; I am Cinna the poet!" pleaded the old man.

The crowd would have none of it. Someone, who obviously wasn't a fan of Cinna's poetry, even found an excuse to justify the attack. "Tear him for his bad verses. Tear him for his bad verses."

"I am not Cinna the conspirator!" begged Cinna the poet, in a last-ditch effort to save his life.

"It's no matter, his name is Cinna!" yelled the mob.

Cinna was killed and the mob moved on, looking for other conspirators.

Traditional cancer treatments like chemotherapy are like mob justice. They easily confuse normal cells for cancer cells. Cancer, the conspirator, is marked by rapid growth and proliferation but so are many other normal cells of the body. For example, cells that line the body cavities such as bowel, bladder, lungs, mouth, and throat. This is even more so for blood cells, as they not only grow and divide rapidly but also move around the body like metastatic cancer cells. Anti-cancer drugs are made to target fast-growing, fast-dividing mobile cells, and hence they target them indiscriminately. The mob lynching of normal cells is what makes cancer treatment so toxic. Nausea, vomiting, diarrhoea due to stomach and bowel cell damage are common, as is anaemia, bruising, bleeding, and reduced immunity due to bone marrow damage. Hair thinning and loss due to skin damage is common, too.

Normal cells are everywhere and an easy target for a chemo-mob, whereas cancer cells are often found in deeper organs, and sometimes seek refuge at sites where drugs cannot penetrate easily. Even targeted therapies, which are made to target cancer-specific features (for example cancer receptors and enzymes) can confuse cancer and normal cells. This is because cancer cells are using the same receptors and enzymes that normal cells use, only in larger numbers.

Hence, we need to have a different approach, or more than one approach, for effectively killing cancer. This is the key to curing cancer. And to cure cancer we first need to know cancer, not in parts but as a

---

[175] The famous "I come to bury Caesar, not to praise him". What a lie! He did the exact opposite.

whole. At present, our understanding of this disease is fragmented at best, like a jigsaw puzzle with missing pieces. A neat way of understanding this is through the story of five blind friends and an elephant.

"Know Thy Enemy" (Sun Tzu, The Art of War, 5th century BC): Five Blind Friends and an Elephant

A long time ago, in the land where the mighty river Indus flows[176], five blind friends came across a dead elephant.

The first one grabbed its tail and said to the others, "This animal is like a snake."

The second got hold of a leg and disagreed with the first. "This animal is like a pillar."

The third felt the massive body of the animal and exclaimed, "It's more like a big wall."

The fourth got hold of the trunk and stated, "It's definitely a hose-like animal."

The fifth felt the tusks of the elephant and concluded, "You are all wrong, this animal is made of big round bones."

The five friends took a firm stance and argued all day till they were friends no more. They all believed that they were right and so they were, but they accused each other of being wrong and they were wrong to do so. Each one of them had found a piece of the truth but did not know the whole truth.

Cancer is like the metaphorical elephant that we are trying to understand by focusing on its different parts. Experts are often focused, too focused, on one particular aspect of this disease and can't see the whole picture. We need more collaboration and sharing of data between different research departments and centres across the globe. For example, we still don't know why and how a particular type of cancer behaves so differently among different patients of the same or different race, age, sex, and socio-economic groups, and more importantly how it can behave differently in the same patient from one day to another. I have seen aggressive cancers on a rampage come to halt for no apparent reason and staying quiescent for years, and indolent slow-growing tumours turning wild and violent. It's not the rule but exceptional behaviours like these may hold the key to understanding and curing cancer. These are the missing pieces of the jigsaw that need to be found so we can see the whole picture.

---

[176] In present-day Pakistan, before the colonial rule during which jungles were cut down to make farmland to grow and export grain, there were an abundance of wild elephants, lions, tigers, leopards, rhinoceros, and even cheetahs. The latter are still found in isolated pockets in the semi-desert Baluchistan province west of the country.

And here's my humble plan on how (God willingly, touch wood, fingers crossed) it can be achieved.

Let's call it …

THE KHAN PLAN

1. Clarify the Confusion

As explained in section 1.1, there is much confusion in the use of terminology surrounding cancer. There is a dire need to rationalise this, so we all understand what we are talking about.

2. Give Nicotine the Respect It Deserves

'Stop smoking' is easier said than done, so I won't say it[177]. But it is almost certainly one of the best ways of reducing the cancer burden on society.

So, here's a radical suggestion. Nicotine is a drug, addictive and difficult to quit, so why don't we treat it like one?

Only morphine/heroin is more difficult to quit than tobacco. Cocaine, cannabis, amphetamines, LSD, alcohol, and all other drugs are easier to quit than cigarettes. So, while respecting free will and an individual's right to smoke, this doesn't necessarily mean that tobacco companies should be able to sell this highly addictive and dangerous drug to *non-smokers*, getting them hooked on to it. OK, it's true that in many parts of the world, supply is regulated (over 18s, ban on advertising) but tobacco is otherwise freely available.

So, here's my proposal. And it's going to ruffle a lot of feathers.

Cigarettes should be a prescription-only drug.

Why? Well, smokers can still access their favourite tobacco. Online repeat prescriptions could make life straightforward for them. But my proposal has several other features that might make the switch to prescription useful.

Firstly, for example, the first five cigarettes per day could be at a standard price (maybe even relatively inexpensive). For the next five, the price doubles, and so on. The extra money would be channelled directly to cancer research and, in the UK for example, the Cancer Drug Fund, to provide free or subsidised anti-cancer treatment (some are extremely expensive, and not always available through national healthcare

---

[177] Cutting down on smoking is usually a more realistic approach, and over time this can lead to a complete cessation.

provision). This way, smokers would see it as a health fund investment that they might benefit from one day.

And there are added advantages. In my proposal, they wouldn't be available to pregnant women, saving their unborn babies from the toxic effects. I would also anticipate such an approach resulting in a sharp decline in the number of new smokers. Imagine a non-smoker walking up to a general physician and asking for a prescription. You know it won't happen; well, not as often as popping into your local grocery store or tobacconist.

And why stop with cigarettes.

Let's do the same for all other addictive drugs. Cocaine, cannabis, heroin – all can be regulated and safely prescribed to those who are addicted to them in full confidentiality. We are already dispensing sterile syringes so why not also provide unadulterated drugs to go with them? And also give the choice to the patients for detox and rehab services.

The big aim of this plan is to reduce the numbers of new addicts. Also, when there is a reliable drug supply available to patients[178], they will be less compelled to commit crime to get their next fix.

OK, I know it's radical, and there are bound to be problems, not least the willingness of the medical profession to 'prescribe' something so potentially harmful, but awareness campaigns and health initiatives have only gone so far in bringing about a decline in tobacco use. Time to think outside the box, maybe. Get a debate going.

3. A Licence to Drink

I know, you can already guess where I'm heading with this one! We should all (adults, that is) have a licence to drink. Or combine it with an existing licence, driving licence, or passport or that National Insurance Number card, which is the most useless piece of plastic ever invented (when is the last time you ever used one, or looked for it, or shouted out "Honey have you seen my NI card?"). Even better, make a mobile app and get registered.

Why a licence, you ask?

---

[178] Please don't call them 'addicts'; they deserve respect. No child grows up wanting to be one and who knows what me and you could have ended up with if we were in their shoes.

It's simple. You buy your weekly quota of alcohol, 14 units that is, on the licence at the normal price. If you want to drink more, go ahead, but the price should be double for the next 14 units and the extra money should go to health promotion and disease prevention programs, especially cancer research and the Cancer Drug Fund[179], a sort of investment or insurance, just like a health insurance company charges you more if you smoke or drink more.

If you want to buy for the whole family, use their licences too.

Buying for a party? Get a party licence or phone app that generates a party group, and you send invites. People join in from their phones and you can buy for everyone on their account.

But, I hear you say, what if I am hosting a wild party? One going above 14 units per person. It's going to cost more! Allow me to answer that question with another one. When was the last time anyone saved money by throwing a party? At least part of this party cost is going to a good purpose.

The key is to preserve the personal freedom to drink but also have the provision of a fund raised by alcohol pricing that would help one in the future.

Right now, most of that tax money generated from alcohol and cigarettes often ends up bailing out banks. What good is it to you and me unless we are on their board of directors (the lower staff get the axe, not the bail-out package).

Most importantly, with a licence to drink we (society) could discourage the sale of alcohol to pregnant women and save the unborn babies from alcohol-induced genetic damage.

The concept here is to encourage drinking in moderation.

Before you shriek in horror and tear this book to shreds, stop a moment and consider that this idea isn't as 'new' as you might think. With the deregulation of gambling in the UK, and the explosive growth in online gambling apps, there has been growing concern about the rise in gambling addiction, resulting in much financial hardship and decline in mental health for those involved. One of the industry's responses to this is to add features to their apps to allow punters to place limits (individual bets, daily, weekly etc.) on their stakes as an aid to 'responsible gambling'. The principle isn't so very different.

---

[179] CDF, or the Cancer Drug Fund, is a fund created by the UK government to provide money for expensive cancer treatment that is not covered by the general health system. I consider it an excellent initiative by the British government which should be an inspiration for other governments. However, as with all good things, there is a fear that we might lose it in the future due to budgetary cuts.

4. Create Awareness of STCs

Sexually transmitted cancers, STCs, is a term most people have not heard of before, unless you've read this book, where I have introduced it for the first time.

STC awareness is important because these cancers often strike us in the prime of our life and are 100% preventable.

The commonest culprit, human papilloma virus (or HPV for short), has been successfully prevented by use of HPV vaccination, and barrier contraceptives significantly reduce the rates of HPV-induced cancers, especially cervical cancer, as a result of avoiding infection.

HPV vaccination for children is becoming the norm. Initially, some governments were reluctant to offer it to boys and only included girls for the immunisation programme. Then some clever expert explained to the politicians that the act of copulation involves more than one person, and might involve different sexes too. So, they eventually buckled to the pressure and extended the scheme to both sexes. But one-off immunisation is like a tick-box exercise. A comprehensive health plan should monitor antibody levels and offer booster doses to high-risk groups.

An important piece of information to note and impart to the public is that sexually transmitted diseases and cancers are not always a case of promiscuity versus abstinence. In any monogamous relationship one can't guarantee a partner's fidelity past, present, or future, and sadly no amount of chastity secures one against rape and sexual assault.

Awareness programmes especially need to target teenagers, who think having a sexually transmitted disease (STD) is a sign of sexual prowess, not knowing that an STD can lead to an STC later in life.

5. Exercise, the Key to Health

In section 10.5 we briefly looked at how exercise is gradually becoming a more formal aspect to our approach to treating and preventing cancer. For this reason, I've made regular exercise sessions a key element to my plan. But as we learned, most of us don't exercise enough, lack the motivation (because of the absence of immediate rewards), and our hectic daily lives and schedules often (and rather too conveniently) get in the way.

To address this, my plan recommends that exercise should be incorporated into every job plan. Every job should be linked with exercise sessions at least three times a week within the 'paid' working hours, whether at the start, middle, or end of the working shift.

Why not have 'Exercise Breaks' just like lunch and coffee breaks, and make them part of the employees' contract.

To incentivise (and provide that reward), a small percentage of pay should be linked to attending and completing exercise sessions in a similar manner to attendance or work targets. To miss the exercise sessions, one should need to follow the same rules which apply to normal work; that is, apply for an exemption for exceptional circumstances (sickness etc.) or lose that component of pay.

The level of exercise should be customised to the individual (just like we make reasonable adjustments at work for workers of different capabilities) with options to go for higher levels of fitness, possibly linked with a bonus in pay. Why would companies do this, you ask? Well, apart from enhancing performance and productivity, this component of pay might be made reclaimable or tax-deductible.

The right and need to exercise should be enshrined in the constitution as a basic human right because we all have a right to live a healthier, happier, and longer life.

Is this practical? Well, the concept of exercise at work isn't new. Many Chinese companies begin the day with exercises. And many larger companies also provide their staff with sports facilities/clubs already. Provision of facilities by local authorities is often patchy, and often subject to cuts in funding during tough economic times, and this needs to change. It should become a priority, as should be maintaining open spaces in cities and towns.

OK, OK, I know. You're screaming at me about the long-distance lorry driver or self-employed person. How could it work for them? Tricky. Maybe another way is to make use of sports facilities free, 24/7, and have a system whereby people can 'log' sessions and, provided they keep up a minimum, they get a tax rebate if in work, or maybe extra tax credits if they don't.

I guess my emphasis is along the lines of the old saying, *Where there's a will, there's a way*, just that we need a little more encouragement regarding the will to change.

6. Have a Break

Although this might seem the complete opposite of the last point, it isn't – it's complimentary. Take rest when needed, especially after a meal. The Spanish do it on a national level. They siesta, that is take a post-lunch nap in the afternoon. Lunch breaks in Spain can be two hours long for this purpose. Although, the last time I was in Spain, trying to get my booked and pre-paid rental car, it seemed to go into the next day[180]!

Having a break is important for health and happiness. It helps us recharge our batteries. When we eat food the blood rushes to the gut to help with digestion and retrieve nutrition from the food. The heavier the meal in terms of calorie content, the more blood required. This leaves very little blood for other parts of the body, such as the brain and muscles. It's the reason why we slow down after a lunch break and need brain stimulants like tea and coffee to stay alert.

Studies have shown that taking a nap even during work can improve energy levels and mental alertness. The message has not been lost on the corporate world. Google has installed 'Nap Pods' at their workplace where workers can take a sleep break and recharge their energy levels. Nike's headquarters in Portland, Oregon has rooms where employees can sleep or meditate. Ben & Jerry's has had nap rooms at their headquarters for more than 10 years now.

And the best part is that their employees get paid for sleeping on the job.

Now that's a future we all would be looking forward to.

7. We Must Learn from Others, from Nature, and the Past

Experience is something that you gain when you don't need it anymore.

M.M. Khan

Key to human success is learning from others' experiences. Our own experiences mostly serve those who follow us, usually the next generation. Cumulative knowledge and information are the key to understanding and combating cancer, especially when it comes to prevention. We need to learn from those who have experienced cancer up close and personal: patients, cured or uncured, treated or untreated, their families, and professionals who have been treating the disease.

Unless, and until, we make these stakeholders part of the decision-making process and policy formation, we cannot make rapid and realistic progress.

Our ancestors had a lot of knowledge, not to mention 10% larger brains. Ancient wisdom gave birth to the Great Wall of China and the Pyramids. OK, they never managed to finish Stonehenge, but we shouldn't

---

[180] But that might be just my luck, or lack of it.

hold it against them. Nobody's perfect. And builders' contracts are sometimes not worth the paper they are written on.

When it comes to health and treating disease, our ancestors had some very successful strategies. Unfortunately, we have either lost or ignored most of the cumulative knowledge that was passed down generations. For example, smallpox vaccination was used by Chinese in the 16th century and was commonly practiced by the Turks, Persians, and North Africans by the 18th century. Europe ignored it for hundreds of years, at the cost of many lives, before taking it up.

Similarly, many modern medical practices were already standardised and successfully employed by the Arab and Persian physicians a thousand years ago. Ibn Sina was using surgery, herbal chemotherapy, and heat to treat cancers effectively when European physicians were adamant on (unsuccessfully) treating it with a single modality therapy, purgation – the act of vigorous evacuation of the bowels using laxatives.

Ancient literature is full of treatments and cures waiting to be rediscovered.

While we in the West have been arrogantly ignoring ancient wisdom and insisting on reinventing the wheel, other nations like the Chinese have been exploring ancient texts and making valuable discoveries. In 1971, for example, they isolated a herbal compound, 'artemisinin', from a Chinese herb called *qinghaosu*, mentioned in an ancient book called, *A Handbook of Prescriptions for Emergencies* (*Zhou Hou Bei Ji Fang*), written by the scholar Ge Hong in 340 AD. Ge Hong used it for treatment of malaria and today it is the mainstay of treatment against multi-drug resistant malaria.

The search for effective treatments including cancer by exploring ancient texts and folk wisdom continues in China today. They have learnt an important lesson: the future of treating diseases, including cancer, often lies in the past.

Cirencester is a town nestled among the rolling Cotswold Hills in the southwest of England. West of the town lies the Bathurst Estate, seat of Earl Bathurst, and site of one of the finest landscape gardens in England. Three hundred years ago, the first baron and later earl, Allen Bathurst, lovingly created these gardens, and in 1712 AD planted a semi-circular yew hedge around his mansion. Today, this has grown into the oldest and largest yew hedge in the world, 40 feet high and 150 feet wide. Every year it takes 12 days, two men, and a cherry picker to trim it back. The cuttings are not wasted but sent to a pharmaceutical firm that uses it to produce docetaxel, an anti-cancer drug used for treating breast, stomach, prostate, lung, head, and neck cancers. This highly effective drug was first patented in 1986 and approved for medical use in 1995.

But it was no chance finding. In fact, scientists had deliberately looked for an anti-cancer chemical in the leaves from the European yew tree, known by its botanical name as *Taxus baccata* (hence the name 'docetaxel' for the drug).

The inspiration came from across the Atlantic Ocean in America, where the Native Americans had been brewing the leaves of the Pacific yew tree (*Taxus brevifolia*) for centuries, using it to treat fever and arthritis. Researchers from the National Cancer Institute managed to extract paclitaxel, another anti-cancer drug, from its leaves in the 1960s. It has been used since to treat ovarian, breast, lung, cervical, pancreatic, bladder, prostate, and oesophageal cancers, along with melanoma and Kaposi's sarcomas.

In the same decade, research was focused on a flowering plant from Madagascar known as Catharanthus roseus, or the 'Madagascan periwinkle'. The flower had been used as a folk remedy for centuries, and in the 1950s scientists had found it to contain 120 active chemicals known as 'alkaloids'. In July 1963, the United States Food and Drug Administration (FDA) approved one of them, vincristine, to treat cancer. More than 50 years later, it is still an effective drug for treating lung cancer, neuroblastomas, acute myeloid leukaemia, and acute lymphocytic leukaemia.

Vincristine has a sister drug called 'vinblastine', also extracted from the periwinkle flower, which is used in treating melanoma, Hodgkin's lymphoma, lung, bladder, brain, and testicular cancers.

In 1972, the discovery of an antifungal agent from bacteria in the soil of the Polynesian Island of Rapa Nui, known as 'rapamycin', gave us a whole new class of drugs known as 'mTOR inhibitors', which are used to treat kidney, pancreatic, and breast cancers along with a rare brain tumour known as *SEGA* (subependymal giant cell astrocytoma). In fact, mTOR-inhibitor drugs are the only treatment for SEGA and, although not curative, the treatment can shrink the tumours in 65–75%[181] of the patients, keeping them under control for many years.

Nature, it seems, is full of treatments and possible cures for cancer and other diseases. Sadly, we are rapidly losing these wonderful treatments as more and more of our precious forests and ecosystems are replaced by farmland, houses, roads, and concrete jungles. We need to preserve the planet because our survival depends on it in more than one way. At the time of writing, it is reported that the total weight of all manmade structures (concrete, buildings, roads etc.) is set to exceed the world's biomass (weight of all living things) for the first time. The human race is destroying the very planet they live in, just like a cancer.

---

[181] Control rates with rapamycin and everolimus, respectively.

8. Killing a Flock with a Single Stone

Prevention is better than cure.

Desiderius Erasmus, 1500 AD

Having a car breakdown service is quite helpful. But even if you have the best breakdown service in the world, you wouldn't actually 'want' to have a breakdown. Same is true for cancer and its treatment. Ask anyone who has been successfully cured of their cancer. If given a chance to go back in time, they would rather not have had it in the first place.

Prevention should be the backbone of every disease management. And, historically, it has been the most effective cure for all diseases. Take infectious diseases, for example. At the turn of the last century, the early 1900s, infectious diseases were the biggest killers of mankind, accounting for almost 50% of deaths. The top three positions for causes of death went to pneumonia plus flu, tuberculosis, and diarrhoea respectively.

Today, infectious diseases only account for 3% of deaths in developed countries.

You might think the credit goes to the discovery of antibiotics, but the reality is very different. Studies from the UK, comparing data from the 1800s and 1900s, reveal that the rates of infections were falling long before antibiotics came into use due to improved sanitation and a better diet. Prevention of infection accounts for 80% of the reduction in deaths, with antibiotics only contributing a humble 20%.

The top three killers now are heart disease, cancer, and lung diseases. All of these are mostly (up to 70%) preventable.

And cancer prevention is the most effective strategy because measures to avoid cancer also help avoid other major health problems such as heart disease, diabetes, lung diseases, and stroke. It's like killing a whole flock of birds with one stone.

9. Increase Awareness and Separating Fact from Fiction

The success of our efforts in treating and curing cancer lies with the people. Without public awareness and support, we cannot win this fight. It is important that the public have a comprehensive understanding of this disease, its causes, prevention, and treatment, and to achieve this, the very first thing we need to do is remove the misconceptions regarding cancer.

We live in the Information Age, a sad time because information is often replacing knowledge. Never in the history of mankind has ignorance and misinformation spread so fast as it does today.

And nowhere is it truer than regarding cancer management. I have even come across websites, webpages, posts, tweets, and messages claiming that cancer is a hoax. Ironically, such contemptuous concepts did not exist even a thousand years ago, in the time of Ibn Sina, when there was much less information but better understanding of this disease. And this is the tip of the ignorance iceberg. When it comes to treating cancer, the amount of dangerously false information is colossal. Unfortunately, such beliefs serve no function except creating depression and delusion among the masses, and they are extremely painful to those who have to deal with cancer every day – patients, families, and professionals.

We need to separate fact from fiction and ensure that such insensitive misinformation is not allowed to propagate and create disillusionment.

10. Regularise Medical Practice

Quackery is a crime, whether committed in public or online.

If you were to open a shop on the High Street selling charcoal to cure cancer, you would be shut within an hour and placed behind bars. However, if you do it online you can easily get away with it and make a lot of money in the process. But it's not just money that motivates people. Fame, all 15 minutes of it, is also a very big incentive.

In my career as an oncologist, I have seen one too many patients falling for fraudulent treatments from coffee enemas to bicarbonate of soda. I don't blame them. We all tend to clutch at straws in desperation. The saddest part is that pursuit of false hope leads them away from evidence-based, time-tested effective treatment, and by the time they realise their mistake, the window of opportunity for treating cancer has been missed.

Don't get me wrong, I have an open mind about alternative therapies. It is quite possible that, someday, someone might find an effective treatment or even a cure for one or more types of cancer by using unconventional methods of treatment. But this won't happen randomly, because any remedy will need to be scientifically tested before it can be used safely. Erratic use of any treatment can cause more harm than good.

Unfortunately, most people who propagate miracle cures shy away from providing any evidence for their efficacy or safety. I have come across a few 'renowned healers' who claim to have a cure for cancer and many other ailments that plague mankind. But whenever I have offered them an option to test their remedies in a trial setting, they have never availed themselves of the opportunity.

If anyone has an effective treatment for any disease, including cancer, they should get it registered under propriety rights and test its efficacy by scientific trials[182] in accordance with international standards. Until they are able to do so and prove the effectiveness of their treatment, they should not be allowed to propagate it.

Having said that, we also need to get the big pharma to cut down the price of anti-cancer drugs. They always reason that a lot of money goes into research and the cost needs to be recovered, but the reality is not that simple. The basic principle of big corporations is to charge not what it costs but as much as the customer can pay (the concept of willingness to pay). For example, thalidomide, a drug used in the treatment of a type of blood cancer (multiple myeloma), was made in the 1950s and costs *less than* $0.07 per capsule but is sold to the patients for around $197.20. It's no surprise that patients are clutching at straws and drawn like a magnet to cheaper, fraudulent treatments.

11. The Past, Present and Future, It's in Our DNA

Cancer is a disease of genes. Mutated genes to be very exact. It cannot be cured until and unless we target it at the genetic level. Otherwise, we will only be managing and controlling it in the short term. Our understanding of genes and their function has increased tremendously over the last 20 years. The year 2003 was a landmark, being when we completed the Human Genome Project, a collaborative effort of 20 universities and research facilities across the globe from Japan to the United States.

But there's still a lot we don't know. An unbelievable chunk of our DNA, 97% to be exact, is still labelled as 'junk DNA', not because it's useless but because we can't make sense of it.

Professor Robert Pollack, an American biologist says in his book, *Signs of Life: The Language and Meanings of DNA*, that if we were to join all the DNA in our body into a single strand it would stretch up to 10 billion miles, all the way to the edge of the solar system, beyond the planets. It's quite obvious that

---

[182] Usually, new drugs are first tested in the laboratory and through animal models. Next, they are tested among humans in three phases. Phase 1 trials involve a small number of subjects to check, dose, safety, side effects, and formulations. Phase 2 trials have a larger number of patients to assess the efficacy and dosage, and even larger, 'pivotal', Phase 3 trials compare the new treatment against established ones or a placebo to prove the effect is clinically and statistically valid. So, the next time you hear that 'a new drug for treating cancer is in the pipeline' and wonder why it is taking it so long, its undergoing rigorous testing in these phases.

our body has gone to a lot of trouble to make all this DNA. There must be a purpose to it – one which we are unable to fully comprehend.

I believe that the answer to curing cancer and many other secrets of our life lies in this 97% dark matter of DNA which alludes us at present.

An important aspect of genes is that in addition to being inactive by damage (mutations) they can also be switched on and off by environmental stimuli.

This was first demonstrated in the 1940s by Jacques Monod, a French biologist, who was working with a particular type of bacteria known as *Escherichia coli* (also known as *E. coli* for short) often found in the human colon (large bowel). Some variants of *E. coli* can cause human infections, including diarrhoea.

Monod, however, was more interested in the eating habits of E. coli. The bacterium carries genes coding for enzymes that can metabolise glucose and lactose, two types of sugars. When the environment had glucose available, the bacterium switched on the gene for the enzyme needed for glucose while switching off the lactose enzyme gene, and it did the opposite when lactose was provided instead.

Human genes are switched on and off all the time[183]. The part of DNA which acts as the 'power switch' to turn a gene on or off can lie within the gene or in the so-called 'junk DNA', and can sometimes be found in another gene which may act as a master switch for one or more genes. Whole gene cascades have also been identified where one gene switches another one and the latter activates or deactivates another gene, and so on and so forth.

Sometimes, we can even feel the process. Fear, happiness, sorrow, and excitement are all the result of chemicals[184] released in the brain and body due to activation of different genes.

The same happens when we experience something new, be it a different cuisine for the first time or exposure to a new, disease-causing bacteria.

Cancer, too, is a result of different genes switching on and off either by environmental stimuli or damage (mutations). Some are suppressed, like DNA repair genes, while others go into hyperdrive mode, like growth promotor genes. Knowing this fact, scientists have tried to modify these genes in order to control

---

[183] For example, when we are exposed to toxic metals, our cells switch on a gene known as *MT* (metallothionine) which helps to deal with these poisonous metals.

[184] You might argue that in some instances, such responses to stimuli represent a triggered release of chemicals that have already been produced. However, these chemicals are a product of genes that have been switched on or gone into hyperdrive in anticipation of and response to the stimuli.

cancer. You would imagine they would look for natural stimuli to manipulate the genes, but instead they have been trying for decades to replace these genes by using viruses to sneak in replacement genes, like the Greeks used the Trojan horse to get their warriors into the city of Troy. Unsurprisingly, it hasn't worked in most cases so far but, more surprisingly, they haven't given up on the idea.

Another method that has been used, with mixed results, is targeting the products of faulty genes in an attempt to block or neutralise them. These include enzymes and chemicals which drive cell growth and formation of new blood vessels for the cancer cells.

But no matter how successful we are in blocking them, the root cause of cancer, faulty genes, is not addressed.

Now you might be wondering, "What good is switching a gene on or off when it is already damaged/mutated?"

And my answer to your very valid question is that genes don't work in isolation. Their functions and downstream pathways are often. if not always, interlinked. When we block one overactive cancer growth gene by use of drugs, the cancer stops growing and might even shrink at first, but soon after it switches on new growth genes and starts using new pathways, avoiding and bypassing the blockade caused by the drugs.

We need to learn more about this strategy and use it against the cancer itself.

What we need is a method to switch genes on or off by using or manipulating the natural stimuli which have existed all along. I call this the 'MKKM gene switch' and believe that this has an important role to play in the prevention, treatment, and cure of cancers. By reversing the stimulus that turns a gene on or off, one could achieve the desired results without the need for Trojan viruses to deliver replacement genes. The stimuli are all round us: physical, chemical, emotional, diet, or even activity like exercise to name a few. They can be used alone or in combination to get the desired effects.

After all, *E. coli*, a common bowel bug, has shown us how easily and effectively it can be done, on demand, without the need of fancy lab equipment. Last, but not least, you might get a sense arising from this section of a certain cynicism towards gene therapy and the 'Trojan horse' approach. Nothing could be further from the truth. I love horses, including jumbo wooden variants. The techniques devised to sneak in 'good genes' to replace the 'bad' ones are nothing less than marvellous, but they have to be used in combination with other strategies and should not be the sole focus.

We need to launch a thousand ships *and* look for that vulnerable heel of cancer too.

12. Looking Outside the Box

How to catch a monkey and how not to be one. Take a metal jar with a narrow neck. Put in some nuts. Chain it to a tree or a pole, near a monkey habitat.

Wait!

Before long a peckish monkey will come by and put his hand in the jar. Once he has grasped the nuts, his fist will be stuck in the jar but, in his greed and stubbornness, the monkey will not let go of the nuts and so continues trying to pull them out.

Your monkey is ready for you to collect.

This time-tested method has been successfully used for centuries. The method hasn't changed because the monkeys haven't modified their behaviour. If only they would try something different, like turning the jar upside down so they can get to the nuts and avoid capture. Monkeys, it seems, are not quite as bright as squirrels.

But I guess when it comes to retrieving nuts from a jar, the monkeys are sure their methods will one day bear fruit.

Sometimes, we humans also find it difficult to let go of our instinctive behaviour. Like trying to kill cancer after it is born, or using treatments to combat cancer that we are familiar with. Monkeys need to learn from other species like humans (or squirrels) how best to get nuts out of a jar.

Humans need to learn from other species how to prevent cancer.

Both need to learn to let go of antiquated methods that have never worked.

So, let's learn from others who have succeeded in defeating cancer.

Fighting Cancer with Capybaras

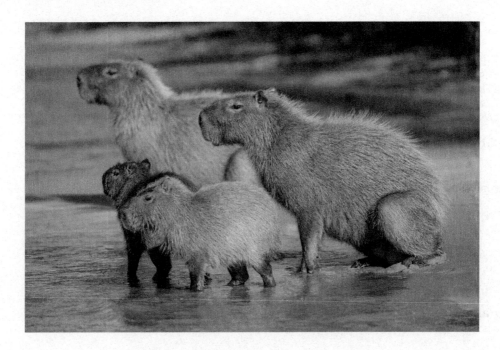

Capybaras, the world's largest living rodents.

Capybaras are an iconic South American animal belonging to a group of rodents known as *Caviomorpha*. Sixty times heavier than its closest modern relative, this is the world's largest living rodent, roughly the size of a small adult human. It looks like a cute guinea pig/hippopotamus mashup. Capybaras spend their day munching grass along the riverbanks of South America. Their ancestors evolved in Africa around 80 million years ago and arrived in South America some 40 million years ago. Rodents generally tend to be tiny so they can hide better. However, at the time the capybaras arrived in South America, the region was almost completely devoid of predators, allowing them to grow bigger and bigger.

But the question was, what genetic mutations enabled them to grow so big? A team of scientists from Columbia, Sweden, and the United States looked at the capybaras' DNA and found a growth system on overdrive. This rang alarm bells, as a growth system on overdrive would also put an animal at increased risk of developing cancer.

However, capybaras had developed an anti-cancer mechanism.

They all have a unique form of insulin. Besides regulating blood sugar, insulin also tells cells to divide and is known to encourage cancer growth. Researcher Santiago Herrera-Alvarez and his colleagues found that the capybaras do not make more insulin but instead have a type of insulin that does the job more effectively and in lesser amounts. Also, they have devised an additional tactic to counter cancer. Immune surveillance! The capybara immune system is far better at detecting and destroying cells that are dividing too rapidly, like cancer cells.

In other words, capybaras have evolved their own form of cancer immunotherapy.

This is a novel approach and gives rise to hope that a more-effective immune system in humans can similarly prevent cancer from developing in future. Already there are immune therapy drugs that increase the efficacy of human immune cells in detecting and destroying cancer cells. With more research and development, we can further refine this strategy and one day become more resistant to cancer, despite being heavy and sluggish like our chubby rodent cousin.

The Big and Beautiful: Bowhead Whales

Unlike humans, other large species have different evolutionary mechanisms for protection against cancer. The bowhead whale is a large creature which can live for more than 200 years. That gives it very good reasons (large number of dividing cells and a long time for mutations to occur) to develop cancers but its rates of cancer are extremely low.

Scientists have even tried to induce cancerous changes in cells taken from bowhead whales and failed spectacularly.

Preliminary data from genetic studies show that it has a unique variant of its DNA repair genes, giving it longevity and reducing the risk of cancer. By studying these genes and their mechanism of DNA repair, we may discover methods of protecting and repairing human DNA before it mutates into a cancer.

The Small Survivor

At the other end of the spectrum to the bowhead whales, small subterranean naked mole rats live longer and are more cancer resistant compared with laboratory mice. In fact, studies carried out over decades have failed to show a single case of cancer among them.

So, what's the key to their success?

They seem to have developed a different mechanism for reducing cancer rates. Their cells stick to each other much better due to a special molecule that prevents tumour formation. This is a sugary chemical called hyaluronan, which fills the gaps between cells and sticks them together tightly. Even if the cells have mutated, this gluey chemical stops them from progressing further.

Humans also make this chemical, but our version is of a slightly different formula and, hence, not as effective as that found in the naked mole rat.

But this is an unexplored territory when it comes to cancer research. I suspect human cancer cells have defective hyaluronan, the sticky glue which keeps cell stuck together, and if we can identify the genetic defect which causes the change in glue composition, we can correct it and prevent an important step in the development of cancer cells, just like the nude … I mean, naked … mole rat.

Forty Reasons Why You'll Wish You Were an Elephant

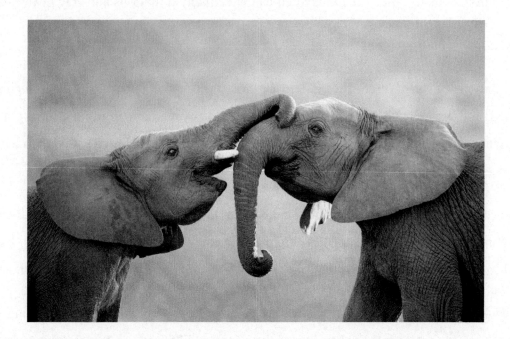

As explained earlier in this book, elephants, the lucky pachyderms, have 40 copies of one type of tumour suppressor gene, called *p53*, while we, in contrast, have only two. And that's not the only type they have, either. One might wonder if having a lot would be possibly helpful. And that's what led some scientists to try it out in mice.

In 2002, scientists tried to produce many copies of p53 genes in lab mice, but the results were not, let's say, very desirable. The mice did become resistant to cancer but also aged very rapidly and their fertility was also affected. In 2007, they tried again, creating lab mice with only one extra copy of p53 gene and it worked like a charm.

It's yet to bet seen what our lucky number is when it comes to p53 genes. One thing we know for sure, it's not the number two (our present copy number).

Elephants have more tumour suppressor genes than us because they have been around for much longer than us. Their bodies developed them in response to increasing environmental and internal (endogenous) carcinogens. One day, we will probably have more too, but it will take time because evolution is a slow and steady process. We already have adequate tools to deal with our earlier 'natural environment and lifestyle'. The trouble has arisen because we live in an unnatural environment with hundreds of thousands of chemicals, and we generally lead inactive lives. Evolutionary changes struggle to catch up with our fast-changing world of progress and the pace of development. We need to slow down.

It's Not Just the Mutation but Its Location That Matters

Not every mutation leads to cancer. A human cell can have many mutations and stay healthy and alive.

Some mutations are lethal, and cells don't survive them.

Non-lethal mutations can be of three types. There are those that happen in parts of DNA which are dormant and never used, and which hence have no effect on the body. Some happen in functional genes; this can make them defective or sometimes better (this is the driving force for evolution). And then there are those that happen in cancer-causing genes.

Not every cancer is a killer. Even when cancer-causing mutations happen, the cells don't always show an aggressive behaviour. Up to 80% of men develop prostate cancer by the age of 80 but it is contained, and many live a healthy, normal life unaware of the disease. Most men die with this cancer rather than of it.

What we need to identify is the mutation that drives a cancer from a contained disease to an invasive one. In my opinion, the usual suspect is the Pandora of the genome, TP53, which triggers the cancer to unleash its aggressive behaviour. Instead of chasing all mutations, we need to focus on this gene and its downstream pathways which are involved in almost every cancer known to mankind. Even when the TP53 is undamaged (in 50% of cancers), its function is found to be defective. Preventing, detecting, and treating this weakest link in the chain of events leading to an aggressive cancer could be the key to controlling and curing this disease.

Customise Prevention Strategies & Treatment

We are all individuals with individual strengths and weaknesses. This cannot be truer when it comes to cancer prevention. A person with a defective or less-effective alcohol metabolising gene is at higher risk of alcohol-induced cancers than others. For such an individual, the general limit of 14 units (for males) or seven units (for females) of alcohol per week is probably too high. And we have all heard of people who chain-smoked for decades and did not get lung cancer, and those who smoked a few for some years and got one. The reason in most cases is an individual variation for detoxifying the carcinogens in cigarette smoke. In others, it might be due to additional risk factors, like recurrent chest infections or exposure to radon gas, in addition to their smoking.

There is a dire need to identify individual variations and customise cancer prevention strategies accordingly. At present, we are offering a blanket cover based on statistics derived from selective populations, which fails to address the individual needs.

Cancer prevention is not the only area where customised healthcare is neglected. When it comes to cancer treatment, our data is driven from trials based on relatively younger, fitter, and healthier populations of patients in developed countries.

Data from around the world is increasingly showing that treatment response is variable depending on a person's age, sex, race, socio-economic group, diet, co-morbidities, and even mental health.

Add to that our individual variations in metabolising drugs and you have a spectrum of treatment responses from highly effective to almost ineffective, all using the same drug. Sometimes there are even variations of drug action in the same patient from one day to another, depending on their environment and general health.

One of my personal areas of interest has been the variable response to anti-cancer treatments in diabetic and non-diabetic patients. Over the last two decades it has become evident that cancer behaves differently in diabetic patients, and the treatment outcomes also vary. Some cancer therapies are more effective in diabetics compared to others. Medication used for controlling blood glucose levels can also affect anti-cancer treatment. A drug called 'metformin', for example, has shown to enhance the effects of anti-cancer treatment in breast-cancer patients.

Despite all these findings, there is a lack of research in customising cancer care to patients' individual need and response.

Unless and until we adopt a holistic approach in treating cancer, our efforts will fail to bear the fruits that we desire.

Cancer Surveillance: New and Improved Techniques

Traditionally, cancer surveillance has been fairly simple and non-specific. For example, after curative surgery for breast cancer, the method to check for recurrence is a low-dose X-ray known as a 'mammogram', the same method which is employed for diagnosing the cancer.

This is about to change, and it will be a change for good. An important development in the surveillance of breast cancer is measuring the circulatory tumour DNA (ctDNA[185]). A study published online in August 2015 in the *Science Translational Medicine* journal showed that women with early-stage breast cancer who had been treated with chemotherapy and surgery could be monitored by measuring the ctDNA in blood samples as early as two to four weeks post-surgery, and the majority of the women testing positive for ctDNA went on to experience a relapse of cancer.

The finding opens a window of opportunity to treat patients earlier in order to prevent cancer metastases and suggests that a non-invasive blood test may one day help identify cancer patients at a higher risk of recurrence, guiding treatment-targeted therapy tailored for these individuals.

However, there are many other unexplored avenues of detecting cancer which need to be utilised. It has been known for a long time that cancers love to feed on glucose. This characteristic has been used to detect them with special scans[186] but it's often ignored that cancer cells do not feed on glucose like normal cells. Normal cells break down glucose in the mitochondria, releasing 36 packets of energy (known as *ATP molecules*) for every one glucose molecule broken down. Cancer cells do it outside the mitochondria and break glucose in a primitive way, releasing only two packs of ATP energy and converting the rest as acid. This acid is toxic to normal cells and the environment around cancer cells is high in acid. Detecting these micro-acidic spots can help detect cancer cells in an early stage, too.

You might wonder why use such an inefficient way of using glucose when they need and spend more energy than normal cells. The answer is simple. Mitochondria are like a kitchen with a chef, cooking glucose in a slow and efficient way to release more energy. But this takes time. Cancer cells are in a rush to grow, multiply, invade, and colonise. They bypass the kitchen and opt for 'fast food' glucose with little processing and quick consumption. For more energy they just use more glucose, and in doing so create a shortage for other body cells.

This opens a new avenue for detecting them. A reduced mitochondrial activity in a cluster of cells using glucose as a fast food and generating a lot of waste in the process should flag up the possibility of a cancer-in-making.

---

[185] ctDNA refers to broken pieces of DNA that have leaked out of damaged tumour cells and are found in the blood.
[186] PET CT scans (positron emission Test CT) which detects an increased uptake of glucose in the body.

Let's Get Addicted (to the Right Things)

Humans have a tendency to get addicted. And there's nothing wrong with it if we can find the right addiction for ourselves. This is what Mr C. Unnikrishnan, a tea shop owner in the village of Marottichal in the state of Kerala, South India, found. Since the 1960s, his village had suffered from alcohol and gambling addiction, which often go hand-in-hand.

But Mr Unnikrishnan had a different kind of addiction, chess, and the villagers had a pet name for him, 'Chess Maaman' (*maaman* means 'uncle' in the local Malayalam language). He decided to share it with the rest of the village and started giving free chess lessons. Today, the village is known as the 'chess village', with 90% of its inhabitants from school children to octogenarians hooked on the game. As chess addiction increased, the community saw a steep drop in alcohol and gambling addiction. Apparently, chess is more addictive than alcohol and gambling.

It doesn't have to be chess for you and me. There is always some sort of advantageous addiction that could be our cup of tea.

Have a Laugh

When it comes to happiness, having a laugh works both ways. It is an expression of joy and also makes us happy.

In addition, it lowers blood pressure, reduces risk of stroke and heart attack, reduces levels of stress hormones, exercises our muscles, triggers release of endorphins, increases dopamine action in the brain, and boosts immunity against diseases, including cancer. So, watch or listen to something funny and laugh off disease.

Ancient wisdom has known this for centuries. In the fertile plains of Punjab (Pakistan) there are whole tribes of professional comedians called *bhands* who have a full-time job of making people laugh for a small fee. They have done so generation after generation for centuries and their skills are passed down from father to son. The profession is supported and patronised by the local community. In other cultures and countries, this essential luxury was only available to royalty, who had court jesters, but the Punjabis brought it to the masses, realising that happiness and health go hand-in-hand and are a basic human right.

Be Grateful or Find a Reason To Be So

When Glenn Fox, a neuroscientist at University of Southern California Marshall School of Business, decided to carry out a study of how gratitude manifests in the human brain, people scoffed at the idea.

Fortunately, this did not dissuade Mr Fox from his mission, and what he and other experts in this field have found so far is nothing less than amazing.

Feeling grateful causes the release of a chemical called *oxytocin* in the brain that helps promote social ties. This is the same chemical which plays an important role in mother-child relationship and bonding.

Gratitude makes us sleep better, reduces depression, makes us more generous, and less angry. Unsurprisingly, it makes us develop a more positive attitude, but what does come as a surprise is the fact that people who are grateful for all things big and small in life feel less pain on injury, heal quicker, have lower blood pressures, better kidney function, less heart disease, lower levels of stress hormones, and better immune systems. The last bit, a more effective immune system, is critical to surveillance and early detection of cancer cells by the body, which result in destroying them, nipping cancer in the bud.

Now that's a good enough reason for being grateful.

The Khan Philosophy

Everything in moderation including moderation[187].

It may sound confusing, but it isn't really.

It's good to play it safe most of the time, but every now and then we need to take calculated risks and test our limits.

We need periodic (not regular) stress to function normally.

It's the reason why lungs have three times the normal capacity needed to live a life on the sofa, our liver can regrow 20% if damaged, and although we can live on one kidney, our body is blessed with two.

Occasional stress is good and necessary – no pain, no gain – but regular or continuous stress has debilitating and devastating effects. It's in our nature to live at the edge, every now and then. Living continuously at the edge is dangerous, not to mention the obvious risk of falling off.

---

[187] The Doric (an ancient Greek dialect) maxim of 'Nothing in excess' (Μηδὲν ἄγαν, known to the West as the 'Golden Mean' or the 'Golden Middle Way') is literally carved in stone on the front of the Delphi temple. In my opinion it needs to be updated to 'Nothing in excess including moderation'. At times, we need to stretch the boundaries and reach for the extremes to challenge our body and soul before we come back to the golden middle way.

A monotonous life, devoid of challenges, is a recipe for depression and makes us reach for the TV remote or the refrigerator door. For a healthy life, we need to find small challenges that can be overcome with a bit of effort, and which give us a sense of achievement.

Occasional, acute stress releases relaxing chemicals in the body such as anandamide, which is the reason why we feel a certain relief after an exciting activity like running or taking a joy ride at the amusement park. It's blissful. But continuous and chronic stress is a torture and torment[188].

Having an occasional crisis in life is not bad for us, either. Every crisis comes with opportunity. Crises are a blessing in disguise, nudging us to do things differently, and for that reason they have played an integral part in our development and survival.

Let's look at it in a historic perspective.

When it poured with rain, we sought shelter in a cave, and when the cave flooded, we made outdoor caves called 'houses'. When our feet were sore walking on rough ground, we made shoes, and when shoes felt cold, we made socks.

Crisis is a trigger for evolution, both biologically and socially. Don't avoid it; look forward to it, because it is the harbinger of new opportunities and change. Ever had that feeling of being pushed to your limits? Congratulations, you are fulfilling the purpose of your life.

Change is good, it's exciting and, as long as it's positive, it enriches our life. Finding new aims in life helps preserve mental faculties and avoid dementia. Scientific studies have shown that people who have a purpose in life live healthier and longer lives.

Learn something new every day, at least one new thing[189] and do something regular in a different way, even if it is taking a new path to your usual destination. This will help switch on some new genes and neurons, and rest the old ones.

Try a new diet, a new cuisine, exotic food, or travel somewhere new but avoid the usual deep-frying, fast-food franchises selling the same old greasy burgers. Our planet is blessed with a wide variety of edibles, and each one has unique nutritional and health benefits. Don't enslave yourself to monotony.

---

[188] Ever wondered why the joy ride operators look so glum and uninterested?
[189] An ancient Arabic saying attributed to the Prophet Mohammad (may peace be upon him).

If you're bored in life, an exciting prospect is to get a pet. It's known to reduce stress levels, help combat depression, improve immunity, and promote good health.

Yes, There Are Some Magic Pills

Aspirin and metformin.

There you go, I have blurted it out without creating any suspense.

Aspirin, which was first discovered in the bark of the willow tree, is known to reduce the risk of heart disease, stroke, and cancer, especially bowel cancer, and also helps in controlling some cancers, such as prostate cancer.

Metformin is an anti-diabetes drug derived from a flowering plant known as 'goat's rue' (or *Galega officinalis* for those who like the Latin/Greek names). In addition to reducing blood glucose levels, it also helps to lose weight. Yes, you heard it right, it's very effective in helping reduce weight. If that isn't good-enough news, it also inhibits a cancer cell growth pathway known as *mTOR* and pushes cancer cells towards a natural death through apoptosis.

So, why don't we use them all the time?

The reason is twofold. Firstly, the benefits are there but not enormous, and on their own these drugs cannot control, let alone cure, cancer. The same goes for their other beneficial effects, like weight loss with metformin. They need to be used in conjunction with other drugs. Secondly, they have side effects and need to be taken under the advice and supervision of a doctor. Drugs related to metformin (phenformin and buformin) derived from the same plant were so toxic that they had to be banned. Moral of the story: not everything from nature is totally safe to use.

Avoid Too Much Sun

Especially children. Use sun protection (clothing, sunscreens etc.) and do not use sunbeds. Beards, on the other hand, keep the skin moist and avoid flaking of skin. However, growing a thick beard is not a practical possibility for everyone. Whether a face mask would offer the same benefit has not yet been studied.

In The Workplace, Protect Yourself

Protect yourself in the workplace against cancer-causing substances and risk factors (such as carcinogenic chemicals in the petroleum industry). Check your local guidelines and follow the recommended health and safety instructions.

Find Out if You Are Being Exposed to Radiation

For example, from naturally high radon levels in your home. If so, take action to reduce levels. You don't have to wait for expert reports or recommendations. Just open the windows for a few hours every day and ventilate the home, getting rid of any radon gas that has accumulated inside.

Breastfeed Babies

Breastfeeding is good for both the baby and the mother. It reduces a mother's risk of breast cancer.

Limit Hormone Replacement Therapy In Women, if and when Possible

Hormone replacement therapy increases the risk of certain cancers. Limit its use and avoid it altogether if possible. Speak to your doctor.

Take Part in Organised Cancer Screening Programmes

Such as those for bowel cancer (men and women), breast cancer (women), and cervical cancer (women), especially if there is a family history of these disease and/or there has been exposure to risk factors. Also, look out for new screening programmes regarding other cancers, and ask your doctor to assess if you fall into a high-risk category for any cancers and can benefit from screening.

Don't Bother Buying Bottled Supplements (Usually)

Vitamins, supplements, nutrients, and minerals work better when taken in their natural form, i.e., fruits, vegetables, honey, and nuts. Synthetic or bottled forms at worst don't work and at best don't work well. For example, vitamin C can easily denature when made into a tablet or powder, or on exposure to room temperature or heat. However, if taken in its natural form, like citrus fruits, it is better absorbed.

It is also suspected that synthetic vitamins are less readily absorbed because they lack the combination of other natural chemicals found in their original sources, like fruits and vegetables, which help in getting them absorbed by the body.

Scientific trials of people taking natural sources of vitamins (like fruits and vegetables) have shown a reduction in risk of cancer and other diseases, especially heart disease.

Ironically, when the same studies were done on people taking synthetic vitamins as supplements, it was found that they did not reduce the risk. In fact, many of these trials showed an increase in the risk of cancer and even heart disease.

So, save that money for a holiday instead of buying bottled stuff. Take naturally packaged vitamins, minerals, nutrients, and supplements in the form of fruit, vegetables, nuts, grains, and honey.

However, as always, if your doctor has instructed you to take vitamin or mineral supplements then do so because if you are deficient then your diet and lifestyle are not providing enough. Also, occasionally, more general health authority advice recommends certain supplements in certain groups. For example, in the UK, it is currently recommended that the over 50s take vitamin D supplements during the winter months, when exposure to natural daylight is restricted.

Say 'Goodbye' to Your Breakfast Bacon

Having bacon, salami, and sausages for breakfast increase the risk of cancer, especially cancer of the bowel. These foods are rich in carcinogenic nitrosamines and tend to have their worst effects when consumed first thing in the morning.

The best way to have a healthy breakfast is to include fruits, fibres, and wholegrain products in your diet.

Avoid Inflammation

Our ancient ancestors were familiar with cancers and closely observed their behaviour. More than a thousand years ago, the famous polymath, physician, and philosopher Abu Ali Sina (Avicenna) had recognised cancer as an inflammatory disease that does not heal. Today, modern science has identified that an inflammatory environment is essential to cancer's survival and growth. More importantly, many cancers are also born, not just bred, in the cradle of inflammation. Chronic infections and inflammatory states like autoimmune diseases can result in a multitude of cancers such as stomach, liver, bladder, bowel, ovarian, and cervical cancers.

Avoiding chronic inflammatory diseases is an important method of stopping cancer. It is even more important to treat and control inflammatory conditions if they cannot be avoided. Chemicals produced in the process of long-term inflammation inhibit apoptosis, the natural process of killing cancer cells.

I would like to take forward Ibn Sina's theory of cancer by suggesting that inflammation can be both a cause and effect of cancer. Based on my experience and knowledge, cancers which are associated with more inflammation are more aggressive and those with less inflammation are less lethal[190]. Having pro-

---

[190] Studies done at Glasgow Hospital, Scotland, have shown that cancer patients with the lowest levels of inflammatory markers are more likely to live longer than this with higher levels.

inflammatory elements like smoking, alcohol, and a diet rich in toxic chemicals is like adding fuel to a fire when it comes to cancer.

Beware of the Canproms

Have you heard of the *Canproms*?

Congratulations, you are one of the first to know of them.

Don't worry about googling the word. It's not yet made it to the lexicon because the concept is being first introduced by yours truly.

We have all heard of DNA-damaging chemicals and factors that can start a cancer, aka carcinogens, which I prefer to call 'canstarts'[191] because they can start a cancer. Then there are 'canstops'[192], known to the rest of the world as 'antioxidants' or substances that can stop a cancer from being born. But the most important and yet-to-be-acknowledged are the 'canproms'[193], the promotors of cancer which help it grow. These are the (yet) unacknowledged and least recognised contributors to the cancer pandemic.

Canproms are not mutagenic; they do not cause mutations by damaging DNA. They are mitogenic[194], causing increased growth and proliferation (mitosis) of cancer cells.

So far, I have discovered four categories of canproms.

Category 1 have a direct and an indirect effect on cancer growth. For example, glucose, which can directly feed the cancer cells and promote their growth and also cause release of other canproms such as insulin and IGF1, which are growth stimulants for cancer cells.

Category 2 only have a direct effect on promoting cancer growth. These include chemicals like insulin and IGF1.

Category 3 contains chemicals that need to undergo a chemical change to release a canprom, such as sugar (sucrose) or high-fructose corn syrup, which contains glucose, a category 1 canprom. Their strength would be determined by how quickly and in what amount they can release the canprom. In the case of glucose-containing chemicals, this would be measured by the glycaemic index (GI). For example, table sugar is a

---

[191] In an attempt to simplify cancer terms and make them more relatable and sensible.

[192] Another one for the dictionary.

[193] Guilty as charged. It is another one of the novel concepts brought to you by this book.

[194] I had half a mind to call them 'mitogens' but resisted the temptation for two reasons. Firstly, it goes against the basic principle of using simple terms, and, secondly, the term is already used to describe chemicals (peptides) that help a cell to start dividing (by triggering signal transduction pathways).

stronger canprom (GI=65) than lactose (GI=46) or honey (GI around 20 depending on the type). Milk is a complex category 3 canprom that contains glucose (combined with galactose as lactose, the milk sugar), insulin, IGF1, and other growth-enhancing hormones.

Category 4 has substances which can promote cancer growth when taken in a high concentration, such as synthetic vitamins and minerals.

Canproms not only help newly born cancers to grow and survive; they also play an important role in the survival and spread of established cancers, making their treatment less effective.

The importance of canproms will become evident as our understanding of cancer and its behaviour improves. This is an area of research that we have been oblivious to so far. Ironically, cancer promotors play an important part in the lifestyle that makes us prone to developing cancer. Our team is studying this phenomenon more closely so we can prevent, treat, and cure cancer more effectively.

Beware of the Unseen and the Unknown Electromagnetic Radiation

It's all around us, emitted by our gadgets and devices, especially mobile phones, and we are yet to find out what impact it has on our body and environment.

There are some precautionary measures which can significantly reduce the intensity of these radiation waves, especially when it comes to mobile phones, but the rule also applies in general to other devices emitting these rays.

1. If you have children below the age of 12, don't let them use a mobile a lot. At this age they are very vulnerable to any damaging factors which can have long-term consequences on their health.

2. Do not use mobiles or devices when travelling because they keep switching between different transmission sources and this increases the amount of radiation. Place on an aeroplane (flight/offline) mode or switch them off completely.

3. When making a phone call, use a hands-free or Bluetooth. Aim to keep the mobile or device at least two feet away from you.

4. At night, when going to sleep, turn the phone and gadgets off (you won't need them in your sleep anyways) and keep them as far away from you, preferably in another room, but at least two feet away.

Good News and More Good News

Every day, numerous cancer cells are born in our body, and our amazing body kills all of them. And this capacity can be enhanced easily.

If a cancer cell is a seed then the tumour is a tree growing from it. The seed takes years or decades to become a full tree. Its survival and growth depend on how favourable the soil, our body, is. A healthy body is an unfavourable environment for cancer to grow and it either dies or survives as a stunted plant. So, the best news is that even if and when a cancer cell survives, it does not always become a threat to human life. By the age of 80, almost 80% of men will have cancer cells in their prostate but in many cases they'll show no aggressive behaviour, which is a pleasant surprise. One can say that most men die with prostate cancer rather than of it. Even more amazingly, many if not all prostate cancer patients do not die of their cancer. With treatment, their cancer can be controlled for many years[195] and they live a normal life.

Cancer does not have to be a killer, but most importantly cancer does not have to be (full stop).

Detox, Not Retox

It's preventable, detectable, treatable, and potentially curable, yet we are facing a cancer pandemic, with the disease occurring more frequently and at an earlier age than before. There was a time it was considered a disease of the rich and privileged, but nowadays it is affecting all strata of society. This is not surprising, because most socioeconomic groups are living a similar lifestyle. As human society progresses, so does its rate of cancer. The World Health Organisation (WHO) estimates that up to 80% of cancers are born due to external influences, like lifestyle and environmental factors. I believe it could be close to 100%.

Our body and the environment are full of chemicals that can damage our DNA. We call them o*xidants*. Think of them like 'accidents' causing damage to DNA and other parts of the cell. Some are produced within our body; others enter from outside. Fortunately, our environment and body also produce their nemesis, neutralising chemicals known as *antioxidants*. Antioxidants are 'anti-accident'; they stop damage to DNA and cells by detoxifying and neutralising the accident-causing oxidants. Health is subject to a balance between these two polarising forces. If we can have more antioxidants in our body than the oxidants then we can stay healthier, younger, cancer-free, and live longer.

---

[195] One of my prostate cancer patients has had a good control of his cancer for 26 years and is still going strong.

We live a toxic lifestyle in a polluted world, both very much our own creation. Our ancestors lived in harmony with their environment. Things were never perfect, but they had methods of restoring the natural balance, a concept totally lost on us. Ancient physicians of all medical systems – Ayurvedic, Arab, Greek, or Chinese – stressed the need for detoxification of the human body. And the best place to start is with our diet. So, let's talk about how we can detox our diet by some simple and easy measures, rather than re-toxifying it. And there are added benefits to doing so; not only do you prevent and kill cancer but also stay younger, healthier, and live longer too. If we can use our food as a medicine then we won't end up taking medicine like food. So, let's talk about the Khan Diet Plan.

THE KHAN DIET PLAN

I've come up with an anti-cancer diet plan based on my personal experience and observations, and which has yet to be tested and tried in a prospective trial setting. Our team is aiming to carry out trials in the future. I call it the 'Khan Diet Plan'.

Basic Principles

The aim is to have a healthy diet and a healthy lifestyle.

The main principle is to **detox**, not **retox**.

An important concept unique to the Khan Diet Plan is that a healthy diet should not just be based on calorie reduction but also a sensible reduction in nutrients. There is increasing evidence from research and trials showing that an excess of nutrients such as vitamins contributes to the progress of cancer. Excessive nutrition has been known to cause health problems other than cancer, too. For example, an excess of vitamin D in the diet can lead to high levels known as *hypervitaminosis D* that causes heart problems, high blood pressure, muscle weakness, kidney damage, and mental retardation in children.

Our modern lifestyle is one of excess, and this is especially true when it comes to food and nutrients. Our diet is already nutrient rich, based on genetically modified and specially bred plants and animals. In addition, we have myriad supplements and food additives that overwhelm our body with nutrition in excess of our basic health requirements. And cancer is a disease strongly associated with excess and abundance, plethora and surplus. This also holds true for other diseases such as diabetes and heart problems. During World War II, when there was a shortage of meat and dairy, with both items being rationed and people only consuming small amounts of them, there was a substantial reduction in heart disease.

The Khan Diet Plan is based on established ancient and contemporary concepts of optimum nutrition, dieting, and fasting. I recommend starting it in a stepwise fashion. An important thing to remember is that, like every other diet, there is room for failure and strategies to recover. Remember, it's a diet, not a divine decree written in stone.

The plan is not to tell you what to do, but what you can do based on reliable information and knowledge that will empower you to make your own decisions.

HOW TO START

Eat Fresh Food

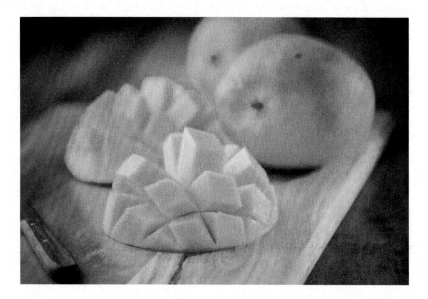

Here's something that you are aware of but possibly never realised. We eat dead things. Be it meat or fruit, vegetables or nuts, it's technically necrophagia[196]. Food, especially dead food, starts to rot as soon as it dies. The cause is microorganisms, especially bacteria, which, like us, feed on dead food and beat us to it. The process of decay, 'rotting' in simple English, reduces the levels of nutrition as the good stuff is eaten by the bugs and is replaced by toxins (bacterial excrements), some of which are carcinogenic. The longer the period between the demise of our food and us consuming it, usually the less nutritious and more toxic it becomes.

There are ways to slow down the rotting process, a bit like the Egyptians did to embalm and mummify bodies, preserving them in salts and oil, removing moisture by drying them out, and adding chemicals that kill bacteria or slow their growth, like chillies, spices, and synthetic preservatives. The latter, modern preserving compounds can sometimes be more toxic and carcinogenic than those that bacteria produce. Even if the preservative chemicals are not carcinogenic, they will engage the liver in metabolising them, thus reducing the liver's ability to detoxify cancerous chemicals. So, the next time you see a cucumber sandwich with 17 ingredients and a three-week shelf life, ask yourself two questions:

1. Would any self-respecting cucumber hang around for so long even if attached to its vine in the garden?

---

[196] Eating the dead; *necro* ('dead)' and *phagia* ('eating').

2. Are the manufacturers adding all these chemicals because they feel generous towards you or because they want to maximise their profit and minimise wastage?

Not all modern methods are evil. Refrigeration and freezing are fairly safe, as are natural preservatives like oil, spices, and chillies, but they but they don't stop the clock on rotting food, only slow it down.

Eating fresh is the best way to gain nutrition and avoid exposure of our body to toxic chemical that can cause cancer. It takes more effort – not a lot, just a little more – to prepare fresh food, but the advantages of consuming fresh (freshly dead to be precise) food far outweighs the trouble taken to make it.

STEP ONE

To Eat or Not to Eat, and How To Do Both

The secret to health, happiness, youth, and longevity is in knowing what, when, and how not to eat.

Mohammad Muneeb Khan

The biggest dilemma one faces, whether 'one' happens to be a connoisseur of fine food or a gifted glutton, is the temptation of food. When facing the inevitable dilemma of eating or not eating, my simple solution is to do both. Here's how it's done.

You come across a delicious piece of cake and ask yourself the question whether to eat it or not. The solution is simple: eat half of it and leave the rest for another time. But be wary of the 'time'. It's dead food and will be slowly rotting away. If left for too long, even in a refrigerator or freezer, return it back to nature in an environmentally friendly way by making compost out of it.

Apply the same rule to all of your regular food items. Your favourite sugar-rich can of cola? Don't drink the whole can or a glass-full, have a small teacup-full instead. Leave the rest for later and when coming back to it tell yourself, "It's no good now because it's flat" and get rid of it in an environmentally friendly way without any guilt. The usual slice of bread? Cut it into half and eat only one (right or left, it doesn't matter). Feed the rest to the birds (add chilli seeds so the rats don't get to it first. Birds can't taste the chilli and would happily gobble up the seeds with the bread). And what to do with the feeling of emptiness left behind, I hear you ask. Fill it, I say, with fruits and nuts. So, you can achieve both, to eat and not to eat, and save yourself the ignominy of noble mental suffering[197].

To Avoid Temptation First Know Your Enemy

The evil of temptation, especially the sweet craving for carbohydrates, attacks us from four directions: front, back, left, and right. The frontal attack is the obvious temptation, like the 3,845 calorie-containing sundae with 18 scoops of ice cream sitting on a foundation of four waffles topped with chocolate bars, syrups, sauces, fresh fruit[198], and pieces of chocolate fudge brownie, retailing in Cardiff for £32.95. It's the type of 'in your face' temptation that is easy to see if not easy to avoid.

---

[197] My sincerest apologies to Shakespearian fans for the heinous parody.

[198] In a vain attempt to hide your guilt.

The backstabbers come in many forms, most commonly as canned or bottled carbonated drinks. A famous brand which doesn't taste very sweet is known to have 54 grams of sugar. That's *thirteen and a half* sugar cubes, which you would never want to stuff your mouth with but are keen to consume in a few gulps.

The attack from the left is pure evil, like the one shot (45 ml) of 190 proof rectified spirit with 285 calories. It's unashamedly bad and has no qualms about it. One look and you know what you are getting yourself into. Pure trouble.

The most serious and devious temptation comes from the right. Evil masquerading as the virtuous. This is the 'pure fruit juice' which is full of sugar, minus all the nutrients found in the pulp' the 'healthy' breakfast cereal that is loaded with glucose and fructose; the fresh salad and fruits that have been washed in chemicals to extend their shelf life (rinse them well before eating). These are the Trojan horses that hide the enemy and let it sneak on you unannounced.

Last but not least, beware of the sugar iceberg, because you only see the tip.

There's a lot more sugar than we see in this world. We tend only to count the spoonfuls that willingly, yet reluctantly, add to the cup, but food manufacturers load their products with it for the sake of flavour and to preserve it.

STEP TWO

Know Thyself

And I don't mean self-consciousness in the pantheistic metaphysical sense, but keeping it real.

Know your tolerances and intolerances to food, especially lactose intolerance, which plagues the majority of the human race and presents as a plethora of symptoms which can easily get one labelled as a hypochondriac.

This is the key to a healthy and happy life.

The human body is not designed to overeat. We are the healthiest and functionally best when remaining slightly under-filled and hungry. Stop eating while you are still hungry. Our body tricks us into eating more, running on a primitive instinct when food was scarce and not in regular supply. The mechanism of tricking us into overeating is simple. The stomach does not tell the brain when it is full. In fact, we get filled up much before (16–20 minutes estimated by one study) our mind knows it's full.

Beware of enzymatic deficiencies such as those which metabolise alcohol and put one at increased risk of alcohol toxicity and cancer.

If you are aware that you're eating too much or too little, get medical help. Your doctor may want to check your thyroid gland's function. Thyroid function is also a helpful test if you are failing to gain weight or shed it. Having your blood glucose levels checked is also important, especially if you have been putting on weight for a long time (especially around the waist).

Also get to know your hunger and psyche. For most of us, we confuse thirst with hunger. Whenever feeling hungry, please drink some water first. You will be surprised how often it was your thirst which made you reach out for the food.

Break free from the compulsive eating behaviours. Why do we have to eat a full bar of chocolate or full bag of crisps? Why can't we stop halfway?

And discover the real purpose of night; it's sleep, not heading for the fridge[199]. Raiding the refrigerator is not a natural part of our circadian rhythm.

---

[199] Eating at night is associated with increased risk of obesity.

STEP THREE

The Diet Plan

Early Morning

1) Stop cancer in 30 seconds by D.A.N (Doing Absolutely Nothing). Yes, you heard me right. You can detox every cell in your body within 30 seconds without any effort. All you have to do is rise and shine, literally. Here's how it works. When the human eyes are exposed to early-morning light (after sunrise, ideally before 9 AM), the near-infrared part of the light spectrum (NIR light, which is normally felt as warmth and not really seen) falling on the back of our eyes[200] sends a signal to the brain which, in turn, tells every cell in our body to start producing a magical chemical known as *melatonin*. Melatonin is a powerful detox chemical (antioxidant) which neutralises toxins (aka oxidants) in the cell. If not neutralised, these oxidant toxins can damage cell structures, especially DNA, which can lead to mutations and cancers. Now you might be thinking that melatonin was supposed to be made in the brain[201] in response to darkness, and you would be right. However, the latest research has shown that this only accounts for less than 5% of total body melatonin. The majority of the melatonin, more than 95%, is made inside the cells in these small organelles we talked about earlier, the mitochondria. The best time is soon after sunrise, but we need to have exposure to the near infrared rays of the sun to trigger it. You don't have to look at the sun. In fact, you must not look at it, as that could harm your eyes. All you have to do is bask in the direct or indirect sunlight. Even the sunlight bouncing off the trees and grass is rich in the NIR (near-infrared rays) and would stimulate the detox process in your body. And all it takes is 30 seconds and every cell in your body will produce enough melatonin to kick-start the daily detox. This will not only reduce the risk of cancer but also help reduce depression, aggression, stress, and even your blood pressure. Now this is what I call a 'Good Morning'.

This potent natural detox has been a part of our life since the dawn of human civilisation. Technically, we are daytime creatures (the scientific term is 'diurnal'; night creatures are called 'nocturnal') and we need exposure to the morning sunlight to kick-start our daily (circadian) cycle. We need this essential 'Good Morning' to lead to a good day. Morning light also helps with the release of other daytime hormones in our body essential for a healthy mind and body.

It's no surprise, then, that most cultures and religions have advocated this behaviour over the centuries.

---

[200] Lower part of the retina, to be precise.

[201] A particular area of the brain known as the *pineal gland* or *pineal body*.

Taoist and Buddhist monasteries established early-morning exercises like Tai Chi, and Islam strongly recommended that Muslims did not go to sleep after their morning prayer (which is before sunrise). The 17th-century Hindu saint, Samarth Ramdas, popularised it as a part of his yoga rituals, aptly naming it Surya Namaskar, which means 'saying hello to the sun'.

Ironically, modern lifestyles often do not take this essential light therapy into account. Most of us are unaware of it and often miss this detox. An average American spends 93% of his/her time indoors (87% in a building, house, office, shop etc., and 6% in a car). Very few of us make a concerted effort to go out after sunrise and expose our eyes to the sunlight. Many are trapped in high-rise buildings and flats.

This brings us to the two important questions.

Firstly, does the sunlight coming through a window or windscreen have the same effect? And the answer is, no. The intensity of sunlight (measured in units called 'lux') is very weak through glass, somewhere around 50 lux, whereas venturing outside or sticking your head out of a window will expose you to somewhere between 10,00 and 130,000 lux. Now that is a LOT of lux difference.

Secondly, what about an overcast day? Would 30 seconds still be enough? And the answer once again is no. But 30 minutes would suffice on the most overcast day of the year. So anywhere between 30 seconds to 30 minutes, depending on the brightness of the sun, and we can detox each and every cell of our body against cancer-causing chemicals by Doing Absolutely Nothing[202].

The benefits of melatonin don't stop there. Experimental and observational studies have shown that it has the ability to inhibit cancer cells by reducing their growth, spread (metastasis), and even killing them kindly by apoptosis. Future research will enable us to utilise its potent detox and anti-cancer properties more effectively.

* * *

2) Welcome back. Now that you have detoxed every magnificent cell of your body to reduce the risk of cancer, depression, anxiety, and stress, let's start with breaking your overnight fast, aka breakfast[203]. Take one or half a small spoon of honey (contains essential nutrients, vitamins, and minerals). Don't

---

[202] I have coined this term 'D.A.N Doing Absolutely Nothing' so you may not find it elsewhere in case you are looking for references. However, you don't have to be totally inactive; you can go for a walk or stroll in the shade. My favourite advice to people is "Just stand there and look pretty", which is easily achievable when you are glowing in the morning sunlight.

[203] There is a reason it's called 'breakfast'. The human body by nature needs to fast overnight and eating late at night can lead to weight gain, obesity, poor memory function, acid reflux, difficulty sleeping, poor metabolism and impaired immunity, making one prone to infections.

mix it with hot water, as heat destroys most of the beneficial ingredients. Try to find unprocessed, natural honey as the process of heating to extract honey also destroys most of its nutrients.

3) Drink a glass of water (not hot, just normal temperature). This helps flush out toxins that have accumulated overnight, via the kidneys.

4) Take one to two spoons of extra virgin olive oil (another source of essential vitamins, minerals, nutrients, omega-3 fatty acids, and antioxidants).

5) Eat two fruits of your choice (e.g., apple or banana). Fruits and vegetables are best eaten before the main meal, when your gut is full of enzymes ready to extract vitamins and minerals from them. Eating them after a main meal is the least beneficial because most of the enzymes have already been consumed.

6) Your usual/normal breakfast might not be a good idea. The traditional modern breakfasts are not the healthiest of choices and most of us are unaware of it. Consider the ubiquitous egg, an essential part of most breakfasts. Humans have consumed them for thousands of years but not on a regular daily basis. They were difficult to transport due to their fragility, and mass production is a fairly recent phenomenon. A wild version of the modern chicken would only lay a dozen eggs in a year during the breeding season. The modern, selectively bred chicken with their modified feed enables a typical egg factory to produce 12 million eggs in a week. In January 2019 alone, the United States produced 9.41 billion eggs, enough to reach the Moon if stacked one on top of the other.

Eating eggs every day may be a less-risky diet for children of growing age but for an adult consuming more than four eggs a week has shown to increase the risk of cancers, especially those of the breast, ovary, and prostate. This shouldn't come as a surprise as eggs are full of nutrients which promote growth of cells and excessive amounts of these growth promotors can enhance the growth of cancer cells.

7) Similarly, the modern tradition of eating processed meats like bacon at breakfast can increase the risk of cancer. A study of more than 200,000 women showed that eating processed meat increased the risk of breast cancer by 21%.

8) So, it's 'Wakey-Wakey, No Eggs, No Bakey'. (Please note that we are omitting bacon/processed meat altogether but only avoiding the 'eggs' in the plural sense; it's OK to have an egg on alternate days to keep within the weekly safe maximum of four eggs.)

9) Last but not least, wash the eggs before cooking. Most producers don't do so because it reduces their freshness and shelf life.

10) Please make sure the bread you consume is wholemeal and not fortified with artificial vitamins, and the cereals are free of sugar, salt, added vitamins, and preservatives.

11) If you are thinking tea or coffee? The answer is, preferably, coffee. It's definitely better than tea when it comes to reducing weight, detoxing the body and reducing the risk of cancer. Tea comes in as the second-best option.

12) Make sure you avoid dairy or keep it to a minimum (up to one cup per day) and have dairy-free days every now and then if you tend to overindulge.

Lunch

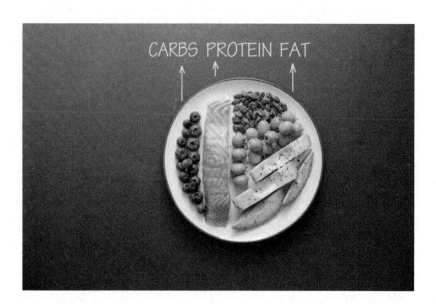

1) Drink one glass of water.

2) Eat two fruits. If possible, stop here and skip lunch every few days. You can double up on the fruits or add some nuts. Skipping a full lunch every now and then will help you keep the weight in check and reduce the spikes of insulin and other growth factors in your bloodstream which can fuel growth of cancer cells.

3) Have a balanced and healthy lunch with protein, fibre, fat, and carbohydrates. Minimise the carbs, especially refined and processed carbohydrates, and include reasonable amounts of healthy fats (olive oil, coconut oil, animal fat, and butter) and proteins.

4) Incorporate olive oil and vinegar in your food. Both have shown to help reduce weight and blood glucose levels.

Dinner

1) Drink one glass of water.

2) Eat two fruits of your choice.

3) Have a balanced and healthy dinner with protein, fibre, fat, and carbohydrates. Minimise the carbs and use reasonable amounts of healthy fats and proteins. Keep the dinner lighter than lunch (if you have had a full lunch) and eat it at least 2–4 hours before you sleep.

Before Going to Bed

1) Take one or more spoonfuls of olive oil[204].

2) Eat one or two fruits of your choice if feeling peckish. Make sure there is a gap of 2–3 hours before you sleep. If not, just fill yourself with water and give it 1–2 hours before hitting the sack.

3) Floss after the last snack and brush at least an hour after. Brushing soon after eating wears off dental enamel. Flossing is a must, as brushing-only leaves 30–70% of the teeth surface unclean, depending on the brushing technique. Not brushing or flossing leaves bacteria to overgrow and produce toxins all night. Don't forget to brush your tongue. Stick it out and brush it. Look in the mirror while you do so; it is a funny and humbling experience at the same time.

4) Avoid bright lights like those from mobile and appliances after sunset. Our natural world has bright light from the sky during the day, and warm low lights from the horizon and ground in the evening and night (think sunsets, campfires, and fireplaces). When our eyes see bright lights above the ground level at night, it sends confusing signals to the brain which changes our normal body rhythm (circadian rhythm), and the body secretes daytime chemicals and hormones. This abnormal pattern has an adverse effect on our health and, in the long run, can increase the risk of chronic diseases, including cancer. So, treat the night time as it should be. Use table lamps instead of ceiling lights, read a book rather than the mobile screen, and go to sleep sooner than later.

---

[204] A good source of minerals and vitamins helps regulate bowel activity, too.

STEP FOUR

The Dos and Don'ts of Life

What to Drink

1) Water. It's essential for life, and 60% of us is water anyway. It helps us detox by flushing out toxins via our kidneys. Add it to juices and milk, especially if you are fond of (expensive) skimmed milk, though there is an easier and cheaper way, i.e., take some whole milk, add water to taste and voila, instant skimmed milk.

2) Coffee. As much as reasonably possible; best if freshly ground and black with no added sugar or milk. Arabica beans are better than robusta, which are only favoured because of being cheaper and easier to produce.

3) Tea, black or green. Loose tea is better than teabags as the paper adds unnecessary and undesirable chemicals to the water, and also makes it taste funny. Green tea has polyphenols which are powerful antioxidants. One of them, known as 'EGCG' (epigallocatechin-3-gallate), also helps kill cancer cells by apoptosis and has shown to enhance the effects of radiotherapy on cancer cells. Black tea has less polyphenols than green tea. It is made by fermenting green tea and this process destroys most of the beneficial polyphenols. For best results, tea needs to be brewed or steeped in boiling water for ten minutes.

4) Skip the usual breakfast items like jams; jellies; conserves; fruit slices preserved in syrup; sweetened drinks; fruit juices, especially from concentrates (eat fruit instead); potatoes, white bread; refined flour products such as bagels, croissants, and muffins; sugar (or food with added sugar); and syrups such as maple and corn syrup. If you can't avoid them completely, please try to keep them to a minimum and choose any one item from the above list on a given day.

What Not to Drink (or at Least Drink Less of)

1) Alcohol (certainly consume in moderation)

2) Carbonated drinks with or without sugar

3) Fruit juices (they are rich in sugars; better to eat fruits)

4) Any drinks with sugar (glucose or other forms of fast-release carbohydrates)

What to Eat

1) Any **food without added sugar or fructose**, preservatives, synthetic multivitamins, and salts. Make sure you consume less carbohydrates, and that those you take are unrefined and unprocessed, such as wholemeal bread. High levels of glucose and insulin (which is produced in response to glucose in the body) are associated with an increased risk of cancer. Cancer rates have started to rise in line with the addition of large quantities of highly refined sugar in our diet since the Second World War. The link doesn't just stop here. Studies of animals with cancer have shown that feeding them a high-sugar diet makes chemotherapy less effective.

2) **Food without artificial sweeteners**, because they trick the body into thinking you are consuming sugar, and the body reacts by secreting sugar-digesting chemicals such as insulin. This not only has a growth stimulating effect on all cells (including cancer cells) but also makes us crave more calories. Hence, we end up eating more.

3) **Good fats and oils**, especially those rich in omega-3 fatty acids. Olive oil is a good source; extra virgin cold press is best. Other sources of omega-3 are fish, strawberry, kiwifruit, chia, linseed, fig, hempseed, hazelnut, walnut, pecan, butternut, lean red meat, turkey, chicken, and eggs from hens fed a diet of greens, not grains. Canola and flaxseed oil are also good sources.

4) **Good proteins**. There are many sources; don't stick to one – diversify. Fish, poultry, beef, mutton, turkey, lentils, fruits, vegetables, nuts – the list goes on. Choose organic, naturally fed and grown sources which are not exposed to chemicals like insecticides and pesticides. Have a moderate meat consumption with alternate meat-free days. Aim for red meat consumption around 300 grams per week or less, with a maximum 500 grams. If you can, balance it with fruits and vegetables.

5) Choose **good sugars** which release their sweetness slowly (low glycaemic index) like wholegrain cereals, multigrain bread, oats, millet, lentils, fruits, and vegetables.

6) **Good vegetables** – natural, organic, insecticide, and pesticide-free. Wash well before use. Best results are achieved when they are combined with other vegetables and cooked. This must be the reason why 'mixed vegetables' are part of almost every cuisine worldwide. Some vegetables must be cooked to release their beneficial elements. Tomatoes, for example, have a chemical with anti-cancer properties called 'lycopene' but it's only released when they are cooked in oil.

Cabbages, cauliflower, and broccoli contain the anti-cancer molecules sulforaphane and indo-3-carbinols (I3Cs), which not only help kill cancer cells and block their growth by stopping them from developing new blood vessels (anti-angiogenesis) but also give a boost to the immune cells (NK or natural killer cells) which are experts in killing cancer. But boiling them destroys these chemicals, so it's best to steam them or fry in olive oil.

Garlic reduces blood pressure and the risk of cancer. It is more effective when crushed and fried in oil.

7) **Good fruits** – natural, organic, free from insecticides and pesticides. Wash well before use. Fruits are full of anti-cancer antioxidants. For example, raspberries and strawberries contain ellagic acid which detoxifies cancer-causing chemicals. Cherries contain glucaric acid, another strong detoxing substance. Blueberries are even better. They contain chemicals called 'anthocyanidins' and 'proanthocyanidins', which can kill cancer cells by apoptosis. Cranberries also contain proanthocyanidins, as does dark chocolate and the spice cinnamon. Berries retain their anti-cancer chemicals even when frozen, but it is better to consume fresh ones.

Citrus fruits have detoxifying molecules known as 'flavonoids' which also inhibit cancer cell growth and spread and kill them by inducing apoptosis.

Pomegranates have antioxidant detoxifying properties and can slow down the growth and spread of existing cancers.

Mangos are my favourite, especially the chaunsa variety from Pakistan[205]. They are rich in vitamin C and other antioxidants. They also contain mangeferin, an anti-cancer compound that inhibits cancer growth and spread. They also boost immunity and are a good source of vitamin B6, vitamin A, and minerals. And if that was not enough, they also delay aging and keep you young for longer. What else could one ask for?

Peaches, plums, and nectarines are also rich in antioxidants, as are almost all other fruits. The main aim should be to have at least five portions of fruit a day.

The list can go on forever and would probably need a book of its own. For best results mix and match, and have different types of fruits on different days.

8) **Nuts** – natural, organic, insecticide and pesticide-free.

9) **Seeds** – natural, organic, insecticide and pesticide-free.

10) **Herbs** – natural, organic, insecticide and pesticide-free. Coriander, mint, basil, thyme, parsley, oregano, celery, and many more herbs are full of antioxidants which are available in a higher

---

[205] Unarguably the best tasting mango in the world and hence its title, 'King of the fruits'.

351

concentration to be absorbed by the body when chopped and mixed with oil. Seaweed has chemicals that kill cancer cells by apoptosis, and which also assist the immune system (natural killer cells) to hunt down cancer cells. It can be added to soups or salads, or fried.

11) **Spices** – natural, organic, insecticide and pesticide-free. And here's the trick – spices work best in combination. For example, turmeric (which contains curcumin, a chemical with anti-cancer properties) is absorbed two thousand times more when combined with pepper. So, for best results, combine the different spices and herbs (turmeric absorption also increases with ginger) and heat them in olive oil while cooking food to release the beneficial chemicals and increase their absorption.

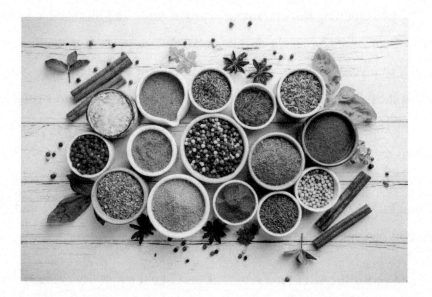

12) **Chillies** – natural, organic, insecticide and pesticide-free. You can find more details in the dedicated section on chillies and spices (7.13).

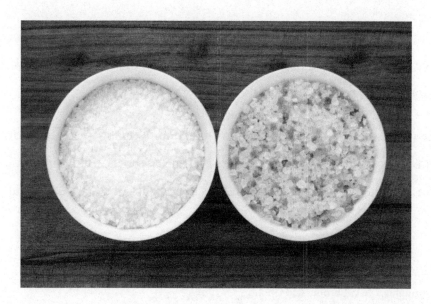

Pink Himalayan Salt (on the right) discovered by Alexander the Great and his horse in Pakistan.

13) **Safe salt**. We take table salt for granted but historically it was one of the rarest commodities in food. Traditionally, it was produced by evaporation of seawater (and still is), but the seawater nowadays is contaminated, and the salt produced from it has been found to have microplastics[206] and, sometimes, toxins produced by fungi, so best to avoid it.

Salt is essential to our health and diet. Due to its rarity, it was used as currency. People were paid in salt rather than cash and such payments were known as 'salary'[207], a term which has survived through the ages.

In some parts of the world, it was exchanged for gold[208].

So, when you found rocks containing salt you literally struck gold. And this is what happened to Alexander the Great in 326 BC on his visit to present-day Pakistan. While passing through a mountain range, his horse, Bucephalus, fell in love with the rocks and started licking them, refusing to move. This intrigued Alexander dismounted the horse and had a lick himself (hopefully not the same rock as Bucephalus) and thus discovered one of the largest rock salt reserves on Earth; mountain after mountain of pure pink Himalayan salt known as the 'Salt Range'. It has been mined for more than 2,100 years and is still producing enough for global consumption. The mines are massive, with 22 floors, underground lakes (where things don't sink, just float), train tracks, buildings made of salt bricks, and even a salt hospital where asthmatic patients can spend hours to treat their disease.

So, skip the sea salt and go for the safer option of rock salt like the pink Himalayan version.

Best is to buy it as ungrounded pellets and grind for use at home using a simple manual grinder like the one used for black pepper and other spices (it only takes a few seconds of extra effort).

14) **Olives** are awesome antioxidants. Black are better than green, and cold-pressed extra-virgin olive oil is the best source of phenolic antioxidants and dietary oil that man can have. Cook, fry, or take it neat. But don't overdose on it – remember the rule of moderation.

15) **Dark chocolate** (more than 70% cocoa) contains many antioxidants that help prevent cancer and can slow the growth of existing tumours. However, mixing chocolate with sugar and milk cancels the benefits and can even help promote cancer due to the effects of glucose, insulin, and other growth factors.

---

[206] Especially sea salt from the USA, Europe, and China.

[207] From the Roman word *sal*, meaning 'salt'.

[208] This was a common practice till the early decades of the last century in the northern gold-rich valleys of Pakistan, where salt was a rarity.

What Not to Eat (or at Least Eat Less of)

1) Anything with added sugar or fructose.

Make sure you consume less carbohydrates, and that those you take are unrefined and unprocessed, such as wholemeal bread. Refined sugars release glucose rapidly and in a high quantity. It's not just the quantity of glucose but the rate at which it is released by food which is important in preventing and controlling cancer. This is measured in terms of the glycaemic index. It is a simple and straightforward system of numbers from 0 to 100. Pure glucose has a glycaemic index of 100 (maximum). Foods with a glycaemic index of 0-55 are very good sources of carbohydrates. These include honey, nuts, seeds, whole grains, most vegetables, and fruits. These are the safest carbohydrates.

Any food with a glycaemic index between 56–69 needs to be consumed in small amounts. These include our commonest foods such as wheat, bread, rice, white sugar, ice cream, fruit juices, raisins, and prunes etc. A glycaemic index between 70–100 is rated as high and such foods are best avoided; these include glucose, high-fructose corn syrup (which is almost half glucose), white bread, white rice, corn flakes, some breakfast cereals, and potatoes. Low glycaemic-index (GI) natural sugars can be used as an alternative to sugar in moderate amounts. These include honey (acacia honey, for example, has a GI of 30), coconut sugar (GI 30) and agave sector (GI 15–21).

Cancer cells feed on glucose and use insulin and IGF-1 (released by the body in response to glucose) to grow. Our bodies are designed to consume small amounts of sugar and historically our ancestors consumed around 2 kg of refined sugar (usually in the form of honey) in a year. The modern human consumes up to 35 kg or more a year, equal to six 10-pound bowling balls. That's a lot of sugar.

2) Anything with artificial sweeteners, because they trick the body into thinking you are consuming sugar, and the body reacts by secreting sugar-digesting chemicals such as insulin. This not only has a growth stimulating effect on all cells (including cancer cells) but also makes us crave more calories. Hence, we end up eating more.

3) Sweets and candies. Treat them like alcohol (unless one is an alcoholic), and consume them in moderation on special occasions. That is exactly how human society has indulged in highly refined sugar food over the centuries. Cakes, ice creams, and candies were celebratory food, not a part of the regular diet or frequent snacks.

4) Excessive amounts of dairy products, especially if you are lactose intolerant. Even if you are not intolerant, remember milk is loaded with growth-promoting factors – good for growing kids, not too good for grown-ups.

5) Snacks. Avoid snacking except on special occasions or limit it to a few days a week. Every time we snack, the body releases the 'full monty' of hormones and chemicals in anticipation of a complete meal. Remember, your pancreas cannot see the bag of crisps but only sense the glucose entering the body, triggering it to pour its stores of insulin into the bloodstream. The key to weight control and general health is limiting food intake to mealtimes only.

6) Stay away from artificial fats such as margarines and polyunsaturated vegetable oils (read the labels to identify them). The healthiest sources of fats are olive oil, butter, coconut oil, and animal fat. That is the type of fat which keeps us healthy.

An important factor when it comes to fats is the balance between omega-3 and omega-6. Both are essential for health but an imbalance in the two with a high proportion of omega-6 is not good for health. So go for a good blend of omega-3 and omega-6. Our bodies benefit most from an optimal ratio of 2:1 (omega-6:omega-3). Modern methods of food production can result in up to 40 times more omega-6 than omega-3. Let me give you an example. The egg laid by a hen fed on a natural diet will have equal amounts of omega-3 and omega-6 (1:1 ratio), but the same egg laid by a corn-fed hen will have 20 times more omega-6 than omega-3 (20:1 ratio). But one can't tell the difference just looking at them.

Soy, palm, and canola oils are a big source of omega-6 and, to make things worse, they are often hydrogenated to increase their shelf life.

A diet rich in omega-6 and deficient in omega-3 also tends to increase the toxic effects of alcohol by making it more carcinogenic (five to 10 times more production of free radicals). This at least partly explains the difference in cancer risk among the Mediterranean population and the rest of Europe and USA. They consume more omega-3 rich olive oil, which probably offsets the risk incurred by their alcohol consumption.

For a healthy life it is essential that we keep this ratio right and try to incorporate more omega-3 in our diet.

7) Avoid any food with high-fructose corn syrup (HFCS). It's no better than sugar. Sucrose or sugar has 50% glucose and 50% fructose. HFCS has 45% glucose and 55% fructose, hardly any different from common sugar. But it is made to sound different and is added to all kinds of foodstuffs to extend their

shelf life and enhance flavour. It's one of the biggest causes of weight gain and obesity all over the world.

8) Avoid using the microwave. Eat fresh; cook and heat on a stove. Store and serve food in non-plastic containers. Glass is best as it does not react chemically with any contents. Metal, ceramic, and earthenware are also good choices. Plastic containers are best avoided for heating food as there can be reactions between the plastic and its contents.

9) Avoid fish from polluted waters. They accumulate toxins (like dioxin and mercury) in their bodies which can damage the body organs and cause cancer.

10) Junk food is as the name suggests. It's full of sugar, unhealthy omega-6 rich fats, and chemical preservatives, most of which are toxic, plus artificial flavours and lots of salt. Everything is geared at producing a cheap product with a long shelf life to maximise profit. Do yourself a favour and bin it as suggested by the name.

What To Do Every Day

1) Early morning, before eating and after opening your eyes, lie in bed, take a deep breath, and be grateful for being alive.

2) Start the day early by stepping outside and feasting your eyes on morning daylight to generate the magical melatonin in every cell of your body for a detox day.

3) Smile and make a habit of it. This helps release happy chemicals which are good for your mind and body.

4) Laugh. If you can't, find a reason to do so. Get help (watch, read, and listen to funny stuff) if you can't. Once again, this will release the happy chemicals, the body's very own class-one narcotics – cannabis-like cannabinoids (e.g., anandamide) and morphine/opium-like endorphins and enkephalins – which do the same job without the side effects and drug withdrawal. Not to mention that they don't cost a penny.

5) Help someone less fortunate (the more fortunate are already taking advantage of you), even if it is donating a pound or a dollar per day to a worthy cause.

6) Spend time with family and friends, those who make you happy. If you don't have any (could be a blessing in disguise, not all relationships and friendships bring joy), find a pet, like a dog; they don't call them man's best friend for nothing.

7) Exercise for at least 30 minutes each day or one hour every alternate day. Ideally, the kind of exercise that makes you sweat. It's more effective than daily exercise. Humans are designed to walk and run, especially long-distance endurance running. It's part of our survival skills so walking comes to us naturally. You can intensify it by brisk walking or hiking. But remember, intermittent exercise is better than intensive daily exercise. Do stay active every day but carry out high-intensity exercises on alternate days. In my opinion, swimming is one of the best exercises. Being in water takes off 25% of your body weight, putting less stress on your joints, and you get to exercise almost all muscle sets at the same time. Once again, do it intermittently – we are not aquatic creatures and being in water regularly for long periods can be counterproductive.

If you don't feel like exercising, changing your diet can help. Animals with a balanced diet show more will to exercise than those who have an unhealthy diet. Having more vegetables and fruits, and less junk food, can give you more motivation to exercise.

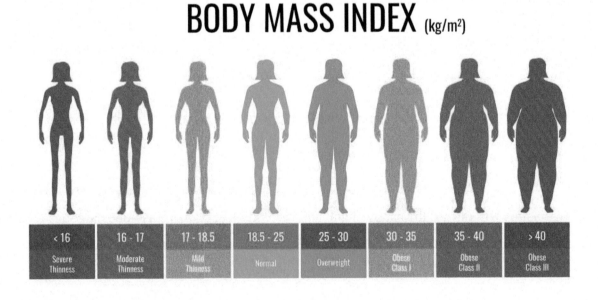

8) Read a good book and reflect on it.

9) Learn one new thing every day. It makes life more interesting.

10) Find a passion and follow it. It could be anything from photography to stamp collecting; anything that floats your boat.

11) Find a purpose in life that is worth living for (accumulating material wealth is not worth it because you will leave it all behind. Even if you build yourself a burial chamber and call yourself 'Tutankhamun' it will probably all end up at a museum in a far-off land).

12) Before sleeping, turn off the lights, lie in bed, reflect on what the good things were in the day, and be grateful for everything – especially for being alive.

STEP FIVE

Time to Go Pro

Congratulations for reaching step five. You are one step short of sainthood. And it's about time you took that final plunge. The ultimate step in dieting is to recreate the environment that our body was designed for. And it is the key to the following principle:

Everything in moderation, including moderation.

Using The Khan Philosophy In Your Diet: Fasting & Feasting

Sounds confusing? It's quite simple. As a general rule, moderation is the principle to live by. Avoid overeating, oversleeping, and overindulgence in anything. At times, however, our body needs to be tested by stretching it beyond its normal limits. This can be achieved by fasting and occasional feasting. This is what we were designed for: living in moderation with occasional exposure to extreme conditions, to train the body for unforeseeable situations. Fasting is the key to detoxifying the human body, fighting ageing, and discouraging cancer cells from developing. It also helps optimise the immune system, keeping it active within a favourable range and avoiding immune suppression or an overdrive that can lead to autoimmune diseases. It also amplifies the effects of exercise. If you exercise for half an hour during a fast (ideally just before breaking the fast) it is better than exercising for many hours on a non-fasting day.

Fasting helps burn fat. In fact, fat is stored in the body to be used on occasions when we have no food available, so let fat realise its potential – give it a chance to burn off. And here's a fun fact. You have been fasting all your life without knowing it; even overlooking the fact that you break your fast by calling it 'breakfast'. Every night our body goes into a natural fasting mode to rest and detoxify itself. It is essential for our health and unnatural feasting at night, like raiding the fridge, is known to cause weight gain, indigestion, and disruption of your normal circadian rhythm.

So, when it comes to fasting, the first thing to do is to preserve our natural fasting routine and not to eat late at night. The longer we are without food between sunset and sunrise, the better it is for our health.

The next step is to fast during daylight hours (from dawn to sunset), at least two days a week and, if possible, a whole month a year, Ramadan style. The method is simple. You eat and drink before dawn breaks, and then don't have any food or water till sunset. It's doable; more than a billion adults do it for a whole month every year as a religious ritual and there have been no reports of risk to life. The reason is that our bodies are designed to withstand absence of food and water for long periods of time, and once you start testing your limits you will be pleasantly surprised how naturally it comes to you.

It's not just Muslims who fast. Buddhists, Orthodox Christians, and Mormons fast too and have done so for centuries. Having said that, fasting is not everyone's cup of tea. Even for Muslims who have the obligatory fasts, Allah has made exceptions. Those who cannot fast can compensate by providing free food to the needy instead of fasting. Some are totally exempted, like children, pregnant or nursing mothers, elderly and the infirm, or those in poor health. So, don't beat yourself about it if you can't fast. You can always try the strategy I suggested earlier, i.e., if in doubt then take both options. Start the day with a fast and when you think you have had enough, break it. This way you have managed a few hours of restraint and reduced the calories for the day. Next time, you can try to stretch it a bit longer and longer, until you can fast the whole day. And if you can't, it's OK.

Some people have devised variations of the typical fasting (I call it 'traditional' or 'true' fasting, which involves abstaining from both food and water) where you are allowed to have water but no food. This is a good alternative for those who are prone to getting dehydrated, like those using diuretic medications. I call it a '**partial fast**'.

There is yet another version, **pseudo-fasting** or '**fake-a-fast**'[209], in which you can drink water and eat a low-carbohydrate and calorie diet, such as a vegetable soup, during the 'fasting hours'. The main purpose is to provide the body a period of time where it can burn calories without consuming more.

Intermittent fasting is a well-established method of losing weight and bringing down insulin levels, both of which help our body stay younger, healthier, and free of cancer.

But be beware that fasting every day is counterproductive. The human body is quick to adapt and if you make fasting a routine, it will get used to it and all the beneficial aspects, such as weight loss and burning calories, will be nullified. So, fasting days have to be followed by feasting days, so the body is challenged with and without food.

The best part of fasting is breaking the fast. Food has never tasted so delicious and water so refreshing than at the end of a fast. You will probably love the experience and ask for more. And, contrary to common belief, it is very difficult to overeat after a fast. Humans are more likely to overeat when they snack all day, because this releases insulin again and again, and insulin is the hormone which drives our hunger instinct.

---

[209] If these terms sound unfamiliar to you, the reason is that I have coined them especially for the purpose of this book, so please save yourself the trouble of googling them.

If you feel apprehensive about intermittent fasting, start during the winter months when the days are shorter. In Northern Europe, the fast starts around 6 AM (you have a breakfast before that) and ends around 3:30 pm at sunset. It's just like having a late lunch on a busy day when you've had no chance to drink water for a long time (most of us do that anyway, especially during days at work).

One of the obvious worries in fasting is the fear of hunger. Surprisingly, one does not feel hungry all the time while fasting. The feeling comes in waves and doesn't last very long. In fact, after the first few waves you feel very comfortable with the fast and the urge to eat subsides.

Last but not least, in all matters of health, especially diet and fasting, consult your doctor first. To every rule there are exceptions, and your physician knows most about the exceptions regarding your health. If your doctor advises against a particular diet or fasting, take it seriously and use another recommendation (like extra exercise and eating fresh[210]) to compensate for it.

And Finally …

The answer to your question is "**Yes**".

By now you must be thinking the very obvious question:

"Would all this advice and recommendations help cancer patients too?"

And fortunately, the answer is yes, as it's never too late to benefit from them.

And the good news doesn't stop there. Major scientific studies done in a dozen European countries over more than a decade have shown that people who adopted a healthier lifestyle not only had a 60% reduction in cancer mortality but were also 14 years younger in terms of their biological age. So, by preventing cancer, you get the bonus of staying younger and living longer.

Coming back to cancer patients, a research article published in the renowned journal *Cancer* many years ago showed that women with breast cancer had a 68% less risk of dying if they undertook better nutrition, physical activity, and stress management along with their conventional treatment.

The mechanism behind this became clear in 2008 when Professor Ornish at the University of California, San Francisco, showed that changes in diet, exercise, and stress can actually modify genes in cancer cells. Samples were taken from patients before and three months after starting a lifestyle modification programme and results showed changes in the functioning of more than 500 genes. Some were more active while others were inhibited. More needs to be known and the international charity I have founded, Killing

---

[210] Once again, consult your doctor before undertaking them. Trust me, I am a doctor.

Cancer Kindly, aims to carry out more research into this mechanism so we can control the cancer-causing genes and modify their behaviour.

Over the last two decades of my medical practice, I have seen cancer behaving differently from one person to another, and more bizarrely from one day to another in the same person. It is the same type of cancer but the rate of growth and effects on health vary. Sometimes (but not often) it would stop growing, start shrinking, and even disappear altogether. In some case I have seen it come back after many years, while others are still under surveillance with no sign of disease. There is no doubt in my mind that the genetic and physical make-up of the cancer remains dynamic and dependent on our environment and lifestyle. However, I must stress that once a cancer has established itself, we need a combination of lifestyle changes and active treatment to control the disease. But when it comes to prevention, lifestyle changes on their own can stop or kill a cancer in its very early stage.

Cancer Is Not Inevitable

Far from it, cancer should be a rarity. This might sound shocking to you, especially given the fact that lifetime risk of cancer is as high as 50% in some parts of the world. The fact is that the natural rate of cancer for humans should be less than 5%.

Cancer is somewhat a disease of excess and modernity.

Some cancers are seven to 60 times more frequent in the developed countries compared to less-developed ones. But it's not genetic, because when people move from one country to another, and adopt the new lifestyle, their cancer risk matches their new homeland within one to two generations. Similarly, adopted children have a cancer risk more similar to their adoptive parents than their biological parents. More interestingly, identical twins who share every gene in their body tend to have a different risk of developing cancer depending on their lifestyle choices.

And you don't have to move countries to alter the risk of cancer. Studies of Aboriginal populations have shown how cancer becomes more common when they adopt a Western lifestyle and soon matches or even exceeds the risk of their colonising countrymen.

Cancer is least dependent on what cards we are dealt and mostly determined by how we play them.

"In life, we are free to make our decisions but obliged to live with their consequences."

M. M. Khan

EPILOGUE

EPILOGUE

363

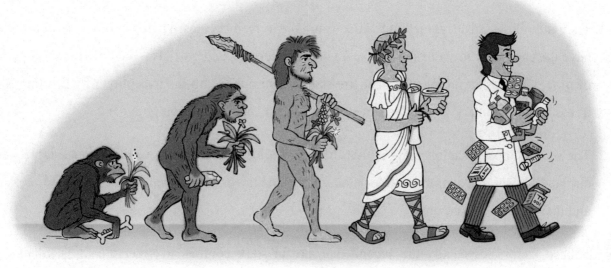

EPILOGUE

Cancer As a Metaphor: Survival of the Weakest

Darwin was wrong. Well, partially. Evolution is _not always_ driven by survival of the fittest. It might be true for almost all creatures, for example great white sharks and Galapagos finches, but it fails to explain the modern human. Let's have an unbiased view of the process from the neutral standpoint of an alien. Imagine, you and I are two aliens who have never been to the planet Earth before and have just landed an exploratory craft from outer space. Among all the creatures that we study, one species stands out from the rest, literally.

HUMANS.

Humans stand out for two major reasons:

1. They literally stand up, something which is unique to their species. There are other creatures which have the capability to stand straight – like bears, meerkats, and gorillas – but only for short periods of time. Humans spend most of their life standing straight (with the exception of when they sleep or assume a voluntary vegetative state, also known as being a 'couch potato').

2. The second most amazing thing is that they have a lot of accessories in life. Chairs, tables, cars, airplanes, boats, ships, mobiles, televisions, wheelchairs, ramps to wheelchairs, roads, refrigerators, and the list goes on and on.

Both of these factors, especially the second one, are in stark contrast to other creatures. Sharks, for example, have been around for 400 million years and have evolved to rule the oceans. It's even believed that they were the driving force which pushed other creatures out of the oceans onto the safety of land and evolve into non-aquatic organisms. 400 million years is a long time, but apart from surviving remarkably well (they survived every mass extinction event since their emergence in the fossil record, even the one that wiped out dinosaurs, and I mean all dinosaurs: land, water, or airborne) they don't have much to show for it. Not a single motorway or road, no cars, planes, or computers, and not even a couch or a bed. The poor creatures have to sleep on the move and faint when flipped upside down, while humans sleep on cosy mattresses and toss and turn without any fear. The same applies to all other creatures. And the reason is obvious.

Every creature has evolved on the Darwinian principle of 'survival of the fittest/ natural selection', except the modern human. We have developed and evolved on the reverse principle, 'survival of the weakest/

unnatural selection'[211]. Our world is designed and developed to ensure the survival of the weakest member of our species. Indoor heating for the vulnerable young and old, running water for those who cannot go to the nearest waterhole to quench their thirst, disabled access for the less abled, cars for those who can't run a marathon, and airplanes for everyone who can't fly.

Survival of the fittest is a rule. To every rule there is an exception. And our survival is an exception to the Darwinian rule. Even among the lesser-known human societies like the primitive aboriginal tribes of the Amazon jungle and Andaman and Nicobar Islands, the least developed of all human groups, there is a significant degree of social evolution based on survival of the weakest. It's in our nature to strive for protecting and nurturing the weakest members of our society. We are the only species whose newborns remain dependent and vulnerable for many years[212]. Compared to us, a foal (baby horse) stands and walks soon after birth and fry (baby fish[213]) swim immediately after hatching. Humans have experimented with survival of the fittest at times, but it has failed spectacularly. The Spartans[214] tried and failed. In the last century it was championed by many in Europe and Americas, but the eugenics programme did not go very well, and the gas chambers failed to win approval by the masses. In conclusion, whether we like it or not, our society and its survival are based on the principle of protecting and safeguarding the weakest.

The human body is also like a human society. The whole body is designed to ensure the survival of its most vulnerable members. For example, the brain's neurons, which give us all our brilliant ideas, are dependent on the stomach, intestines, liver, and pancreas to feed them. Without these organs functioning normally, the brainy brain cells would not survive. Cancer is a rebellion against this basic ideology. Ironically, cancer cells are following the Darwinian principles of survival of the fittest.

Cancerous cells lose their collective function as part of the human body, based on the principle of 'live and help others live', and opt for an independent self-survival strategy at the expense of other (vulnerable)

---

[211] This is my humble theory of evolution so please feel free to agree or disagree.

[212] This can range from 3–5 years in case of a toddler to 35+ for the 'failed fledglings' (who never left the nest) or 'boomerangers' (who left the nest only to come back at a later stage).

[213] Not the fried variety.

[214] Sparta was a militarised Greek city state which was a staunch believer in survival of the fittest long before Darwin. They even carried out state-approved and organised infanticide. When a baby was born, it had to be presented to a council of inspectors and examined for any physical defects. If deemed unfit, the baby was abandoned at a hillside and left to die. Babies who passed the test were brought up in strict discipline (for example, if they cried, they were ignored) and separated from their parents at the age of seven for a state-sponsored training regimen which went on for years and included food deprivation, exposure to cold and pain, and regular floggings in 'contests of endurance' which sometimes resulted in death. And Spartans had to keep fit all their life. Overweight citizens were publicly ridiculed and were at risk of being banished from the state if remaining unfit. Ironically, the state did not survive the attacks by less fit and more lazy Romans, who took over their country and made the super fit Spartans flog each other to death in amphitheatres for their entertainment.

cells of the body. They are the rebels of the society whose driving motive is personal greed, and they satisfy it at the expense of their fellow members and the environment. The result is a disaster.

In the short run they appear to survive and prosper but this is a Pyrrhic[215] victory. In doing so they are destroying the very being they are exploiting, eventually spelling their own demise. No cancer has ever outlived its host[216].

There is a lot we can learn from cancer and preventing cancer. Especially when it comes to individual and collective survival. If only they (cancer cells) had the insight, they would live and let live. Be a benign bump or lump, if not a functional member of the body they would stop their rebellion, and everyone would live happily ever after. But they are blinded by their endless greed.

If only we (humans) had the same insight to live and let live. It's our culture of endless greed that creates an environment of social disparity where a few thrive at everyone else's cost. Our rapacity is destroying not only the society but also the environment we live in. Just like cancer, we are on a path of self-destruction, cutting the very branch we sit on. If this self-destructing selfishness is not stopped, it will spell the end of our society and species.

Sometimes survival of the fittest can spell the end for everyone.

Survival of the weakest, or 'unnatural selection' as I call it, has always made us progress while survival of the fittest (natural selection as Darwin coined the term) has led us down the path of death and destruction, be it Nazism, Fascism, genocide, or the greed of the big global corporations.

In the end, I would like to leave you with a story that has fascinated me for a long time. It's the tale of survival against all odds. A survival of the weakest, if you may.

Once upon a time, not too long ago, there lived a young man who was not very fit to survive. In fact, he was so unfit that he spent much of his adult life suffering from ill health. His recurring symptoms included malaise, dizziness, vertigo, muscle spasms, tremors, vomiting, cramps, colic, bloating, headaches, alterations of vision, lethargy, breathlessness, blistering of skin, eczema, fainting, palpitations, ringing in

---

[215] A Pyrrhic victory comes at the cost of a devastating toll for the victor. It is named after the Greek King Pyrrhus of Epirus, who won a battle against the Romans but lost too many soldiers in doing so. When congratulated, he famously said, "One more victory like this and we will be utterly ruined". Not surprisingly, in his next encounter with Romans he lost the battle and the Greeks had to retreat.

[216] With the exception of cancer cells harvested from the patient and grown in test tubes for experiment purposes (for example, HeLa cells, which were taken from the cervical tumour cells of Henrietta Lacks, a 31-year-old African American lady who passed away on 4th October, 1951 but her cancer cells are still kept alive in laboratories). But you won't call that existence a 'life'. Till date, more than 50 million tons of HeLa cells have been grown in the laboratory.

the ears (tinnitus), insomnia, depression, attacks of anxiety, and episodes of inconsolable hysterical crying to name a few. From a very early age, even as a child, he was considered a lost cause; his father predicted that he would be a disgrace to himself and his family. Aged 16 he left school due to poor grades. Later he resumed his studies but dropped out of medical school after two years because he could not stand the sight of human bodies being dissected. Later, he applied for a job on a ship and reluctantly got accepted because others had declined. The ship's captain and crew suspected he would be unfit for the job, and he proved them right by continuously suffering from bouts of sea sickness in addition to his usual ailments. The crew put up with him but made him pay for his food, so he got no salary, and the 'job' was very much self-funded.

According to the philosophy of evolution, that is the survival of the fittest. He had not much going in his favour for either survival or success. But, despite all odds, this young man survived, prospered, and succeeded by the support of his family, friends, and colleagues, becoming one of the most renowned scientists of all time. Today the world knows him as the "father of evolutionary thought" … Mr Charles Robert Darwin.

ACKNOWLEDGMENTS

He who does not thank people has not thanked God.

(Prophet Mohammad, may peace be upon him, 570–632 AD)

I have many people to thank (this list is not exhaustive).

And I would like to start by thanking you for buying (I hope!) and reading this book. I would also like to take this opportunity to add that, aside from learning how best to protect yourself and your loved ones from cancer, a share of proceeds from the sale of this book will go towards research and efforts in preventing and curing cancer, undertaken through the international cancer awareness and education charity I have been proud to establish, Killing Cancer Kindly (Registered Charity Number 1200040). Alongside Killing Cancer Kindly's important work in educating and empowering the public worldwide, it is also my mission in life to provide the most up-to-date knowledge and information for preventing and treating cancer in the form of future editions of this book.

The driving force for this book was the inspiration I received from my patients and their families, whose heroic courage, resilience, and dignity gave me the motivation and strength to pursue this project for 14 years. As with all human efforts, this one is likewise standing on the shoulder of giants, known and unknown. To name but a few, the anonymous author of the Egyptian papyrus written 2,600 years ago with the first mention of cancer; Hippocrates, the 'father of medicine', who named it *carcinos*; Celsus, who translated it to *cancer* in Latin; Galen, who first used the term *oncos*; Abu Ali Sina (Avicenna to the West), who more than a thousand years ago established the principles of cancer treatment which are valid even today; Percival Potts, for taking the first steps to prevent cancer, and many more since then.

I also owe an inestimable debt to my own family, beginning with my late grandparents, who have been role models and a source of inspiration for me and many more.

Similarly, my late father, who passed away in his youth (he was just 38 years old, and I was nine months old) but left me a legacy and very large shoes to fill. I wish I would have known you for longer.

My mother, grandmother, and aunt, who worked selflessly and tirelessly against all odds to bring me up and get me through medical school. I am what I am today all because of them.

My aunts, uncles, and cousins (too many to name individually) for their unconditioned love. I am fortunate to be part of an amazing family full of warmth and benevolence.

Iman Mohammad Khan, the best daughter a father can have, for her kindness, compassion, and concern.

Rania Mohammad Khan, beloved daughter whose untimely death changed my outlook on life forever.

Mohammad Isa Khan, the best son a father can have, for his empathy, care, and love, which is amazing to see at such a young age.

Dr Afroz Khan for bringing these beautiful babies to this world and being such a good mother.

Unreserved thanks should also go to Dr Qazi Mohib ur Rehman Mohib, the first and most altruistic physician I ever met and who inspired me to follow in his footsteps and choose the medical profession. Likewise, his daughter, Mrs Ghazala Mufti, and son, Dr Junaid Bilal Qazi, who continue his altruistic and medical legacy.

Dr Shahid Idris Mufti, the best and kindest cardiologist I have ever known, for his vital support and guidance in writing and publishing this book.

Abdul Latif, Fizza, Noor, and Hamdan for their support and care.

Dr Tahir Masoud and Seham Tahir, for their support and efforts for this mission.

Ilyas Khan and family (Mrs Ilyas, Wasif, Taimur, Zarnigar, and Zahra) – core members of Killing Cancer Kindly (KCK) – for their devotion.

Milana Mereshkova, for her beautiful and perfect Russian translations – not to forget her sincerity and commitment to killing cancer, which is unparalleled.

Fatima Gagieva, for her fabulous ideas and keen concern to make this mission a global success.

Ahmed Gagi, Amina Gagieva, and Ms Asia Mankiyeva, for their quiet but crucial behind-the-scenes efforts.

Mr Mogamedov Gagiev, for his unfailing courtesy and kindness.

Fariza Mankiyeva, for her honest and invaluable criticism and appreciation.

Kashifa Aamir, née Riaz (who is a brilliant psychologist and a doctor, even if she doesn't like to be identified as one), for her unfailing support and encouragement.

Zainab Asad, for her essential work in selecting images and designing the book. She has spent countless hours and attended daily meetings to finalise the manuscript for publication.

Naomi Cropper, and her tireless typing, for the initial draft of this book.

My colleagues, who are more like a family, at multiple hospitals in NHS England., especially Dr Nabil El-Mahdawi and Dr George Bozas for their kind review of the manuscript.

The team at Cornerstone Literary Consultancy (especially Helen, Isobel, Sarah, and Kate) for getting me one of the best mentors and editors in the publishing world, Craig Simpson. I am grateful for his unparalleled, sincere mentoring, fine-tooth combed editing, and meticulous review of the manuscript. This book would not be in its current form if it wasn't for his hard work.

Publicist and proof editor Anthony Harvison and the team at book PR agency Palamedes for their hard work and professionalism. They created the final version of the book you are reading and, perhaps more importantly, they took a deep interest in the mission to kill cancer and went out of their way to help promote it. Anthony, in particular, worked endless hours, including weekends, through health and sickness to meet the deadlines and I never heard him complain even once. His patience is only paralleled by his professionalism and perfect editing skills.

Dr Kiran Munir, née Sana, excellent psychiatrist, amazing psychologist, expert health consultant (probably the one and only doctor with these three qualifications!), and once upon a time my student par excellence. Also known among her patients as "the best doctor in the world" but is too modest to admit it. Twenty years ago, we briefly joined forces against cancer and then 18 years later you came back to rekindle the fire and guide me back to the path. This book and mission would not have been without you, and I would not want it any other way.

And finally, all praise and gratitude are for Almighty ALLAH, who has blessed me with all these wonderful people and many more who have made this book possible.

Last but not the least, thank you once again for choosing to read You'll Wish You Were an Elephant (Killing Cancer Kindly). I hope you enjoy and benefit from it as much as I have in writing it.

REFERENCES

You'll Wish You Were an Elephant (Killing Cancer Kindly):

Selected References

Part One

- Hanahan, D & Weinberg, RA (January 2000). 'The hallmarks of cancer'. *Cell*, 100 (1), pp. 57–70. DOI:10.1016/S0092-8674(00)81683-9. PMID 10647931.
- Hanahan, D & Weinberg, RA (2011). 'Hallmarks of cancer: the next generation'. *Cell*, 144 (5), pp. 646–674. DOI:10.1016/j.cell.2011.02.013. PMID 21376230. Cell 100:59.
- Evan, GI & Vousden, KH (17 May 2001). 'Proliferation, cell cycle and apoptosis in cancer'. *Nature*, 411 (6835), pp. 342–8. Bibcode:2001Natur.411.342E. DOI:10.1038/35077213. PMID 11357141. S2CID 4414024.
- Bryson, B (November 2005). *A short history of nearly everything: special illustrated edition*. Broadway Books. ISBN 0-7679-2322-7.

Part Two

- Van Gent, DC, Hoeijmakers, JH & Kanaar, R (2001). 'Chromosomal stability and the DNA double-stranded break connection'. *Nature Reviews Genetics*, 2 (3), pp. 196–206. DOI:10.1038/35056049. PMID 11256071.
- Frank, SA (2003). 'Somatic mutation: early cancer steps depend on tissue architecture'. *Current Biology*, 13 (7), R261–3. DOI:10.1016/s0960-9822(03)00195-7. PMID 12676101.
- Campisi, J (2005). 'Aging, tumor suppression and cancer: High wire-act!'. *Mechanisms of Ageing and Development*, 126 (1), pp. 51–8. DOI:10.1016/j.mad.2004.09.024. PMID 15610762.
- Michor, F, Iwasa, Y & Nowak, MA (2004). 'Dynamics of cancer progression'. *Nature Reviews Cancer*, 4 (3), pp. 197–205. DOI:10.1038/nrc1295. PMID 14993901.

Reference – Cannabis and Cancer

- 'Special issue: cannabis in medicine*'*. Novack, V (ed.). *European Journal of Internal Medicine,* 49, pp. 1–50 (5 March 2018).

Part Three

- E and Anderson, S (eds.) (1998). *The Chambers dictionary*. London: Chambers.
- Kirkpatrick, EM (ed.) (1992). *Brewer's concise dictionary of phrase and fable*. London: Weidenfeld Nicolson Illustrated.
- Peto, R, Roe, FJC, Lee, PN; Levy, L & Clack, J (October 1975). 'Cancer and ageing in mice and men'. *British Journal of Cancer*, 32 (4), pp. 411–426. DOI:10.1038/bjc.1975.242. PMC 2024769. PMID 1212409.
- Nagy, JD, Victor, EM & Cropper, JH (2007). 'Why don't all whales have cancer? A novel hypothesis resolving Peto's paradox'. *Integrative and Comparative Biology*, 47 (2), pp. 317–328. DOI:10.1093/icb/icm062. PMID 21672841.

Part Four

Cancer Genes: Size Doesn't Matter

- Data from Huntsman Cancer Institute provide one explanation of how large animals have adopted an evolutionary mechanism to address cancer (Dr Mel Greaves, PhD and Luca Ermini, PhD of the Institute of Cancer Research, London).

Part Five

Alcohol General Discussion

- Al.-Hassani, S & Abattouy, M (2008). 'The advent of scientific chemistry'. *Muslim Heritage*.
- Curzon, GN (7 July 2010). 'The history of alcohol in Islam'. *Coming Anarchy*.
- Forbes, RJ (1970). *A short history of the art of distillation*. Brill Publishers. Page 87. ISBN 978-9-00400-617-1.
- Multhauf, R (1966). *The origins of chemistry*. London: Oldbourn. Pages 204–6.
- Hill, DR (1993). *Islamic science and engineering*. Edinburgh: Edinburgh University Press. ISBN 978-0-74860-455-5.
- Hitti, PK (1977). *History of the Arabs from the earliest times to the present* (10th ed.). London: Macmillan Publishers. Page 365. ISBN 978-0-33309-871-4.
- Modanlou, HD (November 2008). 'A tribute to Zakariya Razi (865–925 AD), an Iranian pioneer scholar' (PDF). *Archives of Iranian Medicine*, 11 (6), pp. 673–677. PMID 18976043.
- Schlosser, Stefan (May 2011). 'Distillation – from Bronze Age till today'. 38th International Conference of SSCHE.
- Harper, Douglas. 'Alcohol'. *Etymonline*. MaoningTech.
- Lohninger, H (21 December 2004). 'Etymology of the word "alcohol"'. *VIAS Encyclopedia*.

Alcohol and Cancer

- Maasland, DH, van den Brandt, PA, Kremer, B et al. (2014). 'Alcohol consumption, cigarette smoking and the risk of subtypes of head-neck cancer: Results from the Netherlands Cohort Study'. *BMC Cancer*, 14, p. 187.
- Prabhu, A, Obi, KO & Rubenstein, JH (2014). 'The synergistic effects of alcohol and tobacco consumption on the risk of esophageal squamous cell carcinoma: a meta-analysis. *Am J Gastroenterol,* 109, pp. 822–7.
- Seitz, HK & Stickel, F (2007). 'Molecular mechanisms of alcohol-mediated carcinogenesis'. *Nat Rev Cancer*, 7, pp. 599–612.
- Boffetta, P & Hashibe, M (2006). 'Alcohol and cancer'. *Lancet Oncol*, 7, pp. 149–56.
- Linhart, K, Bartsch, H & Seitz, HK (2014). 'The role of reactive oxygen species (ROS) and cytochrome' P-450 2E1 in the generation of carcinogenic etheno-DNA adducts'. *Redox Biol*, 3, pp. 56–62.
- Baumgardner, JN, Shankar, K, Korourian, S et al. (2007). 'Undernutrition enhances alcohol-induced hepatocyte proliferation in the liver of rats fed via total enteral nutrition'. *Am J Physiol Gastrointest Liver Physiol*, 293, G355–64.
- Acharya, C & Bajaj, JS (2017). 'Gut microbiota and complications of liver disease'. *Gastroenterol Clin North Am*, 46, pp. 155–69.

- Fedirko, V, Tran, HQ, Gewirtz, AT et al. (2017). 'Exposure to bacterial products lipopolysaccharide and flagellin and hepatocellular carcinoma: a nested case-control study'. *BMC Med*, 15, p. 72.
- Kong, SY, Tran, HQ, Gewirtz, AT et al. (2016). 'Serum endotoxins and flagellin and risk of colorectal cancer in the European Prospective Investigation into Cancer and Nutrition (EPIC) cohort'. *Cancer Epidemiol Biomarkers Prev*, 25, pp. 291–301.
- Singletary, KW & Gapstur, SM (2001). 'Alcohol and breast cancer: review of epidemiologic and experimental evidence and potential mechanisms'. *JAMA*, 286, pp. 2143–51.

Smoking and Cancer Part 1 References

- Reitsma, MB, Fullman, N; Ng, M, Salama, JS & Abajobir, A (April 2017). 'Smoking prevalence and attributable disease burden in 195 countries and territories, 1990–2015: a systematic analysis from the Global Burden of Disease Study 2015'. *The Lancet*, 389 (10082), pp. 1885–906. DOI:10.1016/S0140-6736(17)30819-X. PMC 5439023. PMID 28390697.
- Pollard, T (2004). 'The pleasures and perils of smoking in early modern England'. *Smoke: a global history of smoking*. Gilman, SL & Xun, Z (eds.). London: Reaktion Books. Page 38.
- World Health Organisation (2008). *WHO report on the global tobacco epidemic 2008*. Geneva: WHO Press. Pages 267–88.

Smoking and Cancer Part 2 References

- Feng, Z, Hu, W, Hu, Y & Tang, MS (October 2006). 'Acrolein is a major cigarette-related lung cancer agent: preferential binding at p53 mutational hotspots and inhibition of DNA repair'. *Proceedings of the National Academy of Sciences of the United States of America*, 103 (42), pp. 15404–9. Bibcode:2006PNAS..10315404F. DOI:10.1073/pnas.0607031103. PMC 1592536. PMID 17030796.
- Hecht, SS (1999). 'Tobacco smoke carcinogens and lung cancer'. *JNCI Journal of the National Cancer Institute*, 91 (14), pp. 1194–1210. DOI:10.1093/jnci/91.14.1194. PMID 10413421.
- Martell, EA (March 1983). 'alpha-Radiation dose at bronchial bifurcations of smokers from indoor exposure to radon progeny'. *Proceedings of the National Academy of Sciences of the United States of America*, 80 (5), pp. 1285–9. Bibcode:1983PNAS...80.1285M. DOI:10.1073/pnas.80.5.1285. PMC 393580. PMID 6572389.
- Muggli, ME, Ebbert, JO, Robertson, C & Hurt, RD (September 2008). 'Waking a sleeping giant: the tobacco industry's response to the polonium-210 issue'. *American Journal of Public Health*, 98 (9), pp. 1643–50. DOI:10.2105/AJPH.2007.130963. PMC 2509609. PMID 18633078.
- Rego, B (September 2009). 'The polonium brief: a hidden history of cancer, radiation, and the tobacco industry' (PDF). *Isis; an International Review Devoted to the History of Science and Its Cultural Influences*, 100 (3), pp. 453–84. DOI:10.1086/644613. PMID 19960838.
- Office of Research Services, Division of Radiation Safety. 'F. Typical Sources of Radiation Exposure'. United States National Institutes of Health.
- 'Radiation risk for Xray and CT exams – dosage chart'. Associated Radiologists.
- 'Radiation Risks and Realities' (PDF). United States Environmental Protection Agency (16 July 2014).
- Talhout, R, Opperhuizen, A & van Amsterdam, JG (October 2007). 'Role of acetaldehyde in tobacco smoke addiction'. *European Neuropsychopharmacology*, 17 (10), pp. 627–36. DOI:10.1016/j.euroneuro.2007.02.013. PMID 17382522.
- Maneckjee, R & Minna, JD (October 1994). 'Opioids induce while nicotine suppresses apoptosis in human lung cancer cells'. *Cell Growth & Differentiation*, 5 (10), pp. 1033–40. PMID 7848904.
- 'Secondhand smoke'. American Lung Association (June 2007).

Electronic Cigarettes References

- Burstyn, Igor (9 January 2014). 'Peering through the mist: systematic review of what the chemistry of contaminants in electronic cigarettes tells us about health risks'. *BMC Public Health*, 14 (1), p. 18. DOI:10.1186/1471-2458-14-18. ISSN 1471-2458. PMC 3937158. PMID 24406205.
- Brady, Benjamin R, De La Rosa, Jennifer S, Nair, Uma S & Leischow, Scott J (2019). 'Electronic cigarette policy recommendations: a scoping review'. *American Journal of Health Behavior*, 43 (1), pp. 88–104. DOI:10.5993/AJHB.43.1.8. ISSN 1087-3244. PMID 30522569.
- Smith, L, Brar, K, Srinivasan, K, Enja, M & Lippmann, S (June 2016). 'E-cigarettes: how "safe" are they?'. *J Fam Pract*. 65 (6), pp. 380–5. PMID 27474819.
- 'Nicotine without smoke: tobacco harm reduction'. Royal College of Physicians (28 April 2016).
- 'Evidence review of e-cigarettes and heated tobacco products 2018 A report commissioned by Public Health England' (PDF). Public Health England.
- Hartmann-Boyce, J, McRobbie, H, Bullen, C; Begh, R, Stead, LF, Hajek, P & Hartmann-Boyce, J (2016). 'Electronic cigarettes for smoking cessation'. *Cochrane Database Syst Rev.*, 9, CD010216. DOI:10.1002/14651858.CD010216.pub3. PMC 6457845. PMID 27622384.
- Breland, AB, Spindle, T, Weaver, M & Eissenberg, T (2014). 'Science and electronic cigarettes'. *Journal of Addiction Medicine*, 8 (4), pp. 223–233. DOI:10.1097/ADM.0000000000000049. ISSN 1932-0620. PMC 4122311. PMID 25089952.
- Harrell, PT, Simmons, VN, Correa, JB, Padhya, TA & Brandon, TH (4 June 2014). 'Electronic nicotine delivery systems ("e-cigarettes"): review of safety and smoking cessation efficacy'. *Otolaryngology–Head and Neck Surgery*, 151 (3), pp. 381–393.
- 'Electronic nicotine delivery systems' (PDF). World Health Organization (21 July 2014). Pages 1–13.
- Hajek, P, Etter, JF, Benowitz, N, Eissenberg, T & McRobbie, H (31 July 2014). 'Electronic cigarettes: review of use, content, safety, effects on smokers and potential for harm and benefit'. *Addiction*, 109 (11), pp. 1801–10.
- Durmowicz, EL (2014). 'The impact of electronic cigarettes on the paediatric population'. *Tobacco Control*, 23 (Supplement 2), ii41–ii46.
- Ebbert, JO, Agunwamba, AA & Rutten, LJ (2015). 'Counseling patients on the use of electronic cigarettes'. *Mayo Clinic Proceedings*, 90 (1), pp. 128–134.
- Rowell, TR & Tarran, R (2015). 'Will chronic e-cigarette use cause lung disease?'. *American Journal of Physiology. Lung Cellular and Molecular Physiology*, 309 (12), L1398–L1409.
- Hildick-Smith, GJ, Pesko, MF, Shearer, L, Hughes, JM., Chang, J, Loughlin, GM & Ipp, LS (2015). 'A practitioner's guide to electronic cigarettes in the adolescent population'. *Journal of Adolescent Health*, 57 (6), pp. 574–9.
- Caponnetto, P, Russo, C, Bruno, CM., Alamo, A, Amaradio, MD & Polosa, R. (March 2013). 'Electronic cigarette: a possible substitute for cigarette dependence'. *Monaldi Archives for Chest Disease*, 79 (1), pp. 12–19.
- Palazzolo, DL (November 2013). 'Electronic cigarettes and vaping: a new challenge in clinical medicine and public health. A literature review'. *Frontiers in Public Health*, 1 (56), p. 56.
- Glantz, SA & Bareham, DW (January 2018). 'E-Cigarettes: use, effects on smoking, risks, and policy implications'. *Annual Review of Public Health*, 39 (1), pp. 215–235.
- 'Companies cease sales of e-liquids with labeling or advertising that resembled kid-friendly foods following FDA, FTC warnings'. United States Food and Drug Administration (23 August 2018).
- 'E-cigarettes to be regulated as medicines'. National Health Service (12 June 2013).
- Collaco, JM (2015). 'Electronic use and exposure in the pediatric population'. *JAMA Pediatrics*, 169 (2), pp. 177–182.
- Mravec, B, Tibensky, M, Horvathova, L & Babal, P (2019). 'E-cigarettes and cancer risk'. *Cancer Prevention Research*, 13 (2), pp. 137–144.

- Holbrook, BD (2016). 'The effects of nicotine on human fetal development'. *Birth Defects Research Part C: Embryo Today: Reviews*, 108 (2), pp. 181–192.

Cigarette Additives References

- 'Cigarette Ingredients - Chemicals in Cigarettes'. Tri-County Cessation Center. New York State Department of Health Tobacco Control Program. Archived on the Wayback Machine on 21 January 2016.
- Martin, T (15 November 2016) 'Ingredients that can be found in cigarettes'. *Verywell Mind*.
- Rabinoff, M, Caskey, N, Rissling, A & Park, C (November 2007). 'Pharmacological and chemical effects of cigarette additives'. *American Journal of Public Health*, 97 (11), pp. 1981–1991. DOI: 10.2105/AJPH.2005.078014. PMC 2040350.
- BAT (12 December 1986). 'Mutagenic activity of flavour compounds. FN AQ2222, BN 400916808-400916815'. Cited in a health information web page published by BUPA. Archived on the Wayback Machine on 7 June 2007.

Part Six

Infection and Cancer

- Plummer, M, de Martel, C, Vignat, J, Ferlay, J, Bray, F & Franceschi, S (2012). 'Global burden of cancers attributable to infections in 2008: a review and synthetic analysis'. *Lancet Oncol*, 13, pp. 607–615.
- Pisani, P, Parkin, DM, Muñoz, N & Ferlay, J (1997). 'Cancer and infection: estimates of the attributable fraction in 1990'. *Cancer Epidemiol Biomarkers Prev*, 6, pp. 387–400.

Part Seven

References – Diet and Cancer

The Mediterranean Diet

- Zhou, W, Mukherjee, P, Kiebish, MA, Markis, WT, Mantis, JG & Seyfried, TN. (2007). 'The calorically restricted ketogenic diet, an effective alternative therapy for malignant brain cancer'. *Nutrition & Metabolism*, 4 (5). DOI: 10.1186/1743-7075-4-5.
- Weber, DD, Aminazdeh-Gohari, S & Kofler, B (11 February 2018). 'Ketogenic diet in cancer therapy'. *Aging (Albany NY)*, 10 (2), pp. 164–165.

Intermittent Fasting from Dawn to Sunset

- Mindikoglu, AL. et al (2017). 'Impact of time-restricted feeding and dawn-to-sunset fasting on circadian rhythm, obesity, metabolic syndrome, and nonalcoholic fatty liver disease'. *Gastroenterol. Res. Pract.*, 2017. DOI:10.1155/2017/3932491.
- Deng, J et al. 'LATS1 suppresses proliferation and invasion of cervical cancer'. *Mol. Med. Rep.*, 15 (4) (2017), pp. 1654–1660.
- Leber, SL et al. (20170. 'Homer1a protein expression in schizophrenia, bipolar disorder, and major depression'. *J. Neural Transm.* (Vienna), 124 (10), pp. 1261–1273.

High-Fructose Corn Syrup and Cancer

- European Starch Association (10 June 2013). 'Factsheet on glucose fructose syrups and isoglucose'.
- White, JS (2014). 'Sucrose, HFCS, and fructose: history, manufacture, composition, applications, and production'. *Fructose, high fructose corn syrup, sucrose and health, nutrition and health*. Rippe, JM (ed.). New York: Springer Science+Business Media. ISBN 978-1-4899-8077-9.
- US Food and Drug Administration (4 January 2018). 'High fructose corn syrup: questions and answers'.
- The Coca-Cola Company (23 March 2010). 'Coca Cola freestyle dispenser users manual' (PDF). Pages 4 & 13. Retrieved 12 August 2016.
- 'Mexican Coke a hit in U.S.' *The Seattle Times*. Archived from the original on 29 June 2011.
- Mao, W, Schuler, MA, Berenbaum, MR (2013). 'Honey constituents up-regulate detoxification and immunity genes in the western honey bee Apis mellifera'. *Proceedings of the National Academy of Sciences*, 110 (22), pp. 8842–8846.

Sugar and Cancer

- World Health Organization (2015). *Guideline: sugars intake for adults and children*. Geneva: WHO Press. Page. 4. ISBN 978-92-4-154902-8. Archived (PDF) from the original on 4 July 2018.
- Harper, Douglas. 'Sugar'. *Online Etymology Dictionary*.
- Adas, M (January 2001). *'Agricultural and pastoral societies in ancient and classical history'*. Philadelphia, Pennsylvania: Temple University Press. Page. 311. ISBN 1-56639-832-0.
- Kieschnick, J (2003). *The Impact of Buddhism on Chinese material culture*. Princeton, New Jersey: Princeton University Press. ISBN 0-691-09676-7.
- Pariona, A (25 April 2017). 'Top sugar consuming nations in the world'. *World Atlas*. Retrieved 20 May 2018.
- WHO/FAO (2003). *Diet, nutrition and the prevention of chronic diseases: report of a joint WHO/FAO expert consultation* (PDF). WHO Technical Report Series 916. ISBN 92-4-120916-X. Retrieved 25 December 2013.
- Malik, VS, Popkin, BM, Bray, GA, Despres, JP, Willett, WC & Hu, FB (2010). 'Sugar-sweetened beverages and risk of metabolic syndrome and type 2 diabetes: A meta-analysis'. *Diabetes Care*, 33 (11), pp. 2477–83.
- Malik, VS, Pan, A, Willett, WC & Hu, FB (01 October 2013). 'Sugar-sweetened beverages and weight gain in children and adults: a systematic review and meta-analysis'. *The American Journal of Clinical Nutrition*, 98 (4), pp. 1084–1102.
- World Health Organization (2015). *Guideline: sugars intake for adults and children*. Geneva: WHO Press. ISBN 978-92-4-154902-8. Archived (PDF) from the original on 4 July 2018.

Milk and Cancer Part 1

- Echternkap SE, Aad PY, Eborn DR & Spicer LJ (2012). 'Increased abundance of aromatase and folical stimulating hormone receptor mRNA and decreased insulin-like growth factor-2 receptor mRNA in small ovarian follicles of cattle selected for twin births'. *J Anim Sci*, 90, pp. 2193–200.
- 'Managing cow lactation cycles'. *The Cattle Site* (18 May 2015)
- Ganmaa, D & Sato, A (2005). 'The possible role of female sex hormones in milk from pregnant cows in the development of breast, ovarian and corpus uteri cancers'. *Med Hypotheses,* 65, pp. 1028–37.
- Barr, SI, McCarron, DA, Heaney, RP et al. (2000). 'Effects of increased consumption of fluid milk on energy and nutrient intake, body weight and cardiovascular risk factors in healthy older adults'. *J Am Diet Asoc*, 100, pp. 810–7.
- Cadogan, J, Eastell, R, Jones, N & Barker, ME (1997). 'Milk intake and bone mineral acquisition in adolescent girls: randomised, controlled intervention trial'. *BMJ*, 315, pp. 1255–60.
- Zhu, K, Du, X, Cowell, CT et al. (2005). 'Effects of school milk intervention on coritcal bone acceleration and indicators relevant to bone metabolism in Chinese girls aged 10–12 y in Beijing'. *Am J Clin Nutr*, 81, pp. 1168–75.
- Rich-Edwards, JW, Ganmaa, D, Pollaak, MN et al. (2007). 'Milk consumption and the pre-pubertal somatoropic axis'. *Nutr J*, 6, p. 28.

- FAO/WHO/UNU (1985). *Energy and protein requirements: report of a joint FAO/WHO/UNU expert consultation*. WHO Technical Report Series 724. Geneva: World Health Organisation.
- Harrison, Lennon R, Holly, J, et al. (2017). 'Does milk intake promote prostate cancer initiation or progression via effects on insulin-like growth factors (IGFs)? A systematic review and meta-analysis'. *Cancer Causes Control*, 28, pp. 497–528.
- Melnik, BC (2015). 'Milk – a nutrient system of mammalian evolution promoting mTORC1-dependent translation'. *Int J Mol Sci*, 16, pp. 17048–87.
- World Cancer Research Fund/American Institute for Cancer Research (2007). 'Second expert report: food, nutrition, physical activity, and the prevention of cancer: a global perspective'. Washington, DC: AICR.
- Hemenway, D, Azrael, DR, Rimm, EB, Feskanich, D & Willett, WC (1994). 'Risk factors for hip fracture in US men ages 40 through 75 years'. *AM J Public Health*, 84, pp. 1843–5.
- Hegsted, DM (1986). 'Calcium and osteoporsosis'. *J Nutr*, 116, pp. 2316–9.
- Hegsted, DM (2001). 'Fractures, calcium, and the modern diet'. *AM J Clin Nutr*, 74, pp. 571–3.
- Feskanich, D, Bischoff-Ferrari, HA, Frazier, AL. & Willett, WC (2014). 'Milk consumption during teenage years and risk of hip fractures in older adults'. *JAMA Pediatr*, 168, pp. 54–60.
- Ganmaa, D, Li, XM, Wang J. Qin, LQ, Wang, PY & Sato, A (2002). 'Incidence and mortality of testicular and prostatic cancers in relation to world dietary practices'. *Int J Cancer*, 98, pp. 262–7.
- Aune, D, Navarro Rosenblatt, DA, Chan, DS et al. (2015). 'Dairy products, calcium, and prostate cancer risk: a systematic review and meta-analysis of cohort studies'. *Am J Clin Nutr*, 101, pp. 87–117.
- Song, M, Fung, TT, Hu, FB et al. (2016). 'Association of animal and plant protein intake with all-cause and cause-specific mortality'. *JAMA Intern Med*, 176, pp. 1453–53.
- Scientific Committee on Animal Health and Animal Welfare (10 March 1999). 'Report on animal welfare aspects of the use of bovine somatotrophin'.

Milk and Cancer Part 2

- Echternkap, SE, Aad, PY, Eborn, DR & Spicer, LJ (2012). 'Increased abundance of aromatase and folical stimulating hormone receptor mRNA and decreased insulin-like growth factor-2 receptor mRNA in small ovarian follicles of cattle selected for twin births'. *J Anim Sci*, 90, pp. 2193–200.
- Ganmaa, D & Sato, A (2005). 'The possible role of female sex hormones in milk from pregnant cows in the development of breast, ovarian and corpus uteri cancers'. *Med Hypotheses*, 65, pp. 1028–37.
- Barr, SI, McCarron, DA, Heaney, RP et al. (2000). 'Effects of increased consumption of fluid milk on energy and nutrient intake, body weight and cardiovascular risk factors in healthy older adults'. *J Am Diet Asoc*, 100, pp. 810–7.
- Cadogan, J, Eastell, R, Jones, N & Barker, ME (1997). 'Milk intake and bone mineral acquisition in adolescent girls: randomised, controlled intervention trial'. *BMJ*, 315, pp. 1255–60.
- Zhu, K, Du, X, Cowell, CT et al. (2005). 'Effects of school milk intervention on coritcal bone acceleration and indicators relevant to bone metabolism in Chinese girls aged 10–12 y in Beijing'. *Am J Clin Nutr*, 81, pp. 1168–75.
- Rich-Edwards, JW, Ganmaa, D, Pollaak, MN et al. (2007). 'Milk consumption and the pre–pubertal somatoropic axis'. *Nutr J*, 6, p. 28.
- FAO/WHO/UNU (1985). *Energy and protein requirements: report of a joint FAO/WHO/UNU expert consultation*. WHO Technical Report Series 724. Geneva: World Health Organisation.
- Harrison, LR, Holly, J et al. (2017). 'Does milk intake promote prostate cancer initiation or progression via effects on insulin–like growth factors (IGFs)? A systematic review and meta-analysis'. *Cancer Causes Control*, 28, pp. 497–528.
- Melnik, BC (2015). 'Milk – a nutrient system of mammalian evolution promoting mTORC1–dependent translation'. *Int J Mol Sci*, 16, pp. 17048–87.
- World Cancer Research Fund/American Institute for Cancer Research (2007). 'Second expert report: food, nutrition, physical activity, and the prevention of cancer: a global perspective'. Washington, DC: AICR.
- Hegsted, DM (1986). 'Calcium and osteoporsosis'. *J Nutr*, 116, pp. 2316–9.
- Feskanich, D, Bischoff–Ferrari, HA, Frazier, AL. & Willett, WC (2014). 'Milk consumption during teenage years and risk of hip fractures in older adults'. *JAMA Pediatr*, 168, pp. 54–60.
- Ganmaa, D, Li, XM, Wang, J, Qin, LQ, Wang, PY & Sato, A (2002). 'Incidence and mortality of testicular and prostatic cancers in relation to world dietary practices'. *Int J Cancer*, 98, pp. 262–7.
- Song, M, Fung, TT, Hu, FB et al. (2016). 'Association of animal and plant protein intake with all-cause and cause-specific mortality'. *JAMA Intern Med*, 176, pp. 1453–53.
- Scientific Committee on Animal Health and Animal Welfare (10 March 1999). 'Report on Animal Welfare Aspects of the Use of Bovine Somatotrophin'.

Milk and Cancer Part 3

- Lerman, B et al. (14 September 2018). 'Oxytocin and cancer: an emerging link'. *World Journal of Clinical Oncology*, 9 (5), pp. 74–82.
- Whittington, K, Connards, B et al. (1 July 2007). 'The effect of oxytocin on cell proliferation in the human prostate is modulated by gonadal steroid implications for benign prostate hyperplasia and cancer of the prostate'. *Prostate*, 67 (10), pp. 1132–42.
- 'Formaldehyde and cancer risk'. National Cancer Institute, 2011 (IARC Working Group on the Evaluation of Carcinogenic Risks to Humans, 2006, National Toxicology Program, 2011).
- 'Occupational safety and health guidelines for formic acid'. OSHA. USA.
- National Toxicology Program (2011). *Report on carcinogens* (12th ed.). U.S. Department of Health and Human Services, Public Health Services, National Institute of Health. ISBN 9781613442333.
- Bhatti, M – investigative journalist. GNN News Channel, Pakistan.

Part Eight

- Colditz, GA (ed.) (2015). *The SAGE encyclopedia of cancer and society*. Thousand Oaks, California: SAGE Publications.
- International Agency for Research on Cancer/World Health Organization. *IARC Monographs on the Evaluation of Carcinogenic Risks to Humans*. Available at: monographs.iarc.fr.
- Caballero, B et al. (eds.) (2015). *Encyclopedia of food and health*. Amsterdam: Elsevier Science. Page 658. ISBN 978-0-12384-953-3.

It's a Radiant World

How Much Radiation is Safe?

- Koerth-Baker, M (27 August 2010). 'Bananas are radioactive—But they aren't a good way to explain radiation exposure'. *Boing Boing*. Retrieved 25 May 2011. Attributes the title statement to Geoff Meggitt, a former health physicist for the UK Atomic Energy Authority.
- Federal Guidance Report 13, p. 16. United States Environmental Protection Agency, 1999.
- Eisenbud, M & Gesell & TF (1997). *Environmental radioactivity: from natural, industrial, and military sources*. Academic Press, pp. 171–172. ISBN 978-0-12235-154-9.

Measuring Radioactivity with Bananas

- Nain, M, Gupta, M, Chauhan, RP, Kant, K, Sonkawade, RG & Chakarvarti, SK (November 2010). 'Estimation of radioactivity in tobacco'. *Indian Journal of Pure & Applied Physics,* 48 (11), pp. 820–2.
- Abd El-Aziz, N, Khater, AEM. & Al.-Sewaidan, HA (2005). 'Natural radioactivity contents in tobacco'. *International Congress Series*, 1276, pp. 407–8.

Radiation and Cancer

- LaFavore, M (1986). 'Radon: the quiet killer'. *Funk & Wagnalls 1987 Science Yearbook*. New York: Funk & Wagnalls. ISBN 0-7172-1517-2.

Natural Sources of Radon in the Environment

- Mueller Associates, SYSCON Corporation, Brookhaven National Laboratory (1988). *Handbook of radon in buildings: detection, safety, & control*. CRC Press. Pages 28–32. ISBN 978–0-89116-823-2.
- 'The geology of radon'. United States Geological Survey.

History of Radiation Toxicity with Radon

- 'Radon toxicity: who is at risk?'. Agency for Toxic Substances and Disease Registry, 2000.
- Roscoe, RJ, Deddens, JA, Salvan, A & Schnorr, TM. (1995). 'Mortality among Navajo uranium miners'. *American Journal of Public Health*, 85 (4), pp. 535–40.

Health Risks of Radon Gas Radiation

- 'Known and probable carcinogens'. American Cancer Society.
- Rericha, V, Kulich, M, Rericha, R, Shore, DL & Sandler, DP (2007). 'Incidence of leukemia, lymphoma, and multiple myeloma in Czech uranium miners: a case-cohort study'. *Environmental Health Perspectives*, 114 (6), pp. 818–822.

Health Risks in Children

- 'Environmental radon exposure and childhood leukemia'. *Journal of Toxicology and Environmental Health*, 15 (5), pp. 332–347.
- Druzhinin, V, Sinitsky, MY, Larionov, AV, Volobaev, VP, Minina, VI & Golovina, TA (2015). 'Assessing the level of chromosome aberrations in peripheral blood lymphocytes in long-term resident children under conditions of high exposure to radon and its decay products'. *Mutagenesis*, 50 (5), pp. 677–83.

Intentional or Therapeutic Exposure to Radon Gas

- Salak, K & Nordeman, L (2004). '59631: Mining for Miracles'. *National Geographic*. National Geographic Society.

Health Policies for Radon Control

- 'Protecting people and families from radon: a federal action plan for saving lives'. United States Environmental Protection Agency.

National Radon Action Plan

- 'The national radon action plan: a strategy for saving lives.' US Environmental Protection Agency.

Death Toll Attributed to Radon

- 'Radon: a likely carcinogen at all exposures'. *Annals of Oncology*, 12 (10), pp. 1341–51.
- Field, RW, Steck, DJ, Smith, BJ et al. (2000). 'Residential radon gas exposure and lung cancer: the Iowa Radon Lung Cancer Study'. *American Journal of Epidemiology*. Oxford Journals, 151(11), pp. 1091–102.

Radiation Testing for Radon Gas

- Kansas State University. 'National radon program services'. Retrieved 17 October 2017.

Radon Mitigation and Radon Removal

- 'Consumer's guide to radon reduction'. United States Environmental Protection Agency.

Nitrosodimethylamine References

- Tricker, AR & Preussmann, R (1991). 'Carcinogenic N-nitrosamines in the diet: occurrence, formation, mechanisms and carcinogenic potential'. *Mutation Research/Genetic Toxicology*, 259(3–4), pp. 277–289.
- Najm, I & Trussell, RR (2001). 'NDMA formation in water and wastewater'. *Journal American Water Works Association*, 93 (2), pp. 92–99.
- Mitch, WA, Sharp, JO, Trussell, RR, Valentine, RL, Alvarez-Cohen, L & Sedlak, DL (2003). 'N-Nitrosodimethylamine (NDMA) as a drinking water contaminant: a review'. *Environmental Engineering Science*, 20 (5), pp. 389–404.
- 'Nitrosamine impurities'. European Medicines Agency (EMA). Retrieved 11 July 2020.
- Mitch, William A & Sedlak, David L (2002). 'Formation of N-Nitrosodimethylamine (NDMA) from dimethylamine during chlorination'. *Environmental Science & Technology*, 36 (4), pp. 588–595.

All Suspects Big and Small

List of IARC Group 1 Agents - Carcinogenic to humans

- International Agency for Research on Cancer/World Health Organization. 'List of classifications, agents classified by the IARC monographs, volumes 1–124'. *IARC Monographs on the Evaluation of Risk to Humans*.

Part Nine

- 'What is cancer screening?'. National Cancer Institute. 2010-01-13.
- Wilson, JM, Jungner, G (1968). 'Principles and practice of screening for disease' (PDF). Public Health Papers. Vol. 34. Geneva: World Health Organization.

Part Ten

- 'The top 10 causes of death'. World Health Organization. 9 December 2020.
- 'Cancer prevention: 7 steps to reduce your risk' (27 September 2008). Mayo Clinic. Retrieved 30 January 2010.

- Valle, I, Tramalloni, D & Bragazzi, NL (June 2015). 'Cancer prevention: state of the art and future prospects'. *Journal of Preventive Medicine and Hygiene*, 56 (1), E21–7. PMC 4718348. PMID 26789828.
- Anand, P, Kunnumakkara, AB, Kunnumakara, AB, Sundaram, C, Harikumar, KB, Tharakan, ST, Lai, OS, Sung, B & Aggarwal, BB (2008). 'Cancer is a preventable disease that requires major lifestyle changes'. *Pharm. Res.* 25 (9), pp. 2097–116.

Prevention of Cancer

History of Cancer Before Modern Prevention

- 'The history of cancer'. American Cancer Society.
- 'The history of cancer'. Institut Jules Bordet (Association Hospitalière de Bruxelles - Centre des Tumeurs de ULB).
- Skinner, P (2001). 'Unani-tibbi'. *Gale encyclopedia of alternative medicine*. Longe, JL (ed.). Michigan: Gale Group.
- 'Avicenna'. *Encyclopedia Britannica*.

The Components of Cancer Prevention

- Gofrit, ON, Shemer, J, Leibovici, D, Modan, B & Shapira, SC (2000). 'Quaternary prevention: a new look at an old challenge'. *Isr Med Assoc J*, 2 (7), pp. 498–500.

References – Prevention of Cancer

- Leavell, HR & Clark, EG (1979). 'The science and art of preventing disease, prolonging life, and promoting physical and mental health and efficiency'. *Preventive medicine for the doctor in his community* (3rd ed.). Huntington, NY: Robert E. Krieger Publishing Company.
- 'Preventive health care'. *The Lancet*, 345 (8965), pp. 1611–1615. DOI:10.1016/s0140-6736(95)90119-1. PMID 7783540.
- Gofrit, ON, Shemer, J, Leibovici, D, Modan, B & Shapira, SC (2000). 'Quaternary prevention: a new look at an old challenge'. *Isr Med Assoc J*, 2 (7), pp. 498–500.

Chillies and Cancer

- University of California, San Diego (3 August 2014). 'Study: spicy capsaicin can reduce risk of colorectal tumors'. *News-Medical*.

Intermittent Fasting from Dawn to Sunset Part 2 Reference

- Mindikoglu, Ayse L, Abdulsada, Mustafa M, Antrix, J, Min Choi, J et al. (15 April 2020). 'Intermittent fasting from dawn to sunset for 30 consecutive days is associated with anticancer proteomic signature and upregulates key regulatory proteins of glucose and lipid metabolism, circadian clock, DNA repair, cytoskeleton remodeling, immune system and cognitive function in healthy subjects'. *Journal of Proteomics,* 217, DOI: 10.1016/j.jprot.2020.103645.

Prostate Cancer References

- Hurst, R, Hooper, L, Norat, T et al. (2012). 'Selinium and prostate cancer: systematic review and meta-analysis'. *American Journal of Clinical Nutrition*, 96, (1), pp. 111–22.
- Aune, D, Navarro Rosenblatt, DA et al. (2014). 'Dairy products calcium and prostate cancer risk: a systematic review in meta-analysis of cohort studies'. *American Journal of Clinical Nutrition*, 202 (1), pp. 87–117).
- Rodrigues, C, McCullough, ML, Mondul, AM et al. (2003). 'Calcium dairy products and risk of prostate cancer in a prospective cohort of united states men'. *Cancer Epidemiology Biomarkers Prev*, 12, pp. 597–603).

Breast Cancer

- Ferlay, J, Soerjomataram, I, Ervik, M et al. (2015). 'GLOBOCAN 2012 v1.0, Cancer incidence and mortality worldwide. IARC Cancer Base, No. 11' [Internet]. Lyon, France: IARC.
- McPherson, K, Steel, CM & Dixon, JM (2000). 'ABC of breast diseases. Breast cancer epidemiology, risk factors and genetics'. *BMJ*, 321, pp. 624–8.
- 'American Cancer Society (2014). 'Cancer Facts & Figures 2014', Atlanta: American Cancer Society.
- Putti, TC, El-Rehim, DM, Rakha, EA et al. (2005). 'Estrogen receptor-negative breast carcinomas: a review of morphology and immunophenotypical analysis'. *Mod Pathol*, 18, pp. 26–35.

General Risk Factors

Life Events

- McPherson, K, Steel, CM & Dixon JM (2000). 'ABC of breast diseases. Breast cancer epidemiology, risk factors and genetics'. *BMJ*, 321, pp. 624–8.
- MacMahon, B (1993). 'General Motors Cancer Research Prizewinners Laureates Lectures. Charles S. Mott Prize. Reproduction and cancer of the breast'. *Cancer,* 71, pp. 3185–8.
- Berkey, CS, Gardner, JD, Frazier, AL. et al. (2000). 'Relation of childhood diet and body size to menarche and adolescent growth in girls'. *Am J Epidemiol*, 152, pp. 446–52.

Ionising Radiation

- Modan, B, Chetrit, A, Alfandary, E et al. (1989). 'Increased risk of breast cancer after low-dose irradiation'. *Lancet*, 1, pp. 629–31.
- Ronckers, CM, Erdmann, CA & Land, CE (2005). 'Radiation and breast cancer: a review of current evidence'. *Breast Cancer Res*, 7, pp. 21–32.

Medication

- International Agency for Research on Cancer/World Health Organization (2012). *Combined estrogen-progestogen contraceptives (IARC monographs on the evaluation of carcinogenic risks to humans, 100A)*. Lyon, France: IARC Publications/WHO Press. Pages 283–317. ISBN 978-92-832-1318-5.
- GK, Beral, V, Green, J et al. (2006). 'Hormonal therapy for menopause and breast-cancer risk by histological type: a cohort study and meta-analysis'. *Lancet Oncol*, 7, pp. 910–8.

Physical Activity and Breast Cancer

- Sczaniecka, AK, Brasky, TM, Lampe, JW et al. (2012). 'Dietary intake of specific fatty acids and breast cancer risk among postmenopausal women in the VITAL cohort'. *Nutr Cancer*, 64, pp. 1131– 42.110.
- World Cancer Research Fund/American Institute for Cancer Research. 'Breast cancer report 2017'. Washington DC: AICR.
- Hastert, TA, Beresford, SA, Patterson, RE et al. (2013). 'Adherence to WCRF/AICR cancer prevention recommendations and risk of postmenopausal breast cancer'. *Cancer Epidemiol Biomarkers Prev*, 22, pp. 1498–508.
- Howard, RA, Leitzmann, MF, Linet, MS et al. (2009). 'Physical activity and breast cancer risk among pre- and postmenopausal women in the U.S. Radiologic Technologists cohort'. *Cancer Causes Control*, 20, pp. 323–33.

- Suzuki, R, Iwasaki, M, Yamamoto, S et al. (2011). 'Leisure-time physical activity and breast cancer risk defined by estrogen and progesterone receptor status – the Japan Public Health Center–based Prospective Study'. *Prev Med*, 52, pp. 227–33a.
- Wu, Y, Zhang, D & Kang, S (2013). 'Physical activity and risk of breast cancer: a meta-analysis of prospective studies'. *Breast Cancer Res Treat*, 137, pp. 869–82.
- Borch, KB, Lund, E, Braaten, T et al. (2014). 'Physical activity and the risk of postmenopausal breast cancer – the Norwegian Women and Cancer Study'. *J Negat Results Biomed*, 13, p. 3.
- McKenzie, F, Ferrari, P, Freisling, H et al. (2015). 'Healthy lifestyle and risk of breast cancer among postmenopausal women in the European Prospective Investigation into Cancer and Nutrition cohort study'. *Int J Cancer*, 136, pp. 2640–8.
- McTiernan, A (2008). 'Mechanisms linking physical activity with cancer'. *Nat Rev Cancer*, 8, pp. 205–11.

Obesity and Weight

- Schonfeld, SJ, Pfeiffer, RM, Lacey JV, Jr. et al. (2011). 'Hormone-related risk factors and postmenopausal breast cancer among nulliparous versus parous women: an aggregated study'. *Am J Epidemiol*, 173, pp. 509–17.
- Michels, KB, Terry, KL & Willett, WC (2006). 'Longitudinal study on the role of body size in premenopausal breast cancer'. *Arch Intern Med*, 166, pp. 2395–402a.
- Burton, A, Martin, R, Galobardes, B et al. (2010). 'Young adulthood body mass index and risk of cancer in later adulthood: historical cohort study'. *Cancer Causes Control*, 21, pp. 2069–77.
- Wada, K, Nagata, C, Tamakoshi, A et al. (2014). 'Body mass index and breast cancer risk in Japan: a pooled analysis of eight population-based cohort studies'. *Ann Oncol*, 25, pp. 519–24.

Breast Feeding

- Iwasaki, M, Otani, T, Inoue, M et al. (2007). 'Role and impact of menstrual and reproductive factors on breast cancer risk in Japan'. *Eur J Cancer Prev*, 16, pp. 116–23a.
- Kawai, M, Minami, Y, Kuriyama, S et al. (2010). 'Reproductive factors, exogenous female hormone use and breast cancer risk in Japanese: the Miyagi Cohort Study'. *Cancer Causes Control*, 21, pp. 135–45a.
- Palmer, JR, Boggs, DA, Wise, LA et al. (2011). 'Parity and lactation in relation to estrogen receptor negative breast cancer in African American women'. *Cancer Epidemiol Biomarkers Prev*, 20, pp. 1883–91.
- Butt, S, Borgquist, S, Anagnostaki, L et al. (2014). 'Breastfeeding in relation to risk of different breast cancer characteristics'. *BMC Res Notes*, 7, p. 216.

Alcohol and Vitamins

- Trichopoulou, A, Bamia, C, Lagiou, P et al. (2010). 'Conformity to traditional Mediterranean diet and breast cancer risk in the Greek EPIC (European Prospective Investigation into Cancer and Nutrition) cohort'. *Am J Clin Nutr*, 92, pp. 620–5.
- World Cancer Research Fund/American Institute for Cancer Research. 'Breast cancer report 2017'. Washington DC: AICR. Page 107.
- Couto, E, Sandin, S, Lof, M et al. (2013). 'Mediterranean dietary pattern and risk of breast cancer'. *PLoS One*, 8, e55374.
- Zhang, X, Spiegelman, D, Baglietto, L et al. (2012). 'Carotenoid intakes and risk of breast cancer defined by estrogen receptor and progesterone receptor status: a pooled analysis of 18 prospective cohort studies'. *Am J Clin Nutr*, 95, pp. 713–25.
- Bakker, MF, Peeters, PH, Klaasen, VM et al. (2016). 'Plasma carotenoids, vitamin C, tocopherols, and retinol and the risk of breast cancer in the European Prospective Investigation into Cancer and Nutrition cohort'. *Am J Clin Nutr*, 103, pp. 454–64.
- Visvanathan, K, Crum, RM, Strickland, PT et al. (2007). 'Alcohol dehydrogenase genetic polymorphisms, low-to-moderate alcohol consumption and risk of breast cancer'. *Alcohol Clin Exp Res*, 31, pp. 467–76.
- Zhang, SM, Lee, IM, Manson, JE et al. (2007). 'Alcohol consumption and breast cancer risk in the Women's Health Study'. *Am J Epidemiol*, 165, pp. 667–76.
- Suzuki, R, Iwasaki, M, Inoue, M et al. (2010). 'Alcohol consumption-associated breast cancer incidence and potential effect modifiers: the Japan Public Health Center–based Prospective Study'. *Int J Cancer*, 127, pp. 685–95.
- Chen, WY, Rosner, B, Hankinson, SE et al. (2011). 'Moderate alcohol consumption during adult life, drinking patterns, and breast cancer risk'. *JAMA*, 306, pp. 1884–90.
- World Cancer Research Fund/American Institute for Cancer Research. 'Breast cancer report 2017'. Washington DC: AICR.

Tall Stature

- Berkey, CS, Frazier, AL., Gardner, JD et al. (1999). 'Adolescence and breast carcinoma risk'. *Cancer*, 85, pp. 2400–9.

Greater Birth Weight

- Sainsbury, JR, Anderson, TJ & Morgan, DA (2000). 'ABC of breast diseases: breast cancer'. *BMJ*, 321, pp. 745–50.
- Baer, HJ, Colditz, GA, Willett, WC et al. (2007). 'Adiposity and sex hormones in girls'. *Cancer Epidemiol Biomarkers Prev*, 16, pp. 1880–8.
- World Cancer Research Fund/American Institute for Cancer Research. 'Breast cancer report 2017'. Washington DC: AICR.

Increased Intake of Dairy Products

- Trichopoulou, A, Bamia, C, Lagiou, P et al. (2010). 'Conformity to traditional Mediterranean diet and breast cancer risk in the Greek EPIC (European Prospective Investigation into Cancer and Nutrition) cohort'. *Am J Clin Nutr*, 92, pp. 620–5.
- World Cancer Research Fund/American Institute for Cancer Research. 'Breast cancer report 2017'. Washington DC: AICR. Page 107.
- Kesse-Guyot, E, Bertrais, S, Duperray, B et al. (2007). 'Dairy products, calcium and the risk of breast cancer: results of the French SU.VI.MAX prospective study'. *Ann Nutr Metab*, 51, pp. 139–45.
- Lin, J, Manson, JE, Lee, IM et al. (2007). 'Intakes of calcium and vitamin D and breast cancer risk in women'. *Arch Intern Med*, 167, pp. 1050–9.
- Hjartaker, A, Thoresen, M, Engeset, D et al. (2010). 'Dairy consumption and calcium intake and risk of breast cancer in a prospective cohort: the Norwegian Women and Cancer study'. *Cancer Causes Control*, 21, pp. 1875–85.

Increased Calcium in Diet

- Kesse-Guyot, E, Bertrais, S, Duperray, B et al. (2007). 'Dairy products, calcium and the risk of breast cancer: results of the French SU.VI.MAX prospective study'. *Ann Nutr Metab*, 51, pp. 139–45.
- Hjartaker, A, Thoresen, M, Engeset, D et al. (2010). 'Dairy consumption and calcium intake and risk of breast cancer in a prospective cohort: the Norwegian Women and Cancer study'. *Cancer Causes Control*, 21, pp. 1875–85.
- Larsson, SC, Bergkvist, L & Wolk, A (2009). 'Long-term dietary calcium intake and breast cancer risk in a prospective cohort of women'. *Am J Clin Nutr*, 89, pp. 277–82d.

- Abbas, S, Linseisen, J, Rohrmann, S et al. (2013). 'Dietary intake of vitamin D and calcium and breast cancer risk in the European Prospective Investigation into Cancer and Nutrition'. *Nutr Cancer*, 65, pp. 178–87.

Family History

- Pharoah, PD, Day, NE, Duffy, S et al. (1997). 'Family history and the risk of breast cancer: a systematic review and meta-analysis'. *Int J Cancer*, 71, pp. 800–9.
- Collaborative Group on Hormonal Factors in Breast Cancer (2001). 'Familial breast cancer: collaborative reanalysis of individual data from 52 epidemiological studies including 58,209 women with breast cancer and 101,986 women without the disease'. *Lancet*, 358, pp. 1389–99.
- Kharazmi, E, Chen, T, Narod, S et al. (2014). 'Effect of multiplicity, laterality and age at onset of breast cancer on familial risk of breast cancer: a nationwide prospective cohort study'. *Breast Cancer Res Treat*, 144, pp. 185–92.

BRCA Genes – BRCA2

- Gershoni-Baruch, R, Dagan, E, Fried, G et al. (2000). 'Significantly lower rates of BRCA1/BRCA2 founder mutations in Ashkenazi women with sporadic compared with familial early onset breast cancer'. *Eur J Cancer*, 36, p. 983.
- Hodgson, SV, Heap, E, Cameron, J et al. (1999). 'Risk factors for detecting germline BRCA1 and BRCA2 founder mutations in Ashkenazi Jewish women with breast or ovarian cancer'. *J Med Genet*, 36, p. 369.
- Antoniou, A, Pharoah, PD, Narod, S et al. (2003). 'Average risks of breast and ovarian cancer associated with BRCA1 or BRCA2 mutations detected in case Series unselected for family history: a combined analysis of 22 studies'. *Am J Hum Genet*, 72, p. 1117.
- Chen, S & Parmigiani, G (2007). 'Meta-analysis of BRCA1 and BRCA2 penetrance'. *J Clin Oncol*, 25, p. 1329.
- Breast Cancer Linkage Consortium (1999). 'Cancer risks in BRCA2 mutation carriers'. *J Natl Cancer Inst*, 91, p. 1310.
- Kote-Jarai, Z, Leongamornlert, D, Saunders, E et al. (2011). 'BRCA2 is a moderate penetrance gene contributing to young-onset prostate cancer: implications for genetic testing in prostate cancer patients'. *Br J Cancer*, 105, p. 1230.

Breast Cancer Supplementary Information

Level 1 - Primal and Primordial Prevention

- Gillman, MW (2015). 'Primordial prevention of cardiovascular disease'. *Circulation*, 131 (7), pp. 599–601. DOI:10.1161/circulationaha.115.014849.
- Chiolero, A et al. (2015). 'The pseudo-high-risk prevention strategy'. *Int J Epidemiol*, 44 (5), pp. 1469–1473. DOI:10.1093/ije/dyv102.

Level 2 – Primary Prevention

- Katz, D & Ather, A. (2009). 'Preventive medicine, integrative medicine & the health of the public'. Commissioned for the IOM Summit on Integrative Medicine and the Health of the Public.
- Patterson, C.& Chambers, LW (1995). 'Preventive health care'. *The Lancet*, 345 (8965), pp. 1611–1615.

Level 3 – Tertiary Prevention

- Katz, D & Ather, A. (2009). 'Preventive medicine, integrative medicine & the health of the public'. Commissioned for the IOM Summit on Integrative Medicine and the Health of the Public.

Level 4 – Quaternary Prevention

- Leavell, HR & Clark, EG (1979). 'The science and art of preventing disease, prolonging life, and promoting physical and mental health and efficiency'. *Preventive medicine for the doctor in his community* (3rd ed.). Huntington, NY: Robert E. Krieger Publishing Company.
- Chiolero, A et al. (2015). 'The pseudo-high-risk prevention strategy'. *Int J Epidemiol*, 44 (5), pp. 1469–1473.
- Gofrit, ON, Shemer, J, Leibovici, D, Modan, B & Shapira SC (2000). 'Quaternary prevention: a new look at an old challenge'. *Isr Med Assoc J*, 2 (7), pp. 498–500.

Melanoma Risk Factors

- Siegel, RL, Miller, KD & Jemal, A (2019). 'Cancer statistics, 2019'. *CA Cancer J Clin*, 69, p. 7.
- Garbe, C & Leiter, U (2009). 'Melanoma epidemiology and trends'. *Clin Dermatol*, 27, p. 3.
- Aitken, JF, Youlden, DR, Baade, PD et al. (2018). 'Generational shift in melanoma incidence and mortality in Queensland, Australia, 1995-2014'. *Int J Cancer*, 142, p. 1528.
- Lange, JR, Palis, BE, Chang, DC et al. (2007). 'Melanoma in children and teenagers: an analysis of patients from the National Cancer Data Base'. *J Clin Oncol*, 25, p. 1363.

Risk Factors

1) Ultraviolet Radiation

- Gilchrest, BA, Eller, MS, Geller, AC & Yaar, M (199). 'The pathogenesis of melanoma induced by ultraviolet radiation'. *N Engl J Med*, 340, p. 1341.
- Buckel, TB, Goldstein, AM, Fraser, MC et al. (2006). 'Recent tanning bed use: a risk factor for melanoma'. *Arch Dermatol*, 142, p. 485.

2) Timing and Pattern of Sun Exposure

- Nelemans, PJ, Groenendal, H, Kiemeney, LA et al. (1993). 'Effect of intermittent exposure to sunlight on melanoma risk among indoor workers and sun-sensitive individuals'. *Environ Health Perspect*, 101, p. 252.
- Whiteman, DC, Stickley, M, Watt, P et al. (2006). 'Anatomic site, sun exposure, and risk of cutaneous melanoma'. *J Clin Oncol*, 24, p. 3172.
- Holman, CD & Armstrong, BK (1984). 'Cutaneous malignant melanoma and indicators of total accumulated exposure to the sun: an analysis separating histogenetic types'. *J Natl Cancer Inst*, 73, p. 75.

3) Indoor Tanning

- Centers for Disease Control and Prevention (CDC) (2012). 'Use of indoor tanning devices by adults--United States, 2010'. *MMWR Morb Mortal Wkly Rep*, 61, p. 323.
- El Ghissassi, F, Baan, R, Straif, K et al. (2009). 'A review of human carcinogens--part D: radiation'. *Lancet Oncol*, 10, p. 751.
- International Agency for Research on Cancer Working Group on artificial ultraviolet (UV) light and skin cancer (2007). 'The association of use of sunbeds with cutaneous malignant melanoma and other skin cancers: A systematic review'. *Int J Cancer*, 120, p. 1116.
- Boniol, M, Autier, P, Boyle, P & Gandini, S (2012). 'Cutaneous melanoma attributable to sunbed use: systematic review and meta-analysis'. *BMJ*, 345, e4757.
- Vajdic, CM, Kricker, A, Giblin, M et al. (2004). 'Artificial ultraviolet radiation and ocular melanoma in Australia'. *Int J Cancer*, 112, p. 896.

4) *PUVA Therapy*

- Stern RS, PUVA Follow up Study (2001). 'The risk of melanoma in association with long-term exposure to PUVA'. *J Am Acad Dermatol*, 44, p. 755.

5) *Skin Pigmentation and Tanning Ability*

- Gandini, S, Sera, F, Cattaruzza, MS et al. (2005). 'Meta-analysis of risk factors for cutaneous melanoma: III. Family history, actinic damage and phenotypic factors'. *Eur J Cancer*, 41, p. 2040.

6) *Congenital Nevi*

- Vourc'h-Jourdain, M, Martin, L, Barbarot, S & aRED (2013). 'Large congenital melanocytic nevi: therapeutic management and melanoma risk: a systematic review'. *J Am Acad Dermatol*, 68, p. 493.

7) *Atypical Nevi*

- Gandini, S, Sera F, Cattaruzza, MS et al. (2005). 'Meta-analysis of risk factors for cutaneous melanoma: I. Common and atypical naevi'. *Eur J Cancer*, 41, p. 28.

8) *FAMMM Syndrome and Atypical Mole Syndrome*

- Lynch, HT, Frichot, BC 3rd & Lynch, JF (1978). 'Familial atypical multiple mole-melanoma syndrome'. *J Med Genet*, 15, p. 352.

9) *Personal History of Melanoma*

- Bradford, PT, Freedman, DM, Goldstein, AM & Tucker, MA (2010). 'Increased risk of second primary cancers after a diagnosis of melanoma'. *Arch Dermatol*, 146, p. 265.
- Goggins, WB & Tsao, H (2003). 'A population-based analysis of risk factors for a second primary cutaneous melanoma among melanoma survivors'. *Cancer*, 97, p. 639.

10) *Genetic Background*

- Rivers, JK (1996). 'Melanoma'. *Lancet*, 347, p. 803.

11) *History of Non-Melanoma Skin Cancer*

- Marghoob, AA, Slade, J, Salopek, TG et al. (1995). 'Basal cell and squamous cell carcinomas are important risk factors for cutaneous malignant melanoma. Screening implications'. *Cancer*, 75, p. 707.
- Kahn, HS, Tatham, LM, Patel, AV et al. (1998). 'Increased cancer mortality following a history of nonmelanoma skin cancer'. *JAMA*, 280, p. 910.

12) *Immunosuppression*

- Kubica, AW & Brewer, JD (2012). 'Melanoma in immunosuppressed patients'. *Mayo Clin Proc*, 87, p. 991.
- Hollenbeak, CS, Todd, MM, Billingsley, EM et al. (2005). 'Increased incidence of melanoma in renal transplantation recipients'. *Cancer*, 104, p. 1962.

13) *Occupational Exposure*

- Ward, EM, Burnett, CA, Ruder, A & Davis-King, K (1997). 'Industries and cancer'. *Cancer Causes Control*, 8, p. 356.

14) *Dietary Pattern*

- Millen, AE, Tucker, MA, Hartge, P et al. (2004). 'Diet and melanoma in a case-control study'. *Cancer Epidemiol Biomarkers Prev*, 13, p. 1042.

15) *Coffee*

- Liu, J, Shen, B, Shi, M & Cai, J (2016). 'Higher caffeinated coffee intake is associated with reduced malignant melanoma risk: a meta-analysis study'. *PLoS One*, 11, e0147056.
- Wang, J, Li, X & Zhang, D (2016). 'Coffee consumption and the risk of cutaneous melanoma: a meta-analysis'. *Eur J Nutr*, 55, p. 1317.
- Yew, YW, Lai, YC & Schwartz, RA (2016). 'Coffee consumption and melanoma: a systematic review and meta-analysis of observational studies'. *Am J Clin Dermatol*, 17, p. 113.

16) *Citrus Fruits*

- Wu, S, Han, J, Feskanich, D et al. (2015). 'Citrus consumption and risk of cutaneous malignant melanoma'. *J Clin Oncol*, 33, p. 2500.

17) *Smoking*

- Merimsky, O, Inbar, M (1998). 'Cigarette smoking and skin cancer'. *Clin Dermatol*, 16, p. 585.

18) *Oral Contraceptives and Postmenopausal Hormone Therapy*

- Gandini, S, Iodice, S, Koomen, E et al. (2011). 'Hormonal and reproductive factors in relation to melanoma in women: current review and meta-analysis'. *Eur J Cancer*, 47, p. 2607.

19) *Drugs*

- Mariette, X, Matucci-Cerinic, M, Pavelka, K et al. (2011). 'Malignancies associated with tumour necrosis factor inhibitors in registries and prospective observational studies: a systematic review and meta-analysis'. *Ann Rheum Dis*, 70, p. 1895.
- Loeb, S, Folkvaljon, Y, Lambe, M et al. (2015). 'Use of phosphodiesterase type 5 inhibitors for erectile dysfunction and risk of malignant melanoma'. *JAMA*, 313, p. 2449.

20) *Parkinson's Disease*

- Olsen, JH, Friis, S & Frederiksen, K (2006). 'Malignant melanoma and other types of cancer preceding Parkinson disease'. *Epidemiology*, 17, p. 582.
- Inzelberg, R & Israeli-Korn, SD (2009). 'The particular relationship between Parkinson's disease and malignancy: a focus on skin cancers'. *J Neural Transm.* (Vienna), 116, p. 1503.

21) *Endometriosis*

- Kvaskoff, M, Mesrine, S, Fournier, A et al. (2007). 'Personal history of endometriosis and risk of cutaneous melanoma in a large prospective cohort of French women'. *Arch Intern Med*, 167, p. 2061.
- Somigliana, E, Vigano, P, Parazzini, F et al. (2006). 'Association between endometriosis and cancer: a comprehensive review and a critical analysis of clinical and epidemiological evidence'. *Gynecol Oncol*, 101, p. 331.

22)   History of Prostate Cancer

- Li, WQ, Qureshi, AA, Ma, J et al. (2013). 'Personal history of prostate cancer and increased risk of incident melanoma in the United States'. *J Clin Oncol*, 31, p. 4394.

Prevention of Melanoma

- Armstrong, BK & Kricker, A (1993). 'How much melanoma is caused by sun exposure?'. *Melanoma Res*, 3, p. 395.
- Aitken, JF, Youlden, DR, Baade, PD et al. (2018). 'Generational shift in melanoma incidence and mortality in Queensland, Australia, 1995-2014'. *Int J Cancer*, 142, p. 1528.

Pathogenesis of Melanoma

- Wang, SQ, Setlow, R, Berwick, M et al. (2001). 'Ultraviolet A and melanoma: a review'. *J Am Acad Dermatol*, 44, p. 837.

Special Window Glass and Films

- Tuchinda, C, Srivannaboon, S & Lim, HW (2006). 'Photoprotection by window glass, automobile glass, and sunglasses'. *J Am Acad Dermatol*, 54, p. 845.

Using Sunscreen Containing Cosmetics

- Draelos, ZD (2011). 'The multifunctional value of sunscreen-containing cosmetics'. *Skin Therapy Lett*, 16, p. 1.
- de Maleissye, MF, Beauchet A, Saiag, P et al. (2003). 'Sunscreen use and melanocytic nevi in children: a systematic review'. *Pediatr Dermatol*, 30, p. 51.

Nevus (Nevi)

- Egan, KM, Sosman, JA & Blot, WJ (2005). 'Sunlight and reduced risk of cancer: is the real story vitamin D?'. *J Natl Cancer Inst*, 97, p. 161.
- Lim, HW, Gilchrest, BA, Cooper, KD et al. (2005). 'Sunlight, tanning booths, and vitamin D'. *J Am Acad Dermatol*, 52, p. 868.

Tanning Bed Use

- International Agency for Research on Cancer Working Group on artificial ultraviolet (UV) light and skin cancer (2007). 'The association of use of sunbeds with cutaneous malignant melanoma and other skin cancers: A systematic review.' *Int J Cancer*, 120, p. 1116.
- Autier, P & Boyle, P (2008). 'Artificial ultraviolet sources and skin cancers: rationale for restricting access to sunbed use before 18 years of age'. *Nat Clin Pract Oncol*, 5, p. 178.
- Lazovich, D, Isaksson, Vogel R, Weinstock, MA et al. (2016). 'Association between indoor tanning and melanoma in younger men and women'. *JAMA Dermatol*, 152, p. 268.
- Harrington, CR, Beswick, TC, Leitenberger, J & et al. (2011). 'Addictive-like behaviours to ultraviolet light among frequent indoor tanners'. *Clin Exp Dermatol*, 36, p. 33.
- Petit, A, Lejoyeux, M, Reynaud, M & Karila, L (2014). 'Excessive indoor tanning as a behavioral addiction: a literature review'. *Curr Pharm Des*, 20, p. 4070.
- Mosher, CE & Danoff-Burg, S (2010). 'Addiction to indoor tanning: relation to anxiety, depression, and substance use'. *Arch Dermatol*, 146, p. 412.
- Mays, D, Atkins, MB, Ahn, J & Tercyak, KP (2017). 'Indoor tanning dependence in young adult women'. *Cancer Epidemiol Biomarkers Prev*, 26, p. 1636.

Chemo Prevention of Melanoma

- Demierre, MF & Merlino, G (2004). 'Chemoprevention of melanoma'. *Curr Oncol Rep*, 6, p. 406.
- Freeman, SR, Drake, AL., Heilig, LF et al. (2006). 'Statins, fibrates, and melanoma risk: a systematic review and meta-analysis'. *J Natl Cancer Inst*, 98, p. 1538.

Vitamin D

- Caini, S, Boniol, M, Tosti, G et al. (2014). 'Vitamin D and melanoma and non-melanoma skin cancer risk and prognosis: a comprehensive review and meta-analysis'. *Eur J Cancer*, 50 p. 2649.

Non-Steroidal Anti-Inflammatory Agents

- Curiel-Lewandrowski, C, Nijsten, T, Gomez, ML et al. (2011). 'Long-term use of nonsteroidal anti-inflammatory drugs decreases the risk of cutaneous melanoma: results of a United States case-control study'. *J Invest Dermatol*, 131, p.1460.
- Gamba, CA, Swetter, SM, Stefanick, M et al. (2013). 'Aspirin is associated with lower melanoma risk among postmenopausal Caucasian women: the Women's Health Initiative'. *Cancer*,119, p. 1562.

Lipid Lowering Agents

- Freeman, SR, Drake, AL., Heilig, LF et al. (2006). 'Statins, fibrates, and melanoma risk: a systematic review and meta-analysis'. *J Natl Cancer Inst*, 98, p.1538.
- Bonovas, S, Nikolopoulos, G, Filioussi, K et al. (2010). 'Can statin therapy reduce the risk of melanoma? A meta-analysis of randomized controlled trials'. *Eur J Epidemiol*, 25, p. 29.

Oral Nicotinamide (Vitamin B3)

- Chen, AC, Martin, AJ, Choy, B et al. (2015). 'A phase 3 randomized trial of nicotinamide for skin-cancer chemoprevention'. *N Engl J Med*, 373, p. 1618.

Melanoma Screening and Early Detection

- Kang, S, Barnhill, RL, Mihm, MC Jr et al. (1994). 'Melanoma risk in individuals with clinically atypical nevi'. *Arch Dermatol*, 130, p. 999.
- Mar, V, Wolfe, R & Kelly, JW (2011). 'Predicting melanoma risk for the Australian population'. *Australas J Dermatol*, 52, p. 109.
- Fortes, C, Mastroeni, S, Bakos, L et al. (2010). 'Identifying individuals at high risk of melanoma: a simple tool'. *Eur J Cancer Prev*, 19, p. 393.
- Katalinic, A, Eisemann, N & Waldmann (2015). 'A. Skin cancer screening in Germany. documenting melanoma incidence and mortality from 2008 to 2013'. *Dtsch Arztebl Int*,112, p. 629.
- Katalinic, A, Waldmann, A, Weinstock, MA et al. (2012). 'Does skin cancer screening save lives?:An observational study comparing trends in melanoma mortality in regions with and without screening'. *Cancer*, 118, p. 5395.

Recognising Melanoma

- Grob, JJ & Bonerandi, JJ (1998). 'The "ugly duckling" sign: identification of the common characteristics of nevi in an individual as a basis for melanoma screening'. *Arch Dermatol*, 134, p. 103.
- American Academy of Dermatology Ad Hoc Task Force for the ABCDEs of Melanoma, Tsao, H, Olazagasti, JM et al. (2015). 'Early detection of melanoma: reviewing the ABCDEs'. *J Am Acad Dermatol*, 72, p. 717.
- Aitken, JF., Barbour, A, Burmeister, B, Taylor, S, Walpole, E, Australian Cancer Network, Smithers, BM. & Melanoma Guidelines Revision Working Party (2008) 'Clinical practice guidelines for the management of melanoma in Australia and New Zealand'. Sydney, Australia: Cancer Council Australia; Australian Cancer Network; Ministry of Health, New Zealand.

Bladder Cancer

Bladder Cancer

- Ferlay, J, Soerjomataram, I, Ervik, M et al. (2014). 'GLOBOCAN 2012 v1.0, Cancer incidence and mortality worldwide: IARC Cancer Base No. 11' [Internet]. Lyon, France: IARC.

Factors That Increase the Risk of Urinary Bladder Cancer

Arsenic

- FAO/WHO (2006). 'Summary of evaluations performed by the joint FAO/WHO Expert Committee on Food Additives'.

Smoking

- Secretan B, Straif, K, Baan, R et al. (2009). 'A review of human carcinogens--Part E: tobacco, areca nut, alcohol, coal smoke and salted fish'. *Lancet Oncol*, 10, pp. 1033–4.
- Freedman, ND, Silverman, DT, Hollenbeck, AR et al. (2011). 'Association between smoking and risk of bladder cancer among men and women'. *JAMA*, 306, pp. 737–45.

Infection

- International Agency for Research on Cancer (2014). *World cancer report 2014*. Stewart, BW Stewart & Wild, CP (eds.). IARC Publications/WHO Press. ISBN 978-92-832-0429-9.

Occupational Exposure

- Colt, JS, Karagas, MR, Schwenn, M et al. (2011). 'Occupation and bladder cancer in a population-based case-control study in Northern New England'. *Occup Environ Med*, 68, pp. 239–49.

Genetic Mutations

- Garcia-Closas, M, Malats, N, Silverman, D et al. (2005). 'NAT2 slow acetylation, GSTM1 null genotype, and risk of bladder cancer: results from the Spanish Bladder Cancer Study and meta-analyses'. *Lancet*, 366, pp. 649–59.

Healthy Diet

- Padayatty, SJ, Katz, A, Wang, Y et al. (2003). 'Vitamin C as an antioxidant: evaluation of its role in disease prevention'. *J Am Coll Nutr*, 22, pp. 18–35.

Cruciferous Vegetables

- Abbaoui, B, Riedl, KM, Ralston, RA et al. (2012). 'Inhibition of bladder cancer by broccoli isothiocyanates sulforaphane and erucin: characterization, metabolism and interconversion'. *Molecular Nutrition & Food Research*, 56, p. 10.

Tea

- Yang, CS, Wang, H, Li GX et al. (2011). 'Cancer prevention by tea: evidence from laboratory studies'. *Pharmacol Res*, 64, pp. 113–22.31
- World Cancer Research Fund/American Institute for Cancer Research. 'Bladder cancer report 2015'. Washington DC: AICR.

Brain Tumours

- Howlader, N, Noone, AM, Krapcho, M et al. (2015). *SEER cancer studies review, 1975-2012*. Bethesda: National Cancer Institute.
- Braganza, MZ, Kitahara, CM, Berrington de González, A et al. (2012). 'Ionizing radiation and the risk of brain and central nervous system tumors: a systematic review'. *Neuro Oncol*, 14, p. 1316.
- Bowers, DC, Nathan, PC, Constine, L et al. (2013). 'Subsequent neoplasms of the CNS among survivors of childhood cancer: a systematic review'. *Lancet Oncol*, 14, e321.
- Relling, MV, Rubnitz, JE, Rivera, GK et al. (1999). 'High incidence of secondary brain tumours after radiotherapy and antimetabolites'. *Lancet*, 354, p. 34.
- Pearce, MS, Salotti, JA, Little, MP et al. (2012). 'Radiation exposure from CT scans in childhood and subsequent risk of leukaemia and brain tumours: a retrospective cohort study'. *Lancet*, 380, p. 499.
- Piel C, Pouchieu, C, Tual, S et al. (2017). 'Central nervous system tumors and agricultural exposures in the prospective cohort AGRICAN'. *Int J Cancer*, 141, p. 1771.
- Amirian, ES, Zhou, R, Wrensch, MR et al. (2016). 'Approaching a scientific consensus on the association between allergies and glioma risk: a report from the Glioma International Case-Control Study'. *Cancer Epidemiol Biomarkers Prev*, 25, p. 282.
- Ostrom, QT, Adel Fahmideh, M, Cote, DJ et al. (2019). 'Risk factors for childhood and adult primary brain tumors'. *Neuro Oncol*, 21, p. 1357.
- National Research Council (1981). 'The health effects of nitrate, nitrite, and N-nitroso compounds'. Part 1. Washington DC: National Academy Press.
- Huncharek, M, Kupelnick, B & Wheeler, L (2003). 'Dietary cured meat and the risk of adult glioma: a meta-analysis of nine observational studies'. *J Environ Pathol Toxicol. Oncol*, 22, p. 129.

Ionising Radiation

- Braganza MZ, Kitahara, CM, Berrington de González, A et al. (2012). 'Ionizing radiation and the risk of brain and central nervous system tumors: a systematic review'. *Neuro Oncol*, 14, p. 1316.

Children Who Have Been Exposed to Radiation

- Bowers, DC, Nathan, PC, Constine, L et al. 'Subsequent neoplasms of the CNS among survivors of childhood cancer: a systematic review'. *Lancet Oncol*. 2013; 14:e321.

- Relling, MV, Rubnitz, JE, Rivera, GK et al. (1999). 'High incidence of secondary brain tumours after radiotherapy and antimetabolites'. *Lancet*, 354, p. 34.
- Pearce, MS, Salotti, JA, Little, MP et al. (2012). 'Radiation exposure from CT scans in childhood and subsequent risk of leukaemia and brain tumours: a retrospective cohort study'. *Lancet*, 380, p. 499.
- Davis, F, Il'yasova, D, Rankin, K et al. (2011). 'Medical diagnostic radiation exposures and risk of gliomas'. *Radiat Res*, 175, p. 790.

Genetic Factors

- Ostrom, QT, Adel Fahmideh, M, Cote, DJ et al. (2019). 'Risk factors for childhood and adult primary brain tumors'. *Neuro Oncol*, 21, p.1357.

Familial Glioma

- Malmer, B, Iselius, L, Holmberg, E et al. (2001). 'Genetic epidemiology of glioma'. *Br J Cancer*, 84, p. 429.

Neurofibromatosis Type 2

- Rouleau, GA, Merel, P, Lutchman, M et al. (1993). 'Alteration in a new gene encoding a putative membrane-organizing protein causes neuro-fibromatosis type 2'. *Nature*, 363, p. 515.

Diet

- Davis, FG, Preston-Martin, S (1998). 'Epidemiology'. *Russell and Rubinstein's pathology of tumors of the nervous system* (6th ed.). Bigner DD, McLendon RE, Bruner JM (eds.). London: Arnold. ISBN 0-340-58113-1.
- National Research Council (1981). 'The health effects of nitrate, nitrite, and N-nitroso compounds'. Part 1. Washington DC: National Academy Press.
- Huncharek, M, Kupelnick, B & Wheeler, L (2003). 'Dietary cured meat and the risk of adult glioma: a meta-analysis of nine observational studies'. *J Environ Pathol Toxicol Oncol*, 22, p. 129.

Occupation

- Wong, O & Raabe, GK (1989). 'Critical review of cancer epidemiology in petroleum industry employees, with a quantitative meta-analysis by cancer site'. *Am J Ind Med*, 15, p. 283.
- Khuder, SA, Mutgi, AB & Schaub, EA (1998). 'Meta-analyses of brain cancer and farming'. *Am J Ind Med*, 34, p. 252.

Head Injury

- Burch, JD, Craib, KJ, Choi, BC et al. (1987). 'An exploratory case-control study of brain tumors in adults'. *J Natl Cancer Inst*, 78, p. 601.

Infections

- Schuman, LM, Choi, NW & Gullen, WH (1967). 'Relationship of central nervous system neoplasms to Toxoplasma gondii infection'. *Am J Public Health Nations Health*, 57, p. 848.

The Following Factors Are Known to Reduce the Risk of Brain Tumours

Immune Modulation

- Amirian, ES, Zhou, R, Wrensch, MR et al. (2016). 'Approaching a scientific consensus on the association between allergies and glioma risk: a report from the Glioma International Case-Control Study'. *Cancer Epidemiol Biomarkers Prev*, 25, p. 282.
- Scheurer, ME, El-Zein, R, Thompson, PA et al. (2008). 'Long-term anti-inflammatory and antihistamine medication use and adult glioma risk'. *Cancer Epidemiol Biomarkers Prev*, 17, p. 1277.

Suffering From Allergies

- Ostrom, QT, Adel Fahmideh, M, Cote, DJ et al. (2019). 'Risk factors for childhood and adult primary brain tumors'. *Neuro Oncol*, 21, p. 1357.
- Linos, E, Raine, T, Alonso, A, Michaud, D (2007). 'Atopy and risk of brain tumors: a meta-analysis'. *J Natl Cancer Inst*, 99, p.1544.

Suffering from Colds and Flu

- Calboli, FC, Cox, DG, Buring, JE et al. (2011). 'Prediagnostic plasma IgE levels and risk of adult glioma in four prospective cohort studies'. *J Natl Cancer Inst*, 103 p. 1588.

Consuming Food Rich in Vitamin C and Vitamin E

- McCredie, M, Maisonneuve, P & Boyle P (1994). 'Perinatal and early postnatal risk factors for malignant brain tumours in New South Wales children'. *Int J Cancer*, 56, p. 11.

Pre-Natal Vitamin Supplements

- Preston-Martin, S, Pogoda, JM, Mueller, BA et al. (1998). 'Prenatal vitamin supplementation and risk of childhood brain tumors'. *Int J Cancer Suppl*, 11, p. 17.
- Bunin, GR, Kuijten, RR, Buckley, JD et al. (1993). 'Relation between maternal diet and subsequent primitive neuroectodermal brain tumors in young children'. *N Engl J Med*, 329, p. 536.

Colorectal Cancer

- Ferlay, J SI, Ervik, M et al. (2015). 'GLOBOCAN 2012 v1.2, Cancer Incidence and Mortality Worldwide: IARC CancerBase No. 11' [Internet]. Lyon, France: IARC.

Risk Factors Affecting Colorectal Cancer

Smoking

- Liang, PS, Chen, TY & Giovannucci, E (2009). 'Cigarette smoking and colorectal cancer incidence and mortality: systematic review and meta-analysis'. *Int J Cancer*, 124, pp. 2406–15.

Aspirin

- Rothwell, PM, Wilson, M, Elwin, CE et al. (2010). 'Long-term effect of aspirin on colorectal cancer incidence and mortality: 20-year follow-up of five randomised trials'. *Lancet*, 376, pp. 1741–50.

Hormone Therapy

- Vogtmann E, Xiang, YB, Li, HL et al. (2013). 'Fruit and vegetable intake and the risk of colorectal cancer: results from the Shanghai Men's Health Study'. *Cancer Causes Control*, 24, pp. 1935–45.

Whole Grain

- Kyro, C, Skeie, G, Loft, S et al. (2013). 'Intake of whole grains from different cereal and food sources and incidence of colorectal cancer in the Scandinavian HELGA cohort'. *Cancer Causes Control*, 24, pp. 1363–74.
- McCarl, M, Harnack, L, Limburg, PJ et al. (2006). 'Incidence of colorectal cancer in relation to glycemic index and load in a cohort of women'. *Cancer Epidemiol Biomarkers Prev*, 15, pp. 892–6.
- Larsson, SC, Giovannucci, E, Bergkvist, L et al. (2005). 'Whole grain consumption and risk of colorectal cancer: a population-based cohort of 60,000 women'. *Br J Cancer*, 92, pp. 1803–7.
- Fung, TT, Hu, FB, Wu, K et al. (2010). 'The Mediterranean and Dietary Approaches to Stop Hypertension (DASH) diets and colorectal cancer'. *Am J Clin Nutr*, 92, pp. 1429–35.
- Park, Y, Hunter, DJ, Spiegelman, D et al. (2005). 'Dietary fiber intake and risk of colorectal cancer: a pooled analysis of prospective cohort studies'. *JAMA*, 294, pp. 2849–57.

Foods Containing Dietary Fibre

- Aune, D, Chan, DS, Lau, R et al. (2011). 'Dietary fibre, whole grains, and risk of colorectal cancer: systematic review and dose-response meta-analysis of prospective studies'. *BMJ*, 343, d6617.
- Pi-Sunyer, X (2005). 'Do glycemic index, glycemic load, and fiber play a role in insulin sensitivity, disposition index, and type 2 diabetes?'. *Diabetes Care*, 28, pp. 2978–9.

Non-Starchy Vegetables

- Bamia, C, Lagiou, P, Buckland, G et al. (2013). 'Mediterranean diet and colorectal cancer risk: results from a European cohort'. *Eur J Epidemiol*, 28, pp. 317–28.
- Aoyama, N, Kawado, M, Yamada, H et al. (2014). 'Low intake of vegetables and fruits and risk of colorectal cancer: The Japan Collaborative Cohort Study'. *J Epidemiol*, 24, pp. 353–60.

Fruits

- Vogtmann, E, Xiang, YB, Li, HL et al. (2013). 'Fruit and vegetable intake and the risk of colorectal cancer: results from the Shanghai Men's Health Study'. *Cancer Causes Control*, 24, pp. 1935–45.
- Lu, JM, Lin, PH, Yao, Q et al. (2010). 'Chemical and molecular mechanisms of antioxidants: experimental approaches and model systems'. *J Cell Mol Med*, 14, pp. 840–60.

Vitamin C

- Leenders, M, Leufkens, AM, Siersema, PD et al. (2014). 'Plasma and dietary carotenoids and vitamins A, C and E and risk of colon and rectal cancer in the European prospective investigation into cancer and nutrition'. *Int J Cancer*, 135, pp. 2930–9.
- World Cancer Research Fund/American Institute for Cancer Research 'Colorectal cancer report 2017'. Washington DC: AICR. Page 97.
- Park, Y, Spiegelman, D, Hunter, DJ et al. (2010). 'Intakes of vitamins A, C, and E and use of multiple vitamin supplements and risk of colon cancer: a pooled analysis of prospective cohort studies'. *Cancer Causes Control*, 21, pp. 1745–57.
- 'Effects of vitamins C and E on N-nitroso compound formation, carcinogenesis, and cancer'. *Cancer*. 1986; 58: 1842–50.

Red Meat

- Agnoli, C, Grioni, S, Sieri, S et al. (2012). 'Italian mediterranean index and risk of colorectal cancer in the italian section of the EPIC cohort'. *Int J Cancer*, 132, pp. 1404–11.
- Parr, CL, Hjartaker, A, Lund, E et al. (2013). 'Meat intake, cooking methods, and risk of proximal colon, distal colon, and rectal cancer: The Norwegian Women and Cancer (NOWAC) cohort study'. *Int J Cancer*, 133, pp. 1153–63.
- Wie, GA, Cho, YA, Kang, HH et al. (2014). 'Red meat consumption is associated with an increased overall cancer risk: a prospective cohort study in Korea'. *Br J Nutr*, 112, pp. 238–47.
- Egeberg, R, Olsen, A, Christensen, J et al. (2013). 'Associations between red meat and risks for colon and rectal cancer depend on the type of red meat consumed'. *J Nutr*, 143, pp. 464–72.
- Alexander, DD, Miller, AJ, Cushing, CA et al. (2010). 'Processed meat and colorectal cancer: a quantitative review of prospective epidemiologic studies'. *Eur J Cancer Prev*, 19, pp. 328–41.

Food Containing Heam Iron

- Cross, AJ, Ferrucci, LM, Risch (2010), A et al. 'A large prospective study of meat consumption and colorectal cancer risk: an investigation of potential mechanisms underlying this association'. *Cancer Res*, 70, pp. 2406–14.
- Qiao, L & Feng, Y (2013). 'Intakes of heme iron and zinc and colorectal cancer incidence: a meta- analysis of prospective studies'. *Cancer Causes Control*, 24, pp. 1175–83.

Fish

- Spencer, EA, Key, TJ, Appleby, PN et al. (2010). 'Meat, poultry and fish and risk of colorectal cancer: pooled analysis of data from the UK dietary cohort consortium'. *Cancer Causes Control*, 21, pp. 1417–25.

Dairy Products

- Ralston, RA, Truby, H, Palermo, CE et al. (2014). 'Colorectal cancer and nonfermented milk, solid cheese, and fermented milk consumption: a systematic review and meta-analysis of prospective studies'. *Crit Rev Food Sci Nutr*, 54, pp. 1167–79.

Dietary Calcium

- Murphy, N, Norat, T, Ferrari P et al. (2013). 'Consumption of dairy products and colorectal cancer in the European Prospective Investigation into Cancer and Nutrition (EPIC)'. *PLoS One*, 8: e72715.
- Pierre, FH, Martin, OC, Santarelli, RL et al. (2013). 'Calcium and α-tocopherol suppress cured-meat promotion of chemically induced colon carcinogenesis in rats and reduce associated biomarkers in human volunteers'. *Am J Clin Nutr*, 98, pp.1255–62.

Vitamin D

- Skaaby, T, Husemoen, LL, Thuesen, BH et al. (2014). 'Prospective population-based study of the association between serum 25-hydroxyvitamin-D levels and the incidence of specific types of cancer'. *Cancer Epidemiol Biomarkers Prev*, 23: 1220–9.
- Dou, R, Ng, K, Giovannucci, EL et al. (2016). 'Vitamin D and colorectal cancer: molecular, epidemiological and clinical evidence'. *Br J Nutr*, 115, pp. 1643–60.

Multivitamin Supplements

- Gaziano, JM, Sesso, HD, Christen, WG et al. (2012). 'Multivitamins in the prevention of cancer in men: the Physicians' Health Study II randomized controlled trial'. *JAMA*, 308: pp. 1871–80.
- Hutchinson, J, Burley, VJ, Greenwood, DC et al. (2014). 'General supplement use, subsequent use and cancer risk in the UK Women's Cohort Study'. *Eur J Clin Nutr*, 68, pp. 1095–100.
- Park, SY, Murphy, SP, Wilkens, LR et al. (2011). 'Multivitamin use and the risk of mortality and cancer incidence: the multiethnic cohort study'. *Am J Epidemiol*, 173, pp. 906–14.
- Lee, JE, Willett, WC, Fuchs, CS et al. (2011). 'Folate intake and risk of colorectal cancer and adenoma: modification by time'. *Am J Clin Nutr*, 93, pp. 817–25.
- Heine-Broring, RC, Winkels, RM, Renkema, JM et al. (2015). 'Dietary supplement use and colorectal cancer risk: a systematic review and meta-analyses of prospective cohort studies'. *Int J Cancer*, 136, pp. 2388–401.

Alcohol

- Nan, H, Lee, JE, Rimm, EB et al. (2013). 'Prospective study of alcohol consumption and the risk of colorectal cancer before and after folic acid fortification in the United States'. *Ann Epidemiol*, 23, pp. 558–63.
- Everatt, R, Tamosiunas, A, Virviciute, D et al. (2013). 'Consumption of alcohol and risk of cancer among men: a 30 year cohort study in Lithuania'. *Eur J Epidemiol*, 28, pp. 383–92.
- Aleksandrova, K, Pischon, T, Jenab, M et al. (2014). 'Combined impact of healthy lifestyle factors on colorectal cancer: a large European cohort study'. BMC Med, 12, p. 168.

Physical Activity

- Aleksandrova, K, Pischon, T, Jenab, M et al. (2014). 'Combined impact of healthy lifestyle factors on colorectal cancer: a large European cohort study'. *BMC Med*, 12, p. 168.
- Boyle, T, Keegel, T, Bull, F et al. (2012). 'Physical activity and risks of proximal and distal colon cancers: a systematic review and meta-analysis'. *J Natl Cancer Inst*, 104, pp. 1548–61.

Obesity, Waist Circumference, Waist and Hip Ratio, and Adult Attained Height

- Kabat, GC, Heo, M, Wactawski-Wende, J et al. (2013). 'Body fat and risk of colorectal cancer among postmenopausal women'. *CCC*, 24, pp. 1197–205.
- Morikawa, T, Kuchiba, A, Lochhead, P et al. (2013). 'Prospective analysis of body mass index, physical activity, and colorectal cancer risk associated with beta-catenin (CTNNB1) status'. *Cancer Res*, 73, pp. 1600–10.
- Hughes, LA, Simons, CC, van den Brandt, PA et al. (2011). 'Body size and colorectal cancer risk after 16.3 years of follow-up: an analysis from the Netherlands Cohort Study'. *Am J Epidemiol*, 174, pp. 1127–39.
- Levi, Z, Kark, JD, Barchana, M et al. (2011). 'Measured Body Mass Index in adolescence and the incidence of colorectal cancer in a cohort of 1.1 million males'. *Cancer Epidemiol Biomarkers Prev*, 20, pp. 2524–31.
- Yamamoto, S, Nakagawa, T, Matsushita, Y et al. (2010). 'Visceral fat area and markers of insulin resistance in relation to colorectal neoplasia'. *Diabetes Care*, 33, pp. 184–9.
- Li, H, Yang, G, Xiang, YB et al. (2013). 'Body weight, fat distribution and colorectal cancer risk: a report from cohort studies of 134255 Chinese men and women'. *Int J Obes (Lond)*, 37, pp. 783–9.
- Kabat, GC, Xue, X, Kamensky, V et al. (2015). 'Risk of breast, endometrial, colorectal, and renal cancers in postmenopausal women in association with a body shape index and other anthropometric measures'. *CCC*, 26, pp. 219–229.
- Boursi, B, Haynes, K, Mamtani, R et al. (2014). 'Height as an independent anthropomorphic risk factor for colorectal cancer'. *Eur J Gastroenterol Hepatol*, 26, pp. 1422–7.

Endometrial Cancer

- Ferlay, J, Shin, HR, Bray, F et al. 'GLOBOCAN 2008, Cancer Incidence and Mortality Worldwide: IARC CancerBase No. 10'.

Mechanism of Cancer Development

- Amant, F, Moerman, P, Neven, P et al. (2005). 'Endometrial cancer'. *Lancet*, 366, pp. 491–505.
- Hardiman, P, Pillay, OC & Atiomo, W (2003). 'Polycystic ovary syndrome and endometrial carcinoma'. *Lancet*, 361, pp. 1810–2.

Life Events

- Rieck, G & Fiander, A (2006). 'The effect of lifestyle factors on gynaecological cancer. Best practice & research'. *Clinical Obstetrics & Gynaecology*, 20, pp. 227–51.

Medication

- IARC Working Group on the Evaluation of Carcinogenic Risks to Humans (1999). *Hormonal contraception and post-menopausal hormonal therapy (IARC monogr eval carcinog risks hum, 72)*. IARC Publications/WHO Press. ISBN 92-832-1272-X.

Glycaemic Load

- George, SM, Mayne, ST, Leitzmann, MF et al. (2009). Dietary glycemic index, glycemic load, and risk of cancer: a prospective cohort study'. *Am J Epidemiol*, 169, pp. 462–72.
- Cui, X, Rosner, B, Willett, WC et al. (2011). 'Dietary fat, fiber, and carbohydrate intake in relation to risk of endometrial cancer'. *Cancer Epidemiol Biomarkers Prev*, 20, pp. 978–89.
- Gnagnarella, P, Gandini, S, La, VC et al. (2008). 'Glycemic index, glycemic load, and cancer risk: a meta- analysis'. *Am J Clin Nutr*, 87, pp. 1793–801.
- World Cancer Research Fund/American Institute for Cancer Research. 'Endometrial cancer report 2013.' Washington DC: AICR. Page 27.
- World Cancer Research Fund/American Institute for Cancer Research. 'Endometrial cancer report 2013.' Washington DC: AICR. Page 27.

Coffee

- Nilsson, LM, Johansson, I, Lenner, P et al. (2010). 'Consumption of filtered and boiled coffee and the risk of incident cancer: a prospective cohort study'. *Cancer Causes Control*, 21, pp. 1533–44.
- Yu, X, Bao, Z, Zou, J et al. (2011). 'Coffee consumption and risk of cancers: a meta-analysis of cohort studies'. *BMC Cancer*, 11, p. 96.
- Je, Y & Giovannucci, E (2012). 'Coffee consumption and risk of endometrial cancer: findings from a large up-to-date meta-analysis'. *Int J Cancer*, 131, pp. 700–10.
- Bravi, F, Scotti, L, Bosetti, C et al. (2009). 'Coffee drinking and endometrial cancer risk: a metaanalysis of observational studies'. *Am J Obstet Gynecol*, 200, pp. 130–5.

Physical Activity

- Friedenreich, C, Cust, A, Lahmann, PH et al. (2007). 'Physical activity and risk of endometrial cancer: the European prospective investigation into cancer and nutrition'. *Int J Cancer*, 121, pp. 347–55.
- Conroy, MB, Sattelmair, JR, Cook, NR et al. (2009). 'Physical activity, adiposity, and risk of endometrial cancer'. *Cancer Causes Control*, 20, pp. 1107–15.
- Friberg, E, Mantzoros, CS & Wolk, A (2006). 'Physical activity and risk of endometrial cancer: a population-based prospective cohort study'. *Cancer Epidemiol Biomarkers Prev*, 15, pp. 2136–40.
- Gierach, GL, Chang, SC, Brinton, LA et al. (2009). 'Physical activity, sedentary behavior, and endometrial cancer risk in the NIH-AARP Diet and Health Study'. *Int J Cancer*, 124, pp. 2139–47.
- McTiernan, A (2008). 'Mechanisms linking physical activity with cancer'. Nat Rev Cancer, 8, pp. 205–11.
- Kaaks, R, Lukanova, A & Kurzer, MS (2002). 'Obesity, endogenous hormones, and endometrial cancer risk: a synthetic review'. *Cancer Epidemiol Biomarkers Prev*, 11, pp. 1531–43.

Sedentary Habits

- Patel, AV, Feigelson, HS, Talbot, JT et al. (2008). 'The role of body weight in the relationship between physical activity and endometrial cancer: results from a large cohort of US women'. *Int J Cancer*, 123, pp. 1877–82.
- Moore, SC, Gierach, GL, Schatzkin, A et al. (2010). 'Physical activity, sedentary behaviours, and the prevention of endometrial cancer'. *Br J Cancer*, 103, pp. 933–8.
- World Cancer Research Fund/American Institute for Cancer Research. 'Endometrial cancer report 2013.' Washington DC: AICR
- Healy, GN, Wijndaele, K, Dunstan, DW et al. (2008). 'Objectively measured sedentary time, physical activity, and metabolic risk: the Australian Diabetes, Obesity and Lifestyle Study (AusDiab)'. *Diabetes Care*, 31, pp. 369–71.
- Helmerhorst, HJ, Wijndaele, K, Brage, S et al. (2009). 'Objectively measured sedentary time may predict insulin resistance independent of moderate- and vigorous-intensity physical activity'. *Diabetes Care*, 58, pp. 1776–9.

BMI – Body Mass Index

- Bjorge, T, Engeland, A, Tretli, S et al. (2007). 'Body size in relation to cancer of the uterine corpus in 1 million Norwegian women'. *Int J Cancer*, 120, pp. 378–83.
- Lundqvist, E, Kaprio, J, Verkasalo, PK et al. (2007). 'Co-twin control and cohort analyses of body mass index and height in relation to breast, prostate, ovarian, corpus uteri, colon and rectal cancer among Swedish and Finnish twins'. *Int J Cancer*, 121, pp. 810–8.
- Reeves, GK, Pirie, K, Beral, V et al. (2007). 'Cancer incidence and mortality in relation to body mass index in the Million Women Study: cohort study'. *BMJ*, 335, p. 1134.
- Park, SL, Goodman, MT, Zhang, ZF et al. (2010). 'Body size, adult BMI gain and endometrial cancer risk: the multiethnic cohort'. *Int J Cancer*, 126, pp. 490–9.

Waist/Hip Ratio

- Westley, RL & May, FE (2013). 'A twenty-first century cancer epidemic caused by obesity: the involvement of insulin, diabetes, and insulin-like growth factors'. *International Journal of Endocrinology*, 2013, 632461.
- Rexrode, KM, Pradhan, A, Manson, JE et al. (2003). 'Relationship of total and abdominal adiposity with CRP and IL-6 in women'. *Ann Epidemiol*, 13, pp. 674–82.

Adult Attained Height

- Friedenreich, C, Cust, A, Lahmann, PH et al. (2007). 'Anthropometric factors and risk of endometrial cancer: the European prospective investigation into cancer and nutrition'. *Cancer Causes Control*, 18, pp. 399–413.
- Sung, J, Song, YM, Lawlor, DA et al. (2009). 'Height and site-specific cancer risk: A cohort study of a korean adult population'. *Am J Epidemiol*, 170, pp. 53–64.
- Kabat, GC, Heo, M, Kamensky, V et al. (2013). 'Adult height in relation to risk of cancer in a cohort of Canadian women'. *Int J Cancer*, 132, pp. 1125–32.

Gall Bladder Cancer

- Ferlay, J, Soerjomataram, I, Ervik, M, et al. (2014). 'GLOBOCAN 2012 v1.0, Cancer incidence and mortality worldwide: IARC Cancer Base No. 11' [Internet]. Lyon, France: IARC.

Mechanism of Cancer Development (Pathogenesis)

- World Cancer Research Fund/American Institute for Cancer Research (2007). 'Food, nutrition, physical activity, and the prevention of cancer: a global perspective'. Washington DC: AICR.
- Randi, G, Franceschi, S & La Vecchia, C (2006). 'Gallbladder cancer worldwide: geographical distribution and risk factors'. *Int J Cancer*, 118, pp. 1591–602.

Risk Factors Associated with Gall Bladder Cancer

Increased BMI

- Samanic, C, Chow, WH, Gridley, G et al. (2006). 'Relation of body mass index to cancer risk in 362,552 Swedish men'. *Cancer Causes Control*, 17, pp. 901–9.
- Fujino, Y (2007). 'Anthropometry, development history and mortality in the Japan Collaborative Cohort Study for Evaluation of Cancer (JACC)'. *Asian Pac J Cancer Prev*, 8 Suppl, pp. 105–12.

- Schlesinger, S, Aleksandrova, K, Pischon, T et al. (2013). 'Abdominal obesity, weight gain during adulthood and risk of liver and biliary tract cancer in a European cohort'. *Int J Cancer*, 132, pp. 645–57.
- Whitlock, G, Lewington, S, Sherliker, P et al. (2009). 'Body mass index and cause-specific mortality in 900 000 adults: collaborative analyses of 57 prospective studies'. *Lancet*, 373, pp. 1083–96.
- Renehan, AG, Tyson, M, Egger, M et al. (2008). 'Body-mass index and incidence of cancer: a systematic review and meta-analysis of prospective observational studies'. *Lancet*, 371, pp. 569–78.
- Larsson, SC & Wolk, A (2007). 'Obesity and the risk of gallbladder cancer: a meta-analysis'. *Br J Cancer*, 96, pp. 1457–61.

Gastric Cancer

- Ferlay, J, Soerjomataram, I, Ervik, M et al. (2014). 'GLOBOCAN 2012 v1.0, Cancer incidence and mortality worldwide: IARC Cancer Base No. 11' [Internet]. Lyon, France: IARC.
- Ang, TL & Fock, KM (2014). 'Clinical epidemiology of gastric cancer'. *Singapore Med J*; 55, pp. 621–8.
- International Agency for Research on Cancer (2014). *World cancer report 2014*. Stewart, BW & Wild, CP (eds.). IARC Publications/WHO Press. ISBN 978-92-832-0429-9.

Causes of Stomach Cancer

Infection and Infestation

- Ang, TL & Fock, KM (2014). 'Clinical epidemiology of gastric cancer'. *Singapore Med J*; 55, pp. 621–8.
- Ando, T, Goto, Y, Maeda, O et al. (2006). 'Causal role of Helicobacter pylori infection in gastric cancer'. *World J Gastroenterol*, 12, pp. 181–6.
- Ley, C, Mohar, A, Guarner, J et al. (2004). 'Helicobacter pylori eradication and gastric preneoplastic conditions: a randomized, double-blind, placebo-controlled trial'. *Cancer Epidemiol Biomarkers Prev*, 13, pp. 4–10.
- Wu, CY, Kuo, KN, Wu, MS et al. (2009). 'Early Helicobacter pylori eradication decreases risk of gastric cancer in patients with peptic ulcer disease'. *Gastroenterology*, 137, pp. 1641–8.

EBV Infection

- Iizasam, H, Nanbo, A, Nishikawa, J et al. (2012). 'Epstein-Barr Virus (EBV)-associated gastric carcinoma'. *Viruses*, 4, pp. 3420–39.

Genetic Predisposition

- International Agency for Research on Cancer (2014). *World cancer report 2014*. Stewart, BW & Wild, CP (eds.). Lyon, France: IARC Publications/WHO Press. ISBN 978-92-832-0429-9.

Tobacco Use

- International Agency for Research on Cancer (2012). *Personal habits and indoor combustions. A review of human carcinogens (IARC monogr eval carcinog risks hum, 100E)*. Lyon, France: IARC Publications/WHO Press. ISBN 978-92-832-1322-2.
- Tredaniel, J, Boffetta, P, Buiatti, E et al. (1997). 'Tobacco smoking and gastric cancer: review and meta- analysis'. Int J Cancer, 72, pp. 565–73.

Industrial Chemical Exposure

- Welling, R, Beaumont, JJ, Petersen, SJ et al. (2015). 'Chromium VI and stomach cancer: a meta-analysis of the current epidemiological evidence'. *Occup Environ Med*, 72, pp. 151–9.

Low Fruit Intake

- Gonzalez, CA, Lujan-Barroso, L, Bueno-de-Mesquita, HB et al. (2012). 'Fruit and vegetable intake and the risk of gastric adenocarcinoma: a reanalysis of the European Prospective Investigation into Cancer and Nutrition (EPIC-EURGAST) study after a longer follow-up.' *Int J Cancer*, 131, pp. 2910–9.
- Wang Q, Chen Y, Wang X et al. (2014). 'Consumption of fruit, but not vegetables, may reduce risk of gastric cancer: results from a meta-analysis of cohort studies'. *Eur J Cancer*, 50, pp. 1498– 509.

Citrus Fruits

- Freedman, ND, Subar, AF, Hollenbeck, AR et al. (2008). 'Fruit and vegetable intake and gastric cancer risk in a large United States prospective cohort study'. *Cancer Causes Control*, 19, pp. 459–67.

Food Preserved by Salting

- Kurosawa, M, Kikuchi, S, Xu J et al. (2006). 'Highly salted food and mountain herbs elevate the risk for stomach cancer death in a rural area of Japan'. *J Gastroenterol Hepatol*, 21, pp. 1681–6.
- Takachi, R, Inoue, M, Shimazu, T et al. (2010). 'Consumption of sodium and salted foods in relation to cancer and cardiovascular disease: the Japan Public Health Center-based Prospective Study'. *Am J Clin Nutr*, 91, pp. 456–64.
- Galanis, DJ, Kolonel, LN, Lee J et al. (1998). 'Intakes of selected foods and beverages and the incidence of gastric cancer among the Japanese residents of Hawaii: a prospective study'. *Int J Epidemiol*, 27, pp. 173–80.
- Jagerstad M & Skog, K (2005). *Genotoxicity of heat-processed foods*. Mutat Res, 74: pp. 156–72.

Processed Meat

- González, CA, Jakszyn, P, Pera, G et al. (2006). 'Meat intake and risk of stomach and esophageal adenocarcinoma within the European Prospective Investigation into Cancer and Nutrition (EPIC)'. J Nat Cancer Inst, 98, pp. 345–54.
- Iso, H & Kubota, Y (2007). 'Nutrition and disease in the Japan Collaborative Cohort Study for Evaluation of Cancer (JACC)'. *Asian Pac J Cancer Prev*, 8 Suppl, pp. 35–80.
- Zhu, H, Yang, X, Zhang, C et al. (2013). 'Red and processed meat intake is associated with higher gastric cancer risk: a meta-analysis of epidemiological observational studies'. *PLoS One*, 8, e70955.

Alcoholic Drinks

- Sjodahl, K, Lu, Y, Nilsen, TI et al. (2007). 'Smoking and alcohol drinking in relation to risk of gastric cancer: a population-based, prospective cohort study'. *Int J Cancer*, 120, pp. 128–32.
- Everatt, R, Tamosiunas, A, Kuzmickiene, I et al. (2012). 'Alcohol consumption and risk of gastric cancer: a cohort study of men in Kaunas, Lithuania, with up to 30 years follow-up'. *BMC*, 12, p. 475.
- Sung, NY, Choi, KS, Park, EC et al. (2007). 'Smoking, alcohol and gastric cancer risk in Korean men: The National Health Insurance Corporation Study'. *Br J, Cancer*, 97, pp. 700–4.

- Tramacere, I, Negri, E, Pelucchi, C et al. (2012). 'A meta-analysis on alcohol drinking and gastric cancer risk'. *Ann Oncol*, 23, pp. 28–36.

Grilled (Broiled) and Barbequed (Charboiled) Animal Foods

- Ikeda, M, Yoshimoto, K, Yoshimura, T et al. (1983). 'A cohort study on the possible association between broiled fish intake and cancer'. *Gan*, 74, pp. 640–8.
- Kato, I, Tominaga, S & Matsumoto, K (1992). 'A prospective study of stomach cancer among a rural Japanese population: a 6-year survey'. *Jpn J Cancer Res*, 83, pp. 568–75.
- Skog, KI, Johansson, MA & Jagerstad, MI (1998). 'Carcinogenic heterocyclic amines in model systems and cooked foods: a review on formation, occurrence and intake'. *Food Chem Toxicol*, 36, pp. 879–96.

Increased BMI

- O'Doherty, MG, Freedman, ND, Hollenbeck, AR et al. (2012). 'A prospective cohort study of obesity and risk of oesophageal and gastric adenocarcinoma in the NIH-AARP Diet and Health Study'. Gut, 61, pp. 1261–8.
- Hampel, H, Abraham, NS & El-Serag, HB (2005). 'Meta-analysis: obesity and the risk for gastroesophageal reflux disease and its complications'. *Ann Intern Med*; 143: 199–211.

Kidney Cancer

- Ferlay J, Soerjomataram I, Dikshit, R et al. (2015). 'Cancer incidence and mortality worldwide: sources, methods and major patterns in GLOBOCAN 2012'. *Int J Cancer*, 136, E359–86.

Risk Factors For Developing Kidney Cancer

Genetic Factors

- Meister, M, Choyke, P, Anderson, C et al. (2009). 'Radiological evaluation, management, and surveillance of renal masses in Von Hippel-Lindau disease'. *Clin Radiol*, 64, pp. 589–600.

Polycystic Kidney Disease

- Marple, JT, MacDougall, M & Chonko, AM (1994). 'Renal cancer complicating acquired cystic kidney disease'. *J Am Soc Nephrol*, 4, pp. 1951–6.

Medication

- Gago-Dominguez, M, Yuan, JM, Castelao, JE et al. (1999). 'Regular use of analgesics is a risk factor for renal cell carcinoma'. *Br J Cancer*, 81, pp. 542–8.

Smoking

- Gandini, S, Botteri, E, Iodice, S et al. (2008). 'Tobacco smoking and cancer: a meta-analysis'. *Int J Cancer*, 122, pp. 155–64.
- Hunt, JD, van der Hel, OL, McMillan, GP et al. (2005). 'Renal cell carcinoma in relation to cigarette smoking: meta-analysis of 24 studies'. *Int J Cancer*, 114, pp. 101–8.

High Blood Pressure

- Chow, WH, Dong, LM & Devesa, SS (2010). 'Epidemiology and risk factors for kidney cancer'. *Nat Rev Urol*, 7, 245–57.

Increased Weight

- Haggstrom, C, Rapp, K, Stocks, T et al. (2013). 'Metabolic factors associated with risk of renal cell carcinoma'. *P Lo S One*, 8, e57475.
- Parr, CL, Batty, GD, Lam, TH et al. (2010). 'Body-mass index and cancer mortality in the Asia-Pacific Cohort Studies Collaboration: pooled analyses of 424,519 participants'. *Lancet Oncol*, 11, pp. 741–52.
- Renehan, AG, Tyson, M, Egger, M et al. (2008). 'Body-mass index and incidence of cancer: a systematic review and meta-analysis of prospective observational studies'. *Lancet*, 371, pp. 569–78.
- Abdullah, A, Peeters, A, de Courten, M et al. (2010). 'The magnitude of association between overweight and obesity and the risk of diabetes: a meta-analysis of prospective cohort studies'. *Diabetes Res Clin Pract*, 89, pp. 309–19.

Arsenic

- International Agency for Research on Cancer (2012). *Arsenic, metals, fibres, and dusts (IARC monogr eval carcinog risks hum, 100C)*. Lyon, France: IARC Publications/WHO Press. Pages 11–465. ISBN 978-92-832-1320-8.

Factors Reducing the Risk Of Kidney Cancer

Drinking Alcohol

- Lee, JE, Hunter, DJ, Spiegelman, D et al. (2007). 'Alcohol intake and renal cell cancer in a pooled analysis of 12 prospective studies'. *J Natl Cancer Inst*, 99, pp. 801–10.

Hepatocellular Carcinoma – Liver Cancer

- Ferlay J, Soerjomataram, I, Ervick, M at al. (2015), 'GOLBOCAN 2012 v1.2. Cancer Incidence and Mortality Worldwide'. *IARC CancerBase*, No. 11'.

Alcohol

- Pessione, F, Degos, F, Marcellin, P et al. (1998). 'Effect of alcohol consumption on serum hepatitis C virus RNA and histological lesions in chronic hepatitis C'. *Hepatology*, 27, pp. 1717–22.
- Seitz, HK & Stickel, F (2006). 'Risk factors and mechanisms of hepatocarcinogenesis with special emphasis on alcohol and oxidative stress'. *Biol Chem*, 387, pp. 349–60.

Toxins

- Eaton, DL, Ramsdell, HS & Neal, G (1994). 'Biotransformation of aflatoxins'. *The toxicology of aflatoxins: human health, veterinary and agricultural significance*. Eaton, DL & Groopman, JD (eds.). San Diego: Academic Press. ISBN 0-12-228255-8.

Smoking

- Secretan, B, Straif, K, Baan, R et al. (2009). 'A review of human carcinogens-Part E: tobacco, areca nut, alcohol, coal smoke and salted fish'. *Lancet Oncol*, 10, pp. 1033–4.

Obesity

- Alzahrani, B, Iseli, TJ & Hebbard, LW (2014). 'Non-viral causes of liver cancer: does obesity led inflammation play a role?'. *Cancer Lett*, 345, pp. 223–9.

Physical Activity

- Behrens, G, Matthews, CE, Moore, SC et al. (2013). 'The association between frequency of vigorous physical activity and hepatobiliary cancers in the NIH-AARP Diet and Health Study'. *EurJ Epidemiol*, 28, pp. 55–66.

Coffee

- Bohn, SK, Blomhoff, R & Paur, I (2014). 'Coffee and cancer risk, epidermiological evidence and molecular mechanisms'. *Mol Nutr Food Res*, 58, pp. 915–30.

Aspirin

- Simon, Tracy G, Duberg, Ann-Sofi et al. (12 March 2020). 'Association of Aspirin with hepatocellular carcinoma and liver related mortality'. *New England Journal of Medicine*; 382, pp. 1018–28.

Lung Cancer

- Ferlay, J, Soerjomataram, I, Ervik M et al. (2015). 'GLOBOCAN 2012 v1.2, Cancer incidence and mortality worldwide: IARC CancerBase, No. 11' [Internet]. Lyon, France: IARC.
- Lam, WK, White, NW & Chan-Yeung, MM (2004). 'Lung cancer epidemiology and risk factors in Asia and Africa'. *Int J Tuberc Lung Dis*, 8, pp. 1045–57.
- Allemani C, Weir, HK, Carreira, H et al. (2015). 'Global surveillance of cancer survival 1995-2009: analysis of individual data for 25,676,887 patients from 279 population-based registries in 67 countries (CONCORD-2)'. *Lancet*, 385, pp. 977–1010.
- Taylor, R, Najafi, F & Dobson, A (2007). 'Meta-analysis of studies of passive smoking and lung cancer: effects of study type and continent'. *Int J Epidemiol*, 36, pp. 1048–59.

Mechanism of Lung Cancer

- Brenner, DR, Boffetta, P, Duell, EJ et al. (2012). 'Previous lung diseases and lung cancer risk: a pooled analysis from the International Lung Cancer Consortium'. *Am J Epidemiol*, 176, pp. 573–85.
- Sawada, N, Iwasaki, M, Inoue, M et al. (2013). 'Dietary arsenic intake and subsequent risk of cancer: the Japan Public Health Center-based (JPHC) Prospective Study'. *Cancer Causes Control*, 24, pp. 1403–15.

Smoking

- Pesch, B, Kendzia, B, Gustavsson, P et al. (2012). 'Cigarette smoking and lung cancer--relative risk estimates for the major histological types from a pooled analysis of case-control studies'. *Int J Cancer*, 131, pp. 1210–9.
- Bray, FI & Weiderpass, E (2010). 'Lung cancer mortality trends in 36 European countries: secular trends and birth cohort patterns by sex and region 1970-2007'. *Int J Cancer*, 126, pp. 1454–66.

Arsenic

- Chen, CL, Chiou, HY, Hsu, LI et al. (2010). 'Ingested arsenic, characteristics of well water consumption and risk of different histological types of lung cancer in northeastern Taiwan'. *Environ Res*, 110, pp. 455–62.
- Baastrup, R, Sorensen, M, Balstrom, T et al. (2008). 'Arsenic in drinking-water and risk for cancer in Denmark'. *Environ Health Perspect*, 116, pp. 231–7.

Beta Kertatine

- Lin, J, Cook, NR, Albert, C et al. (2009). 'Vitamins C and E and beta carotene supplementation and cancer risk: a randomized controlled trial'. *J Natl Cancer Inst*, 101, pp. 14–23
- Roswall, N, Olsen, A, Christensen, J et al. (2009). 'Source-specific effects of micronutrients in lung cancer prevention'. *Lung Cancer*, 67, pp. 275–81.
- Satia, JA, Littman, A, Slatore, CG et al. (2009). 'Long-term use of beta-carotene, retinol, lycopene, and lutein supplements and lung cancer risk: results from the VITamins And Lifestyle (VITAL) study'. *Am J Epidemiol*,169, pp. 815–28.

Vegetables

- Bradbury, KE, Appleby, PN & Key, TJ (2014). 'Fruit, vegetable, and fiber intake in relation to cancer risk: findings from the European Prospective Investigation into Cancer and Nutrition (EPIC)'. *Am J Clin Nutr*, 100, pp. 394S–8S.
- Gnagnarella, P, Maisonneuve, P, Bellomi, M et al. (2013). 'Nutrient intake and nutrient patterns and risk of lung cancer among heavy smokers: results from the COSMOS screening study with annual low- dose CT'. *Eur J Epi*, 28, pp. 503–11b.

Fruits

- Takata, Y, Cai, Q, Beeghly-Fadiel, A et al. (2012). 'Dietary B vitamin and methionine intakes and lung cancer risk among female never smokers in China'. *Cancer Causes Control*, 23, pp. 1965–75.
- Kabat, GC, Miller, AB et al. (2008). 'Dietary intake of selected B vitamins in relation to risk of major cancers in women'. *Br J Cancer*, 99, pp. 816-21a.

Foods Containing Carotenoids

- Takata, Y, Xiang, YB, Yang, G et al. (2013). 'Intakes of fruits, vegetables, and related vitamins and lung cancer risk: results from the Shanghai Men's Health Study (2002-2009)'. *Nutr Cancer*, 65, pp. 51–61.

Vitamin C in Food

- Terry, P, Lagergren, J, Ye, W, et al. (2000). 'Antioxidants and cancers of the esophagus and gastric cardia'. *Int J Cancer*, 87, pp. 750–4.
- Lee, KW, Lee, HJ, Surh, YJ et al. (2003). 'Vitamin C and cancer chemoprevention: reappraisal'. *Am J Clin Nutr*, 78, pp. 1074–8.

Food with Isoflavones

- Wu, SH & Liu, Z (2013). 'Soy food consumption and lung cancer risk: a meta-analysis using a common measure across studies'. *Nutr Cancer*, 65, pp. 625–32.

Red Meat

- World Cancer Research Fund/American Institute for Cancer Research (2007). 'Food, nutrition, physical activity, and the prevention of cancer: a global perspective'. Washington DC: AICR.

Processed Meat

- Linseisen, J, Rohrmann, S, Bueno-de-Mesquita, B et al. (2011). 'Consumption of meat and fish and risk of lung cancer: results from the European Prospective Investigation into Cancer and Nutrition'. *Cancer Causes Control*, 22, pp. 909–18.
- Tasevska, N, Sinha, R, Kipnis, V et al. (2009). 'A prospective study of meat, cooking methods, meat mutagens, heme iron, and lung cancer risks'. *Am J Clin Nutr*, 89, pp. 1884–94.

Foods Containing Retinol

- Epplein, M, Franke, AA, Cooney, RV et al. (2009). 'Association of plasma micronutrient levels and urinary isoprostane with risk of lung cancer: the multiethnic cohort study'. *Cancer Epidemiol Biomarkers Prev*, 18, pp. 1962–70.

Alcoholic Drinks

- World Cancer Research Fund/American Institute for Cancer Research (2007). 'Food, nutrition, physical activity, and the prevention of cancer: a global perspective'. Washington DC: AICR.
- Jung, EJ, Shin, A, Park, SK et al. (2012). 'Alcohol consumption and mortality in the Korean Multi-Center Cancer Cohort Study'. *J Prev Med Public Health*, 45, pp. 301–8.
- Chao, C, Li, Q, Zhang, F et al. (2011). 'Alcohol consumption and risk of lung cancer in the VITamins And Lifestyle Study'. Nutr Cancer, 63, pp. 880–8.64
- World Cancer Research Fund/American Institute for Cancer Research. 'Lung cancer report 2017'. Washington DC: AICR.
- Kim, MK, Ko, MJ, Han, JT et al. (2010). 'Alcohol consumption and mortality from all-cause and cancers among 1.34 million Koreans: the results from the Korea national health insurance corporation's health examinee cohort in 2000'. *Cancer Causes Control*, 21, pp. 2295–302.
- Ozasa, K (2007). 'Alcohol use and mortality in the Japan Collaborative Cohort Study for Evaluation of Cancer (JACC)'. Asian Pac J Cancer Prev, 8 Suppl, pp. 81–8.

Physical Activity

- Sun, JY, Shi, L, Gao, XD et al. (2012). 'Physical activity and risk of lung cancer: a meta-analysis of prospective cohort studies'. *Asian Pac J Cancer Prev*, 13 pp. 3143–7.

Oesophageal Cancer

- Ferlay, J, Soerjomataram, I, Ervik, M et al. (2014). 'GLOBOCAN 2012 v1.0, Cancer incidence and mortality worldwide: IARC Cancer Base No. 11' [Internet]. Lyon, France: IARC.

Mechanism of Cancer Developing

- Rubenstein, JH & Taylor, JB (2010). 'Meta-analysis: the association of oesophageal adenocarcinoma with symptoms of gastro-oesophageal reflux'. *Aliment Pharmacol Ther*, 32, pp. 1222-7.

Risk Factors for Oesophageal Cancer

Barrett's Oesophagus

- Hvid-Jensen, F, Pedersen, L, Drewes, AM et al. (2011). 'Incidence of adenocarcinoma among patients with Barrett's esophagus'. *N Engl J Med*, 365, pp. 1375–83.

Oesophageal Achalasia

- Leeuwenburgh, I, Scholten, P, Alderliesten, J et al. (2010). 'Long-term esophageal cancer risk in patients with primary achalasia: a prospective study'. *Am J Gastroenterol*, 105, pp. 2144–9.

Tylosis A, Plummer-Vinson Syndrome

- Novacek, G (2006). 'Plummer-Vinson syndrome'. *Orphanet J Rare Dis*, 1, p. 36.

Tobacco Use

- Parkin, DM, Boyd, L & Walker, LC (2011). '16. The fraction of cancer attributable to lifestyle and environmental factors in the UK in 2010'. *Br J Cancer*, 105, Suppl 2: S77–81.
- IARC Working Group on the Evaluation of Carcinogenic Risks to Humans (2004). *Betel-quid and areca-nut chewing and some areca-nut derived nitrosamines (IARC monogr eval carcinog risks hum, 85)*. Lyon, France: IARC Publications/WHO Press. Pages 1–334. ISBN 92-832-1272-X.

Infection with Human Papilloma Virus

- Ludmir, EB, Stephens, SJ, Palta, M et al. (2015). 'Human papillomavirus tumor infection in esophageal squamous cell carcinoma'. *J Gastrointest Oncol*, 6, pp. 287–95.

Vegetables

- World Cancer Research Fund/American Institute for Cancer Research (2007). 'Food, nutrition, physical activity, and the prevention of cancer: a global perspective'. Washington DC: AICR.
- Liu, J, Wang, J, Leng, Y et al. (2013). 'Intake of fruit and vegetables and risk of esophageal squamous cell carcinoma: a meta-analysis of observational studies'. *Int J Cancer*, 133, pp. 473–85.

Fruit

- Liu, J, Wang, J, Leng, Y et al. (2013). 'Intake of fruit and vegetables and risk of esophageal squamous cell carcinoma: a meta-analysis of observational studies'. *Int J Cancer*, 133, pp. 473–85.

Processed Meat

- Choi, Y, Song, S, Song, Y et al. (2013). 'Consumption of red and processed meat and esophageal cancer risk: meta-analysis'. *World J Gastroenterol*, 19, pp. 1020–9.

Mate

- International Agency for Research on Cancer/World Health Organization (1991) *Coffee, tea, mate, methylxanthines and methylglyoxal (IARC monographs on the evaluation of carcinogenic risks to humans. Volume 51)*. Lyon, France: IARC Publications/WHO Press. ISBN 978-92-832-1251-5. Available at: http://monographs.iarc.fr/ENG/Monographs/vol51/mono51.pdf.
- Andrici, J & Eslick, GD (2013). 'Mate consumption and the risk of esophageal squamous cell arcinoma: a meta-analysis'. *DisEsophagus*, 26, pp. 807–16.

Drinking Hot Beverages

- Loomis, D, Guyton, KZ, Grosse, Y et al. (2016), 'Carcinogenicity of drinking coffee, mate and very hot beverages'. *Lancet Oncol*, 17, pp. 877–8

Alcoholic Drinks

- Steevens, J, Schouten, LJ, Goldbohm, RA et al. (2010). 'Alcohol consumption, cigarette smoking and risk of subtypes of oesophageal and gastric cancer: a prospective cohort study'. *Gut*; 59, pp. 39–48.
- Oze,, I, Matsuo, K, Wakai, K et al. (2011). 'Alcohol drinking and esophageal cancer risk: an evaluation based on a systematic review of epidemiologic evidence among the Japanese population'. *Jpn J Clin Oncol*, 41, pp. 677–92.

Physical Activity

- Chen, Y, Yu, C, & Li Y (2014). 'Physical activity and risks of esophageal and gastric cancers: a meta- analysis'. *PLoSOne*, 9, e88082.
- Friedenreich, CM, Neilson, HK & Lynch, BM (2010). 'State of the epidemiological evidence on physical activity and cancer prevention'. *Eur J Cancer*, 46, pp. 2593–604.

Metabolic Syndrome and Insulin Resistance

- Singh, S, Sharma, AN, Murad, MH et al. (2013). 'Central adiposity is associated with increased risk of esophageal inflammation, metaplasia, and adenocarcinoma: a systematic review and meta- analysis'. *Clin Gastroenterol Hepatol*, 11, pp. 1399–412.e7.

BMI

- Merry, AH, Schouten, LJ, Goldbohm, RA et al. (2007). 'Body mass index, height and risk of adenocarcinoma of the oesophagus and gastric cardia: a prospective cohort study'. *Gut*, 56, pp. 1503–11.

Waist Circumference

- Steffen, A, Schulze, MB, Pischon, T et al. (2009). 'Anthropometry and esophageal cancer risk in the European prospective investigation into cancer and nutrition'. *Cancer EpidemiolBiomarkers Prev*, 18, pp. 2079–89.

Central Obesity

- Singh, S, Sharma, AN, Murad, MH et al. (2013). 'Central adiposity is associated with increased risk of esophageal inflammation, metaplasia, and adenocarcinoma: a systematic review and meta- analysis'. *Clin GastroenterolHepatol*, 11, pp. 1399–412.

Waist/Hip Ratio

- Lagergren, J (2011). 'Influence of obesity on the risk of esophageal disorders'. *Nat Rev Gastroenterol Hepatol*; 8, pp. 340–7.

Ovarian Cancer

Mechanism of Ovarian Cancer

- Kufe, D et al. (2003). *Holland-Frei cancer medicine (*6th ed.). Hamilton, Ontario: BC Decker. ISBN 1-55009-213-8.
- Bell, DA (2005). 'Origins and molecular pathology of ovarian cancer'. *Mod Pathol*, 18, Suppl 2, pp. S19–32.

Risk Factors for Ovarian Cancers

Life Events

- Jordan, SJ., Webb & Green, AC (2005). 'Height, age at menarche, and risk of epithelial ovarian cancer'. *Cancer Epidemiol Biomarkers Prev*, 14 (8), pp. 2045–8.

Medication

- International Agency for Research on Cancer (2008). *World cancer report 2008*. Boyle, P & Levin, B (eds.). Lyon, France: IARC Publications/WHO Press. ISBN 978-92-832-0423-7.

Breast Feeding

- Tsilidis, KK et al. (2011). 'Oral contraceptive use and reproductive factors and risk of ovarian cancer in the European Prospective Investigation into Cancer and Nutrition'. *Br. J. Cancer*, 105 (9), pp. 1436–1442.

Body Fat Deposits

- Calle, EE & R, Kaaks (2004). 'Overweight, obesity and cancer: epidemiological evidence and proposed mechanisms'. *Nat Rev Cancer*, 4 (8), pp. 579–91.

Increased BMI

- Brandstedt,, J et al. (2011). 'Anthropometric factors and ovarian cancer risk in the Malmo Diet and Cancer Study'. *Cancer Epidemiol*, 35 (5), pp. 432–437.
- Leitzmann, MF et al. (2009. 'Body mass index and risk of ovarian cancer'. *Cancer*, 115 (4), pp. 812–822.
- Lundqvist, E et al. (2007). 'Co-twin control and cohort analyses of body mass index and height in relation to breast, prostate, ovarian, corpus uteri, colon and rectal cancer among Swedish and Finnish twins'. *Int J Cancer*, 121 (4), pp. 810–818.

Waist Circumference

- Kotsopoulos, J, Baer, HJ & Tworoger, SS (2010). 'Anthropometric measures and risk of epithelial ovarian cancer: results from the Nurses' Health Study'. *Obesity (Silver. Spring)*, 18 (8), pp. 1625–1631.
- Lahmann, PH et al. (2010). 'Anthropometric measures and epithelial ovarian cancer risk in the European Prospective Investigation into Cancer and Nutrition'. *Int J Cancer*, 126 (10), pp. 2404–2415.

Waist/Hip Ratio

- Canchola, AJ et al. (2010). 'Body size and the risk of ovarian cancer by hormone therapy use in the California Teachers Study cohort'. *Cancer Causes Control*, 21 (12), pp.2241–2248.

Adult Attained Height

- Chionh, F et al. (2010). 'Physical activity, body size and composition, and risk of ovarian cancer'. *Cancer Causes Control*, 21 (12), pp. 2183–2194.
- Baer, HJ, Hankinson, SE & Tworoger, SS (2008). 'Body size in early life and risk of epithelial ovarian cancer: results from the Nurses' Health Studies'. *Br J Cancer*, 99 (11), pp. 1916–1922.

Pancreatic Cancer

- Ferlay, J, Shin, HR, Bray, F et al. (2010). 'GLOBOCAN 2008, Cancer Incidence and Mortality Worldwide: IARC CancerBase No. 10' [Internet]. Lyon, France: IARC.

Mechanism of Pancreatic Cancer Development

- Stolzenberg-Solomon RZ, Graubard BI & Chari, S. 'Insulin, glucose, insulin resistance, and pancreatic cancer in male smokers. *JAMA*, 2005, 294, pp. 2872-8.

Risk Factors for Pancreatic Cancer

Red Meat

- Inoue-Choi, M, Flood, A, Robien K et al. (2011). 'Nutrients, food groups, dietary patterns, and risk of pancreatic cancer in postmenopausal women'. *Cancer Epidemiol Biomarkers Prev*, 20, pp. 711–4.

Processed Meat

- Cross, AJ, Leitzmann, MF, Gail, MH et al. (2007). 'A prospective study of red and processed meat intake in relation to cancer risk'. *PLoS Med*, 4, e325.

Foods Containing Fat

- Thiebaut, AC, Jiao, L, Silverman, DT et al. (2009). 'Dietary fatty acids and pancreatic cancer in the NIH-AARP diet and health study'. *J Natl Cancer Inst*, 101, pp. 1001–11.
- Woutersen, RA, Appel, MJ, van Garderen-Hoetmer, A et al. (1999). 'Dietary fat and carcinogenesis'. *Mutat Res*, 443, pp. 111–27.

Coffee

- Nilsson, LM, Johansson, I, Lenner, P et a (2010). 'Consumption of filtered and boiled coffee and the risk of incident cancer: a prospective cohort study'. *Cancer Causes Control*, 21, pp. 1533–44.

Alcoholic Drinks

- Gapstur, SM, Jacobs, EJ, Deka, A et al. (2011). 'Association of alcohol intake with pancreatic cancer mortality in never smokers'. *Arch Intern Med*, 171, pp. 444–51.
- Michaud, DS, Vrieling, A, Jiao, L et al. (2010). 'Alcohol intake and pancreatic cancer: a pooled analysis from the pancreatic cancer cohort consortium (PanScan)'. *Cancer Causes Control*, 21, pp. 1213–25.
- Go, VLW, Gukovskaya, A & Pandol, SJ (2005). 'Alcohol and pancreatic cancer'. Alcohol, 35, pp. 205–11.

Foods and Beverages Containing Sugar Fructose

- Simon, MS, Shikany, JM, Neuhouser, ML et al. (2010). 'Glycemic index, glycemic load, and the risk of pancreatic cancer among postmenopausal women in the women's health initiative observational study and clinical trial'. *Cancer Causes Control*, 21, pp. 2129–36.
- Nothlings, U, Murphy, SP, Wilkens, LR et al. (2007). 'Dietary glycemic load, added sugars, and carbohydrates as risk factors for pancreatic cancer: the Multiethnic Cohort Study'. *Am J Clin Nutr*, 86, pp. 1495–501.

Increased BMI

- Samanic, C, Chow, WH, Gridley, G et al. (2006). 'Relation of body mass index to cancer risk in 362,552 Swedish men'. *Cancer Causes Control*, 17, pp. 901–9.
- Parr, L, Batty, GD, Lam, TH et al. (2010). 'Body mass index and cancer mortality in the Asia-Pacific Cohort Studies Collaboration: pooled analyses of 424,519 participants'. *Lancet Oncol*, 11, pp. 741–52.

Waist Circumference

- Arslan, AA, Helzlsouer, KJ, Kooperberg, C et al. (2010). 'Anthropometric measures, body mass index, and pancreatic cancer: a pooled analysis from the Pancreatic Cancer Cohort Consortium (PanScan)'. *Arch Intern Med*, 170, pp. 791-802.

Waist/Hip Ratio

- Genkinger, JM, Spiegelman, D, Anderson, KE et al. (2011). 'A pooled analysis of 14 cohort studies of anthropometric factors and pancreatic cancer risk'. *Int J Cancer*, 129, pp. 1708–17.
- Arslan, AA, Helzlsouer, KJ, Kooperberg, C et al. (2010). 'Anthropometric measures, body mass index, and pancreatic cancer: a pooled analysis from the Pancreatic Cancer Cohort Consortium (PanScan)'. *Arch Intern Med*, 170, pp. 791–802.

Mechanism of Increased Risk with Increased Body Weight and Fat Deposit

- Calle, EE & Kaaks, R (2004). 'Overweight, obesity and cancer: epidemiological evidence and proposed mechanisms'. *Nat Rev Cancer*, 4, pp. 579–91.

Adult Attained Height

- Berrington, de GA, Spencer, EA, Bueno-de-Mesquita, HB et al. (2006). 'Anthropometry, physical activity, and the risk of pancreatic cancer in the European prospective investigation into cancer and nutrition'. *Cancer Epidemiol Biomarkers Prev*, 15, pp. 879–85.
- Song, YM & Sung, J (2008). 'Adult height and the risk of mortality in South Korean women'. *Am J Epidemiol*, 168, pp. 497–505.

Part Eleven

- US Central Intelligence Agency. 'Life expectancy at birth, country comparison to the world'. *CIA World Factbook*. Archived from the original on 13 June 2007.

- Nuwer, R. 'Keeping track of the oldest people in the world'. *Smithsonian*. Retrieved 13 January 2019.
- Marziali, C (7 December 2010). 'Reaching toward the fountain of youth'. *USC Trojan Family Magazine*.
- Bernstein, A, Willcox, T et al. (2004). 'First autopsy study of an Okinawan centenarian: absence of many age-related diseases'. *Journal of Gerontology: Medical Sciences*, 59A (11), pp. 1195–1199.
- The Okinawa Centenarian Study.
- Stein, R (1 July 2010). 'New study of centenarians links certain genetic variations to a long lifespan'. The Washington Post Company.

Part Twelve

- Reiter, RJ, Rosales-Corral, S, Tan, DX, Jou, MJ, Galano, A & Xu, B (November 2017). 'Melatonin as a mitochondria-targeted antioxidant: one of evolution's best ideas'. *Cellular and Molecular Life Sciences*, 74 (21), pp. 3863–3881
- Reiter, RJ, Mayo, JC, Tan, DX, Sainz, RM, Alatorre-Jimenez, M & Qin, L (October 2016). 'Melatonin as an antioxidant: under promises but over delivers'. *Journal of Pineal Research*, 61 (3), pp. 253–78.
- Bonnefont-Rousselot, D & Collin, F (November 2010). 'Melatonin: action as antioxidant and potential applications in human disease and aging'. *Toxicology*, 278 (1), pp. 55–67.
- Dr Joshua D. Schiffman MD, Huntsman Cancer Institute (HCI), at the University of Utah, Salt Lake City.

Fighting Cancer with Capybaras

- Vincent Lynch – an evolutionary cancer biologist at the University of Chicago.
- Servan-Schreiber, D (2011). *Anticancer: a new way of life*. Revised edition, Michael Joseph. ISBN 978-0-71815-684-8.
- Fung, J (2020). *The cancer code*. HarperCollins Publishers. ISBN 978-0-00843-620-9.
- Lippman, SM et al. (2009). 'SELECT trial'. *JAMA*, 301, pp. 39-51.
- Estrella, V. et al. (1 March 2013). 'Acidity generated by the Tudor microenvironment drives local invasion'. *Cancer Research*, 73, no 5, pp. 1524–35.
- Mi-Young, Kim (24 December 2009). 'Tumor self-seeding by circulating cancer cells'. *Cell*, 139, no 7, pp. 1315–26
- Bodmer, M et al. (2010). 'Long-term metformin use is associated with decreased risk of breast cancer'. *Diabetes Care*, 33, pp. 1304-8.

FIND KILLING CANCER KINDLY ON

IF YOU'RE LOOKING TO STAY UPDATED WITH KCK'S LATEST CONTENT AND CONNECT WITH US ONLINE, YOU CAN FIND US ON THE FOLLOWING PLATFORMS. WE WOULD LOVE TO CONNECT WITH YOU ON THESE PLATFORMS, SO FEEL FREE TO FOLLOW, LIKE, AND SUBSCRIBE TO KCK'S OFFICIAL PAGES. AND IF YOU HAVE ANY QUESTIONS OR COMMENTS, DON'T HESITATE TO REACH OUT THROUGH DIRECT MESSAGES OR COMMENTS ON OUR POSTS. TEAM KCK LOOKS FORWARD TO CONNECTING WITH YOU ONLINE!

Scan to visit our YouTube Channel

Printed in Great Britain
by Amazon

32127797R00218